Emery's
Elements of
Medical Genetics

'Heredity is the last of the fates and the most terrible'
Oscar Wilde

For Churchill Livingstone

Commissioning Editor Mike Parkinson
Project Manager Graham Birnie
Copy Editor Stephanie Pickering
Design Direction Erik Bigland
Project Controller Nancy Arnott
Sales Promotion Executive Marion Pollock

Emery's Elements of Medical Genetics

Robert F. Mueller MB BS BSc FRCP
Department of Clinical Genetics,
St James's Hospital, Leeds, UK

Ian D. Young MD MSc FRCP
Centre for Medical Genetics, Nottingham City Hospital, Nottingham,
UK

Illustrator
Anna Durbin

NINTH EDITION

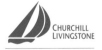
CHURCHILL
LIVINGSTONE

EDINBURGH
HONG KONG
LONDON
MADRID
MELBOURNE
NEW YORK AND
TOKYO
1995

CHURCHILL LIVINGSTONE

Medical Division of Pearson Professional Limited

Distributed in the United States of America by Churchill
Livingstone Inc., 650 Avenue of the Americas, New York,
N. Y. 10011, and by associated companies, branches and
representatives throughout the world.

First edition (University of California Press) 1968
Second edition 1971
Third edition 1974
Fourth edition 1975
Fifth edition 1979
Sixth edition 1983
Seventh edition 1988
Eighth edition 1992
Nineth edition 1995,
    Reprinted 1996, 1997

Standard edition ISBN 0 443 05175 5

International Student Edition of ninth edition 1996
Reprinted 1997
International Student Edition ISBN 0 443 05757 5

British Library Cataloguing in Publication Data
A catalogue record for this book is available from the British
Library.

Library of Congress Cataloging in Publication Data
A catalog record for this book is available from the Library
of Congress.

The
publisher's
policy is to use
**paper manufactured
from sustainable forests**

Produced by Longman Singapore
Publishers (Pte) Ltd
Printed in Singapore

Contents

Preface

In the 27 years which have elapsed since the publication of the first edition of Alan Emery's *Elements of Medical Genetics* there have been many remarkable scientific achievements, most notably in the field of molecular biology. Nowhere have these made a greater impact than in medical genetics. A subject which was once regarded as little more than a curiosity and barely featured in the medical syllabus is now widely accepted as the most exciting and dynamic area of medical research and development.

Throughout these years the *Elements* has succeeded in conveying the excitement and the fascination of this subject without overburdening its many readers with a surfeit of unnecessary information. Mindful of the ever-increasing load imposed on an already over-crowded medical curriculum, we have striven to maintain the principle, established by Professor Emery, that 'the communication of ideas in a subject is more important than the mere acquisition of facts.' Towards this end this edition of the *Elements* has been divided into three sections. The first outlines important basic principles and adheres as far as possible to the recent recommendations of the Royal College of Physicians working party on teaching genetics to medical students. In the second section the horizons of the subject are broadened to show how genetics transcends traditional medical boundaries and is now making a major impact in all areas of medical science. The chapters of the concluding section focus on the practical applications of these new discoveries and how these are being implemented on a widespread basis through the newly developed discipline of clinical genetics.

Whilst aimed primarily at medical undergraduates, we hope that the appeal of the *Elements* will extend beyond the narrow confines of the medical curriculum and be of interest to a wider audience. As practising clinical geneticists we are only too well aware of the challenges imposed on busy scientists and physicians who struggle to keep abreast of rapid advances in molecular biology and a burgeoning medical literature. It is hoped that such individuals will view this book as a resource which can be consulted during all stages of their training and beyond.

Leeds   R.F.M.
Nottingham   I.D.Y.

Acknowledgements

In compiling this edition we are deeply indebted to many colleagues and friends. In particular we would like to thank Professor Alan Emery for his continued support and encouragement and for having nurtured the *Elements* through its first eight editions. We are grateful to many colleagues in Leeds and Nottingham, specifically Mr J. Williams, Cytogenetics Laboratory, St James's Hospital and Mr N. Smith, Cytogenetics Unit, City Hospital, Nottingham for karyotype figures, Mr G.R. Taylor, DNA Laboratory, St James's Hospital, Mr Brian Stephenson, Department of Surgery, Royal Gwent Hospital, Newport and Mr N. Hall, ICRF Genetic Epidemiology Unit, St James's Hospital for substantial help with the chapter on Cancer Genetics, Ms Anna Durbin for inspiration in the illustrations, Mrs Melanie Dakin for painstakingly deciphering I.D.Y.'s hand-written hieroglyphics, the Department of Medical Illustration, St James's Hospital and Professor D.T. Bishop for the use of his printer for the various drafts in preparation of the text.

Finally, we would like to dedicate this book to our respective wives (Pamela and Elizabeth) and children (Katy, Zach, Nick and Andrew) for their forbearance and continued goodwill in the face of husband absenteeism and paternal ill-humour.

R.F.M./I.D.Y.

Plate 1
Fluorescent in situ hybridisation of an interphase nucleus with a centromeric probe to chromosome 21 showing 3 signals consistent with trisomy 21 (courtesy of Mr N. Smith, Cytogenetics Unit, City Hospital, Nottingham).

Plate 2
Fluorescent in situ hybridisation with a probe to the Y chromosome which hybridises to the short of an X chromosome in a 46,XX male (courtesy of Mr N. Smith, Cytogenetics Unit, City Hospital, Nottingham).

Plate 3
Chromosome paint of a Y chromosome (courtesy of Mr N. Smith, Cytogenetics Unit, City Hospital, Nottingham).

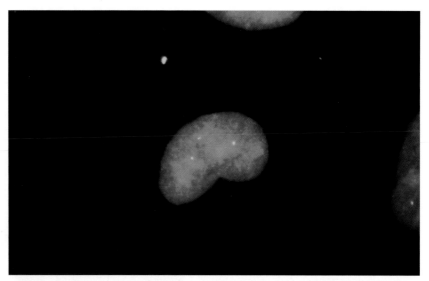

Plate 1 (see p. 28)

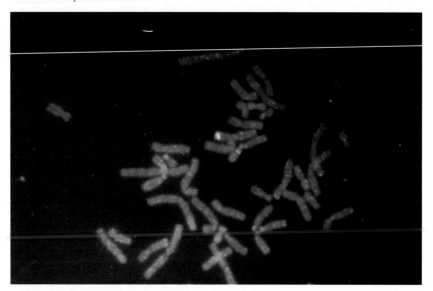

Plate 2 (see pp. 28, 71)

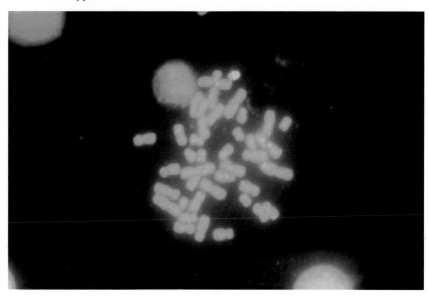

Plate 3
(see p. 28)

Plate 4
A chromosome 8 paint used to identify the material from chromosome 8 attached to the long arm of one of the number 4 chromosomes in a 4;8 balanced translocation (courtesy of Mr N. Smith, Cytogenetics Unit, City Hospital, Nottingham).

Plate 5
Chromosome paint used to identify the origin of a ring chromosome from an X chromosome (courtesy of Mr N. Smith, Cytogenetics Unit, City Hospital, Nottingham).

Plate 6
Heterochromia irides in a person with Waardenburg's syndrome (courtesy of Dr C.P. Bennett, St James's Hospital, Leeds).

Plate 7
Picture of a fundus of a carrier of X-linked ocular albinism showing a mosaic pattern of retinal pigmentation (courtesy of Mr S.J. Charles, The Royal Eye Hospital, Manchester).

Plate 8
Blue sclerae in a child with osteogenesis imperfecta.

Plate 9
Trunk of a female with the X-linked dominant disorder incontinentia pigmenti showing a mosaic pattern of increased skin pigmentation which follows Blaschko's lines.

Plate 10
Oxidation of homogentisic acid excreted in the urine in alkaptonuria imparting a dark colour on exposure to air (courtesy of Dr. J. Wardell, City Hospital, Nottingham).

Plate 11
Dark pigment in ear wax due to alkaptonuria (courtesy of Professor P.S. Harper, Institute of Medical Genetics, University of Wales, Cardiff).

Plate 12
Slit-lamp examination of a person with Wilson's disease showing a Kayser–Fleischer ring at the corneal–conjunctival junction which shows as a rim of brown pigmentation (courtesy of Mr M. Bradbury, Bradford Royal Infirmary).

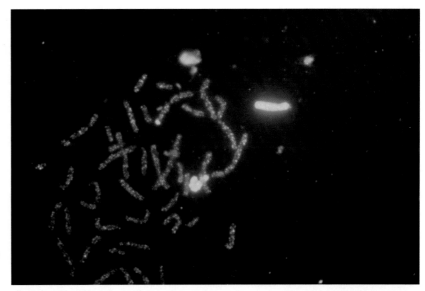

Plate 4 (see p. 28)

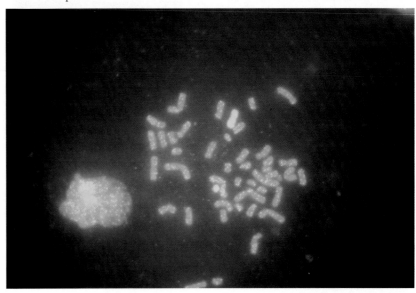

Plate 5 (see p. 28)

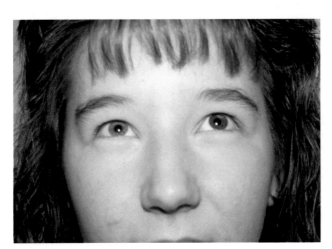

Plate 6 (see p. 69)

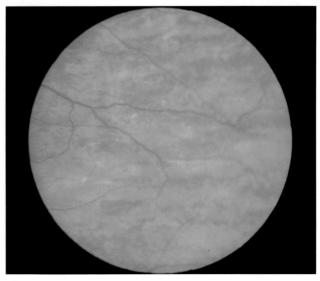

Plate 7 (see pp. 73, 83, 245)

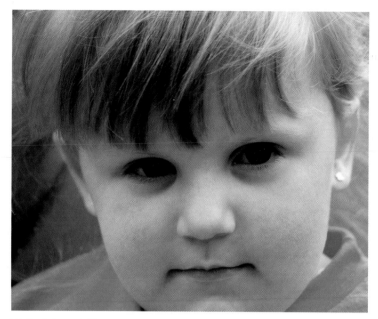

Plate 8 (see p. 77)

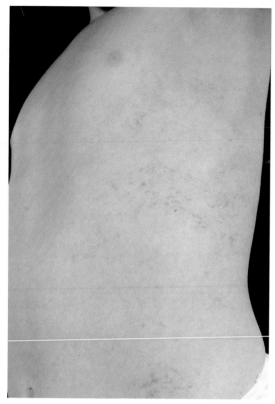

Plate 9 (see p. 85)

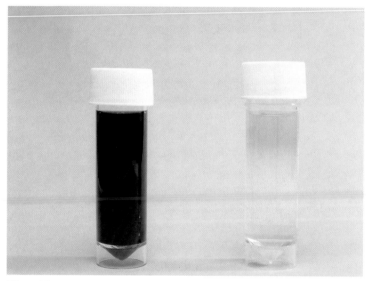

Plate 10 (see p. 130)

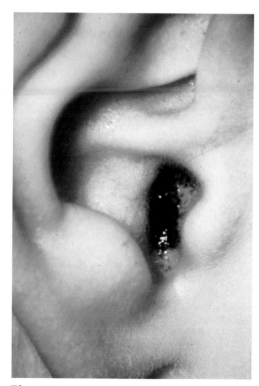

Plate 11 (see p. 130)

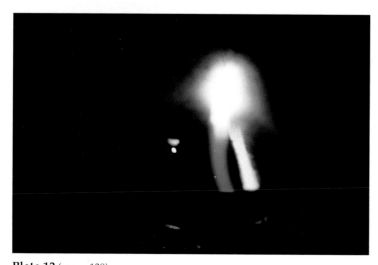

Plate 12 (see p. 139)

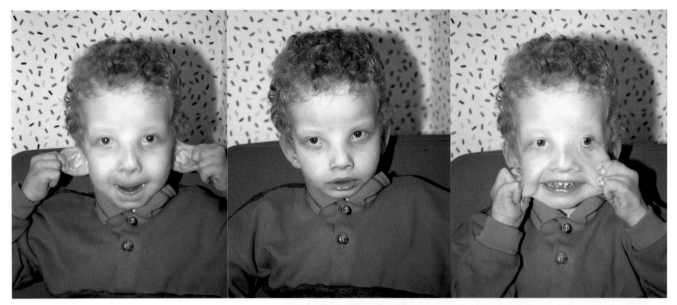

Plate 13 (see p. 208)

Plate 13
Child with one of the Ehlers–Danlos syndromes showing hyperextensible skin of the face.

Plate 14
Mosaic pattern of skin depigmentation on the arm of a person with hypomelanosis of Ito following Blaschko's lines (reproduced with permission from Jenkins D, Martin K, Young I D 1993 Hypomelanosis of Ito associated with mosaicism for trisomy 7 and apparent 'pseudomosaicism' at amniocentesis. J Med Genet 30: 783–784).

Plate 15
Lisch nodules (arrowed) seen in neurofibromatosis type I (courtesy of Mr R. Doran, Dept of Ophthalmology, The General Infirmary at Leeds).

Plate 16
Refractile lenticular opacities in an asymptomatic person with myotonic dystrophy (courtesy of Mr R. Doran and Mr M. Geall, Dept of Ophthalmology, The General Infirmary at Leeds).

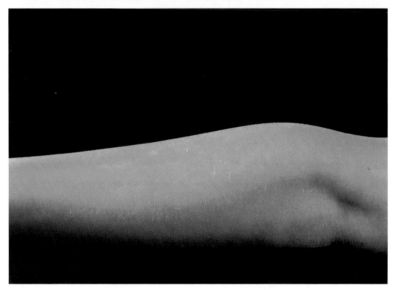

Plate 14 (see pp. 221, 234)

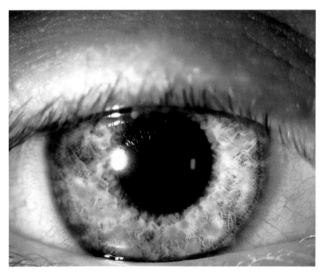

Plate 15 (see p. 248)

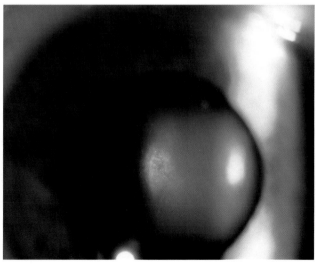

Plate 16 (see p. 249)

SECTION A

PRINCIPLES OF HUMAN GENETICS

The history and impact of genetics in medicine

CHAPTER 1

EARLY BEGINNINGS

Homo sapiens first appeared on this planet approximately 50 000 years ago and it is reasonable to suppose that the first thinking ancestors of humans were just as curious as we are about matters of inheritance. For example, engravings in Chaldea in Babylonia (now Iraq) dating back at least 6000 years show pedigrees documenting the transmission of certain characteristics of the mane in horses. However, any early attempts to unravel the mysteries of genetics would have been severely hampered by a total lack of knowledge and understanding of basic processes such as conception and reproduction.

Early Greek philosophers and physicians such as Aristotle and Hippocrates concluded, with typical masculine modesty, that important human characteristics were determined by semen utilising menstrual blood as a culture medium and the uterus as an incubator. Semen was thought to be produced by the whole body; hence baldheaded fathers would beget baldheaded sons. These ideas prevailed until the seventeenth century when Dutch scientists, such as Leeuwenhoek and de Graaf, recognised the existence of sperm and ova, thus explaining how the female could also transmit characteristics to her offspring.

The blossoming of the scientific revolution in the eighteenth and nineteenth centuries saw a revival of interest in heredity by both scientists and physicians amongst whom two particular names stand out. Pierre de Maupertuis, a French naturalist, studied hereditary traits such as extra digits (polydactyly) and lack of pigmentation (albinism), and showed from pedigree studies that these two conditions were inherited in different ways. Joseph Adams, a British doctor, also recognised that different mechanisms of inheritance existed and published *A Treatise on the Supposed Hereditary Properties of Diseases* which was intended as a basis for genetic counselling.

GREGOR MENDEL AND THE LAWS OF INHERITANCE

Our present understanding of human genetics owes much to the work of the Austrian monk Gregor Mendel who, in 1865, presented the results of his breeding experiments on garden peas to the Natural Science Association in Brunn (now Brno in Moravia). Subsequently Mendel's results were published by this society in their *Proceedings* where they remained largely unnoticed until 1900 when their importance was first recognised. In essence Mendel's work can be considered as the discovery of genes and how they are inherited. In acknowledgement of this major contribution the term *Mendelian* is now applied both to the different patterns of inheritance shown by single gene characteristics and to disorders found to be due to defects in a single gene.

In his breeding experiments Mendel studied contrasting characters in the garden pea using for each experiment varieties which differed in only one characteristic. For example, he noted that, when strains which were bred for a feature such as tallness were crossed with plants bred to be short, all the offspring in the first *filial* or F1 generation were tall. If plants in this F1 generation were interbred, then both tall and short plants resulted in a ratio of three to one (Fig. 1.1). Those characteristics which were manifest in the F1 hybrids were referred to as *dominant*, whereas those which reappeared in the F2 generation were described as being *recessive*.

Mendel interpreted these observations as showing that plant stature (unlike human stature) was controlled by a pair of factors, one of which was inherited from each parent. A Danish botanist, Johannsen, subsequently coined the term *gene* for these hereditary factors. The pure bred plants, with two identical genes, used in the initial cross would now be referred to as *homozygous*. The hybrid F1 plants, each of which has one gene for tallness

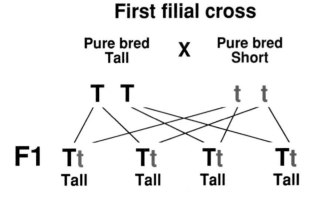

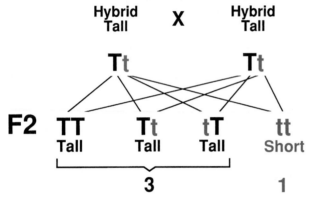

Fig. 1.1
An illustration of one of Mendel's breeding experiments and how he correctly interpreted the results.

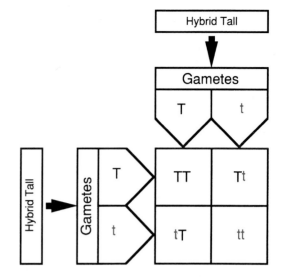

Fig. 1.2
A Punnett's square showing the different ways in which genes can segregate and combine in the second filial cross from Figure 1.1. Construction of a Punnett's square provides a simple method for showing the possible gamete combinations in different matings.

THE LAW OF SEGREGATION

The *law of segregation* refers to the observation that each individual possesses two genes for a particular characteristic, only one of which can be transmitted at any one time. Rare exceptions to this rule can occur when two allelic genes fail to separate due to chromosome non-disjunction in meiosis I (p. 34).

THE LAW OF INDEPENDENT ASSORTMENT

The *law of independent assortment* refers to the fact that members of different gene pairs segregate to offspring independently of one another. In reality this is not always true as genes which are close together on the same chromosome tend to be inherited together, i.e. they are linked (p. 99).

THE CHROMOSOMAL BASIS OF INHERITANCE

As interest in Mendelian inheritance grew, there was much speculation about how it actually occurred. It was also known that each cell contained a nucleus within which there were several threadlike structures called *chromosomes*, so called because of their affinity for certain stains (chroma = colour, soma = body). In 1903, Sutton, a medical student, and Boveri, a German biologist, independently proposed that chromosomes carry the hereditary factors, or genes. These suggestions were prompted by the realisation that the behaviour of

and one for shortness, would be referred to as *heterozygous*. The genes responsible for these contrasting characteristics are referred to as *allelomorphs* or *alleles* for short.

An alternative method for determining *genotypes* in offspring involves the construction of what is known as a Punnett's square (Fig. 1.2). This will be utilised further in Chapter 7 when considering how genes segregate in large populations.

On the basis of Mendel's plant experiments, three main principles were established. These are known as the laws of uniformity, segregation and independent assortment.

THE LAW OF UNIFORMITY

The *law of uniformity* refers to the fact that when two homozygotes with different alleles are crossed, all the offspring in the F1 generation are identical and heterozygous. In other words the characteristics do not blend as had been believed previously, and can reappear in later generations.

chromosomes at cell division provided an explanation for how genes could segregate.

When the connection between Mendelian inheritance and chromosomes was first made, it was thought that the normal chromosome number in humans was 48. The correct number of 46 was not established until 1956. Shortly thereafter it was shown that human disorders could be due to loss or gain of a whole chromosome as well as an abnormality in a single gene. Some chromosome abnormalities, such as translocations, can run in families (p. 35), and are sometimes said to be segregating in a Mendelian fashion.

THE FRUIT FLY

Before returning to historical developments in human genetics, it is worth a brief diversion to consider the merits of an unlikely animal which has proved to be a major tool in genetic research. The fruit fly, *Drosophila*, possesses several distinct advantages for the study of genetics. These are as follows:

1. It can be bred easily in a laboratory.
2. It breeds rapidly and prolifically at a rate of 20–25 generations per annum.
3. It has a number of easily recognised characteristics such as *curly wings* and *yellow body* which show Mendelian inheritance.
4. *Drosophila melanogaster*, the species most frequently studied, has only four pairs of chromosomes each of which has a distinct appearance so that they can be identified easily.
5. The chromosomes in the salivary glands of *Drosophila* larvae are amongst the largest known in nature, being at least 100 times bigger than those in other body cells.

In view of these unique properties, fruit flies were used very extensively in early breeding experiments. Even today their study is proving of great value in fields such as developmental biology for the isolation of genes which are important in embryology and morphogenesis (Ch. 5).

THE ORIGINS OF MEDICAL GENETICS

Mention has already been made of the pioneering studies of far-sighted individuals such as Maupertuis and Adams whose curiosity was aroused by familial conditions such as polydactyly and albinism. Others, such as John Dalton of atomic theory fame, observed that some conditions, notably colour blindness and haemophilia, show what is now referred to as sex- or X-linked inheritance, and to this day colour blindness is still referred to as *Daltonism*. Inevitably these founders of human and medical genetics could only speculate as to the nature of the mechanisms underlying their observations.

The rediscovery of Mendelism in 1900 marks the real beginning of medical genetics and provided an enormous impetus for the study of inherited disease. Credit for the first recognition of a single gene trait is shared by William Bateson and Archibald Garrod who together proposed that alkaptonuria was a rare recessive disorder. In this relatively harmless condition urine turns dark on standing or on exposure to alkali, due to inability on the part of the patient to metabolise homogentisic acid. Realising that this was an inherited disorder involving a chemical process, Garrod coined the term *inborn error of metabolism*. Several hundred such disorders have now been identified giving rise to the field of study known as biochemical genetics (Ch. 10).

During the course of the twentieth century it has gradually become clear that hereditary factors are implicated in many conditions and that different genetic mechanisms are involved. Traditionally, hereditary conditions have been considered under the headings of single gene, chromosomal and multifactorial. Recent discoveries have shown that a fourth category consisting of acquired somatic genetic disease should also be included.

CLASSIFICATION OF GENETIC DISEASE

SINGLE GENE DISORDERS

In addition to alkaptonuria, Garrod suggested that albinism and cystinuria could also show recessive inheritance. Soon other examples followed, leading to an explosion in knowledge and disease delineation. By 1966 almost 1500 single gene disorders or traits had been identified prompting the publication by an American physician, Victor McKusick, of a catalogue of all known single gene conditions. By 1994 when the eleventh edition of this catalogue was published, it contained over 6000 entries (Fig. 1.3). Given that there are likely to be between 50 000 and 100 000 structural genes in the human, it is clear that future editions are likely to be very much larger.

CHROMOSOME ABNORMALITIES

Improved techniques for studying chromosomes led to the demonstration in 1959 that the presence of an additional number 21 chromosome (*trisomy* 21) resulted in Down's syndrome. Other similar discoveries followed

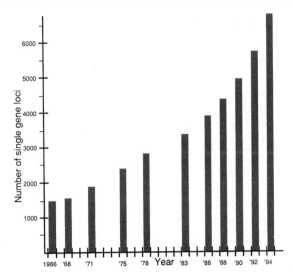

Fig. 1.3
Histogram showing the rapid increase in recognition of conditions and characteristics (traits) showing single gene inheritance (data from McKusick V A).

rapidly. The identification of chromosome abnormalities was further aided by the development of banding techniques in 1970. These enabled reliable identification of individual chromosomes and helped confirm that loss or gain of even a very small segment of a chromosome could have devastating effects on human development.

Most recently it has been shown that several rare conditions featuring mental retardation and abnormal physical features are due to loss of such a tiny amount of chromosome material that no abnormality can be detected using even the most high-powered light microscope. These conditions are referred to as sub-microscopic deletion syndromes (pp. 39, 219).

MULTIFACTORIAL DISORDERS

Francis Galton, a cousin of Charles Darwin, had a long-standing interest in human characteristics such as stature, physique and intelligence. Much of his research was based on the study of identical twins in whom differences in these parameters must be due to environmental influences. Galton introduced to genetics the concept of the regression coefficient as a means of estimating the degree of resemblance between various relatives. This concept was extended to incorporate Mendel's discovery of genes to try to explain how parameters such as height and skin colour could be explained by the interaction of many genes, each of which would exert a small additive effect. This is in contrast to single gene characteristics in which the action of one gene is exerted independently, i.e. in a non-additive fashion.

This model of *quantitative inheritance* is now widely accepted and has been adapted to explain the pattern of inheritance observed for many relatively common conditions (Ch. 8). These include the common congenital malformations such as cleft lip and palate, and acquired disorders such as diabetes mellitus and schizophrenia.

Multifactorial conditions are now believed to make a very major contribution to human morbidity and mortality.

ACQUIRED SOMATIC GENETIC DISEASE

This could seem a contradiction in terms as it could reasonably be thought that all genetic disorders must be due to genetic errors present from conception. However recent research in molecular biology has shown that mutations occur on a regular basis throughout life in somatic cells which have no involvement with the reproductive process. Somatic mutations are believed to account for a large proportion of malignancy and could also be responsible for other events such as senescence and the ageing process.

DEFINITIONS

Before considering the impact of hereditary disease it is necessary to introduce a few definitions.

INCIDENCE

Incidence refers to the rate at which new cases occur. Thus if the birth incidence of a particular condition equals 1 in 1000, then on average 1 in every 1000 new-born infants is affected.

PREVALENCE

Prevalence refers to the proportion of a population affected at any one time. The prevalence of a genetic disease will usually be less than its incidence either because life expectancy is reduced or because the condition shows a delayed age of onset.

FREQUENCY

Frequency is a general term which lacks scientific specificity, although this word is often taken as being synonymous with incidence when calculating gene 'frequencies' (Ch. 7).

CONGENITAL

Congenital means that a condition is present at birth. Not all genetic disorders are congenital in terms of age of onset, nor are all congenital abnormalities genetic in origin.

THE IMPACT OF GENETIC DISEASE

As a result of the improvements in hygiene and health care which have taken place during this century, there has been a steady decline in the contribution of environmental factors to disease in the general population. This decrease in illness due to infections and nutritional deficiency has shifted attention to genetic disorders. Thus, while there is no evidence that taken together these are becoming more common, their relative contribution to both mortality and morbidity is increasing.

An estimate of the overall impact of genetic disease can be made from the following observations.

SPONTANEOUS MISCARRIAGES

A chromosome abnormality is present in at least 50% of all recognised first-trimester pregnancy loss.

NEWBORN INFANTS

2–3% of all neonates have at least one major congenital abnormality. Often these will have been caused by genetic factors (p. 199). 2% of all neonates have a chromosome abnormality or a single gene disorder.

CHILDHOOD

Genetic disorders account for 50% of all childhood blindness, 50% of all childhood deafness and 50% of all cases of severe mental retardation. Genetic disorders and congenital malformations together also account for 30% of all childhood hospital admissions and 40–50% of all childhood deaths.

ADULT LIFE

Approximately 1% of all malignancy is directly due to genetic factors, and 10% of common cancers such as breast, colon and ovary have a strong genetic component. By age 25 years, 5% of the population will have a disorder in which genetic factors play an important role.

The study of genetics and its role in human disease has come a long way from the days of Mendel and Garrod to the point where this subject is now recognised as being amongst the most important in medicine. During the last 30 years the Nobel prize for physiology or medicine has been won on 11 occasions by scientists working in the fields of human and molecular genetics (Table 1.1). Projects such as the sequencing of the human genome (p. 284) will almost certainly lead to the identification of genes which confer susceptibility to common disorders of adult life such as malignancy, hypertension and coronary artery disease. The advent of gene therapy (p. 278) could well be as exciting and revolutionary as were the widespread introduction of immunisation programmes and the development of antibiotics in earlier years. When considered in their broadest context, it is becoming abundantly clear that present and future developments in the fields of human and molecular genetics will impinge increasingly on all areas of medicine.

Table 1.1 Genetic discoveries which have led to the award of the Nobel Prize for Physiology or Medicine 1962–1993

Year	Prize-winners	Discovery
1962	Francis Crick James Watson Maurice Wilkins	The molecular structure of DNA
1965	Francois Jacob Jacques Monod Audree Lwoff	Genetic regulation
1968	Robert Holley Gobind Khorana Marshall Nirenberg	Deciphering of the genetic code
1975	Renato Dulbecco Howard Temin David Baltimore	Interaction between tumour viruses and nuclear DNA
1978	William Arber Daniel Nathans Hamilton Smith	Restriction endonucleases
1980	Baruj Benacerraf George Snell Jean Dausset	Genetic control of immunological response
1983	Barbara McClintock	Mobile genes (transposons)
1985	Michael Brown Joseph Goldstein	Cell receptors in familial hypercholesterolaemia
1987	Tonegawa Susumu	Genetic aspects of antibodies
1989	Michael Bishop Harold Varmus	Study of oncogenes
1993	Richard Roberts Philip Sharp	'Split genes'

ELEMENTS

1 A characteristic manifest in a hybrid (heterozygote) is dominant. A recessive characteristic is expressed only in an individual with two copies of the gene, i.e. a homozygote.

2 Mendel proposed that each individual has two genes for each characteristic: one is inherited from each parent and one is transmitted to each child. Genes at different loci act and segregate independently.

3 Chromosome separation at cell division facilitates gene segregation.

4 Genetic disorders are present in at least 2% of all neonates, account for 50% of childhood blindness, deafness, mental retardation and deaths, and affect 5% of the population by age 25 years.

FURTHER READING

Baird P A, Anderson T W, Newcombe H B, Lowry R B 1988 Genetic disorders in children and young adults: a population study. Am J Hum Genet 42: 677–693
A comprehensive study of the incidence of genetic disease in a large Western urban population.

Emery A E H 1989 Portraits in medical genetics – Joseph Adams 1756–1818. J Med Genet 26: 116–118
An account of the life of a London doctor who made remarkable observations about hereditary disease in his patients.

Garrod A E 1902 The incidence of alkaptonuria: a study in chemical individuality. Lancet ii: 1916–1920.
A landmark paper in which Garrod proposed that alkaptonuria could show Mendelian inheritance and also noted that 'the mating of first cousins gives exactly the conditions most likely to enable a rare, and usually recessive, character to show itself'.

McKusick V A 1994 Mendelian inheritance in man, 11th edn. Johns Hopkins University Press, Baltimore
An exhaustive two-volume catalogue of all known conditions and traits showing Mendelian inheritance.

Sorsby A 1965 Gregor Mendel. Br Med J i: 333–338
A detailed description of Mendel's life and work.

CHAPTER 2

The cellular and molecular basis of inheritance

What is the chain of events which leads from the gene to the final product? This chapter outlines the basic principles of gene structure, the genetic code, gene transcription and gene translation.

THE NUCLEUS

Visible with the light microscope within each cell of the body are the *cytoplasm* and a darkly-staining body, the *nucleus* (Fig. 2.1). The cytoplasm is semifluid in consistency and has within it a complex arrangement of very fine, highly convoluted tubes which open on to the surface of the cell, the *endoplasmic reticulum*. The endoplasmic reticulum is involved in the biosynthesis of macro-molecules and their transportation to the cytoplasm, to other cellular organelles, such as the Golgi apparatus, and to the cell surface. It is particularly well developed in cells involved in *protein* synthesis such as those of the pancreas.

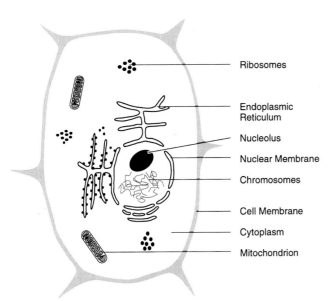

Fig. 2.1
A schematic diagram of an animal cell.

Ribosomes
Endoplasmic Reticulum
Nucleolus
Nuclear Membrane
Chromosomes
Cell Membrane
Cytoplasm
Mitochondrion

Also situated within the cytoplasm are small bodies concerned with cell respiration, the *mitochondria*, and other even more minute structures, the *ribosomes*, involved with protein synthesis. Both of these structures are extremely small and their study only became possible with the advent of the electron microscope.

The nucleus is surrounded by a membrane which separates it from the cytoplasm and within the nucleus are the chromosomes which bear the genes.

DNA: THE HEREDITARY MATERIAL

COMPOSITION

Nucleic acid is composed of a long chain of individual molecules called *nucleotides*. Each nucleotide is composed of a nitrogenous *base*, a sugar molecule and a phosphate molecule. The nitrogenous bases are called *purines* and *pyrimidines*. The purines include adenine and guanine; the pyrimidines include cytosine, thymine and uracil.

There are two different types of nucleic acid. One contains the sugar ribose, and is therefore called *ribonucleic acid* or RNA. The other contains a slightly different sugar called deoxyribose, and is therefore called *deoxyribonucleic acid* or DNA. RNA is found mainly in the *nucleolus* (a structure within the nucleus) and the cytoplasm, there being very little in the chromosomes. DNA, on the other hand, is found mainly in the chromosomes. Both types of nucleic acid contain cytosine and have the same purine bases, but, whereas thymine occurs only in DNA, uracil occurs only in RNA.

STRUCTURE

For genes to be composed of DNA it is necessary that the latter should have a structure sufficiently versatile to account for the great variety of different genes and yet, at the same time, be able to reproduce itself in such a manner that an identical replica is formed at each cell division. In 1953, Wilkins, Crick and Watson, based on

X-ray diffraction studies, proposed a structure for the DNA molecule which fulfilled all the essential requirements.

Watson and Crick suggested that the DNA molecule is composed of two chains of nucleotides arranged in a double helix. The backbone of each chain is formed by sugar-phosphate molecules and the two chains are held together by hydrogen bonds between the nitrogenous bases which point in towards the centre of the helix. Each DNA chain has a polarity determined by the orientation of the sugar-phosphate backbone. The chain end terminated by the 5′ carbon atom of the sugar molecule is referred to as the 5′ end, and the end terminated by the 3′ carbon atom is called the 3′ end. In the DNA duplex the 5′ end of one strand is opposite the 3′ end of the other, i.e. they have opposite orientations and are said to be *antiparallel*.

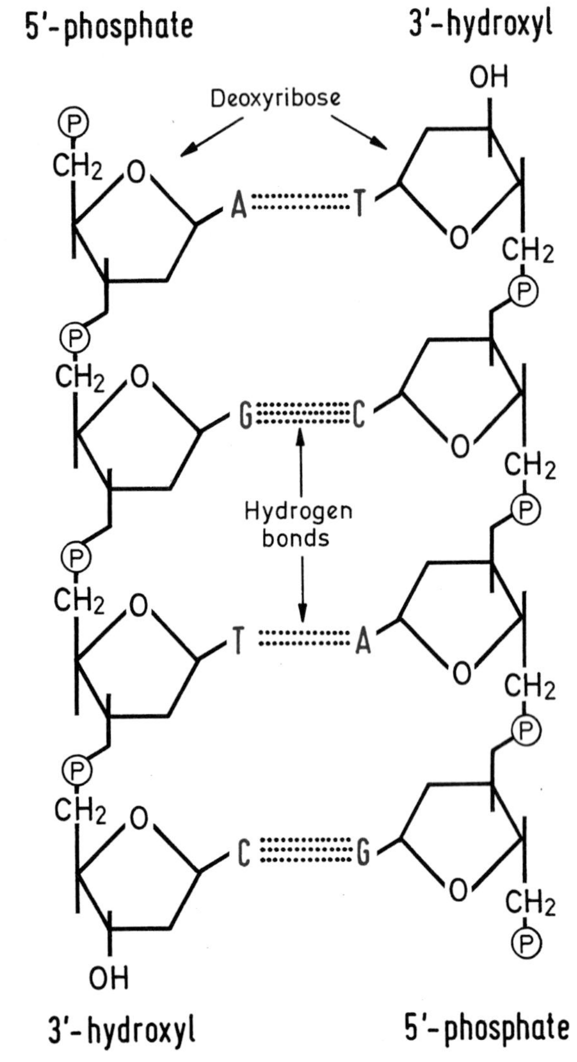

The arrangement of the bases in the DNA molecule is not random: a purine in one chain always pairs with a pyrimidine in the other chain. There is also specific pairing of the *base pairs*: guanine in one chain always pairs with cytosine in the other chain and adenine always pairs with thymine (Fig. 2.2). For their work Wilkins, Watson and Crick were awarded the Nobel Prize for Medicine and Physiology in 1962 (p. 7).

REPLICATION

The Watson–Crick double helix model provides an answer to the question of how genetic information is transmitted from one generation to the next or *replicated*. During nuclear division the two strands of the DNA molecule separate and, as a result of specific base pairing, each chain then builds its complement. In this way, when cells divide, genetic information is conserved and transmitted unchanged to each daughter cell. The process of DNA replication is semi-conservative, as only one strand of the resultant daughter molecule is newly synthesised. DNA replication commences at multiple points in the DNA double helix and progresses in both directions from these points of origin, the *replication forks*, forming a structure referred to as a *replication bubble*, until the replication forks meet an adjacent fork moving in the opposite direction, forming two complete daughter molecules (Fig. 2.3).

CHROMOSOME STRUCTURE

The idea that each chromosome is composed of a single Watson–Crick double helix of DNA is an over-simplification. Firstly, the width of a chromosome is very

Fig. 2.2
Representation of the sugar-phosphate backbone and nucleotide pairing of the DNA double helix (P-phosphate, A-adenine, T-thymine, G-guanine and C-cytosine).

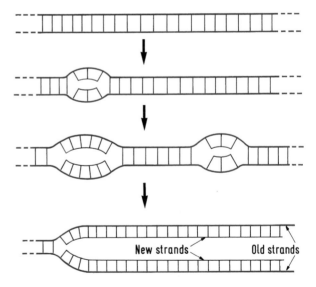

Fig. 2.3
Representation of the multiple points of origin and semi-conservative mode of DNA replication.

much greater than the diameter of a DNA double helix. In addition, the amount of DNA in each nucleus in humans means that the total length of DNA in the chromosomes, if fully extended, would amount to several metres! In fact the total length of the human chromosome complement is less than half a millimetre.

Experimental evidence has shown that there are several orders of DNA coiling in the chromosomes. In addition to the primary coiling of the DNA double helix, there is secondary coiling around the outside of spherical *histone* 'beads' forming what are called *nucleosomes*, tertiary coiling of the nucleosomes forming the chromatin fibres and quarternary coiling in the forms of loops. These loops are further wound in a tight helix to form the chromosome as visualised under the microscope (Fig. 2.4). This is the so-called *solenoid model* of chromosome structure.

Chromosome replication takes place at many thousands of separate sites in different *replication units*, which appear to be activated in a specific sequence, as would be expected given the highly organised structure of chromosomes in humans.

TYPES OF DNA SEQUENCES

Unique DNA sequences

It is estimated that there are some 50–100 000 genes which code for specific proteins in humans, accounting for less than 5% of the DNA of the human *genome*. This means that more than 95% of DNA in humans does not code for proteins. The vast majority of this latter portion, somewhere in the region of 75%, consists of unique or single copy DNA sequences, the function of which is not clear at present.

Satellite DNA

10–15% of the DNA of the human genome consists of short tandemly repeated DNA sequences which code for ribosomal and transfer RNAs, some of which are clustered around the centromeres of certain chromosomes. This class of DNA sequences separates out on density-gradient centrifugation as a shoulder, or 'satellite', to the main peak of DNA and has therefore been referred to as *satellite DNA*.

Interspersed repetitive DNA sequences

10–15% of the human genome is made up of two main classes of *repetitive DNA* sequences that are interspersed throughout the genome. One class is made up of short interspersed repetitive sequences (SINEs), which constitute about 5% of the human genome and consist of in the region of 300 000 copies of a sequence of approximately 300 base pairs. These are called *Alu repeats* because they contain an Alu I restriction enzyme recognition site.

Members of the *Alu* repeat family resemble DNA sequences called transposable elements or *transposons* by being flanked by short direct repeat sequences. Transposons, originally identified in maize by Barbara McClintock (p. 7), move spontaneously throughout the genome from one chromosome location to another and appear to be ubiquitous in the plant and animal kingdoms.

The second class of interspersed repetitive DNA sequences, accounting for about 5% of the DNA of the human genome, is made up of long interspersed repetitive sequences, known as LINEs or the L1 family. These consist of 100 000 or so copies of a slightly longer DNA sequence up to 6000 base pairs in length. The function of these repeat sequences is not clear at present but both the *Alu* and L1 interspersed repetitive DNA sequences have been implicated as a cause of mutation in inherited human disease (p. 234).

There is at present no entirely satisfactory explanation for the vast amount of DNA in the genome which appears to have little or no obvious function and does not appear to contribute to the *phenotype*. It has even been referred to as *selfish DNA*, the implication being that it preserves itself as a result of selection within the genome!

Pseudogenes

Particularly fascinating is the occurrence of genes which closely resemble known structural genes but which are not expressed, so-called *pseudogenes* (p. 117). These are

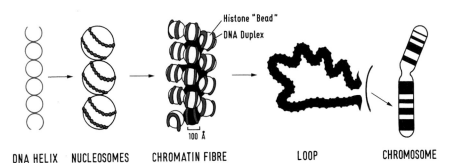

DNA HELIX   NUCLEOSOMES   CHROMATIN FIBRE   LOOP   CHROMOSOME

Fig. 2.4
Simplified diagram of proposed solenoid model of DNA coiling.

thought to be relics of replicated genes which, through acquisition of mutations in coding or regulatory sequences, have become 'silenced' during evolution, rather like a sort of genetic quasar!

Mitochondrial DNA

Nuclear DNA is not the only DNA found in cells. The several hundred mitochondria of each cell possess their own DNA. The mitochondria of the fertilised zygote are inherited almost exclusively from the oocyte.

Mitochondrial DNA, mtDNA, is circular and codes for two types of ribosomal RNA, a number of transfer RNAs (p. 13) and protein subunits of some of the *enzymes*, such as cytochrome b and cytochrome oxidase, involved in the energy producing oxidative phosphorylation pathways. Mitochondrially mediated diseases are in fact now being recognised in humans (p. 89).

GENE STRUCTURE

The original concept of a gene as a contiguous sequence of DNA coding for a protein was turned on its head in the early 1970s by detailed analysis of the structure of the beta globin gene which revealed it to be much longer than the length necessary for the beta globin protein. The gene was found to contain non-coding intervening sequences or *introns* separating the coding sequences or *exons* (Fig. 2.5). It appears to be the exception for genes in humans to consist of uninterrupted coding sequences (pp. 234, 236, 240). The number and size of introns in various genes in humans are extremely variable. Individual introns can be far larger than the coding sequences and some have been found to contain coding sequences for other genes.

MULTIGENE FAMILIES

The numerous copies of genes coding for the various ribosomal RNAs are clustered as tandem arrays on the short arms of the 5 acrocentric chromosomes (p. 23). In addition, the different transfer RNA (p. 13) gene subfamilies are located in numerous clusters interspersed throughout the human genome.

Many genes of closely related DNA sequence are located physically near each other, e.g. the alpha and beta globin gene clusters on chromosomes 16 and 11 (Fig. 2.6). Other examples are the histone protein genes on chromosome 1, the *HLA* major histocompatibility genes on chromosome 6, and the κ and λ light and heavy immunoglobulin chain gene families on chromosomes 2, 14 and 22 (p. 153). It is believed that these are almost certainly derived from duplication of a precursor gene with subsequent evolutionary divergence.

REGULATION OF GENE EXPRESSION

So far we have been discussing what are referred to as structural genes, that is genes responsible for the synthesis of specific proteins and enzymes. In 1961, as a result of their extensive work on the genetics of the bacterium *E. coli*, Jacob and Monod postulated that in addition to structural genes there are genes which are not directly concerned with the synthesis of specific proteins but instead regulate the activity of structural genes determining the amount of gene product, so-called *control* genes.

Jacob and Monod coined the term *operon* for the unit of gene action which consists of an *operator* gene and the adjacent structural genes whose action the operator gene controls. The operator gene in turn is controlled by a *regulator* gene which is not necessarily close to the operator gene. The regulator gene synthesises a substance, a

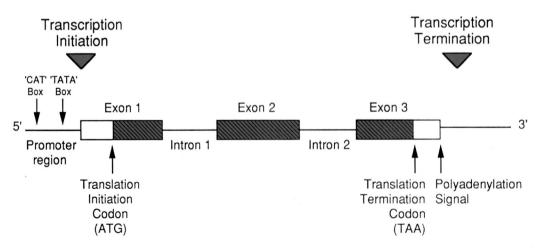

Fig. 2.5
Diagram of the structure of a typical human structural gene.

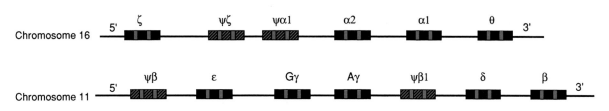

Fig. 2.6
The alpha and beta globin regions on chromosomes 16 and 11.

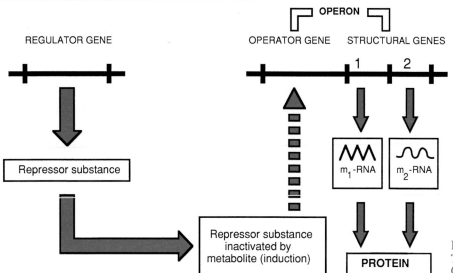

Fig. 2.7
The action of structural and control genes (regulator and operator genes).

repressor, which inhibits the operator gene (Fig. 2.7). Thus, when the regulator gene is functioning, proteins are not synthesised by the associated structural genes. The latter only function when the regulator is 'switched off' by the inactivation of the repressor by a specific metabolite referred to as an *inducer*.

These mechanisms were first demonstrated in lower organisms with no well-defined nucleus, so-called *pro-karyotes*. Analysis of the control of gene expression in higher organisms, *eukaryotes*, has revealed that there could be different factors involved in the regulatory process in humans.

In a 100–300 base-pair *promoter* region located 5' or upstream to the coding sequence of many structural genes in eukaryotic organisms are DNA sequences which control individual gene expression. These include the GGGCGGG *consensus sequence*, the AT-rich *TATA* or *Hogness box*, and the *CAT box*. These so-called *promoter elements*, in conjunction with general transcription factors, are responsible for binding of the enzyme, RNA polymerase II, which is responsible for transcription.

Located at a variable distance from structural genes are DNA sequences, called *enhancers*, which assist with the initiation of transcription. There are also 'negative enhancers' or *silencers* whose normal action is to repress expression.

TRANSCRIPTION AND TRANSLATION

The process whereby genetic information is transmitted from DNA to mRNA is called *transcription* and from mRNA into protein is called *translation*. The information stored in the genetic code is transmitted from the DNA of the gene to a particular type of RNA, *messenger* RNA or mRNA.

Every base in the mRNA molecule is complementary to a corresponding base in the DNA of the gene, i.e. cytosine with guanine, thymine with adenine, but adenine with uracil since the latter replaces thymine in mRNA. The mRNA then migrates out of the nucleus into the cytoplasm where it becomes associated with the ribosomes which are the site of protein synthesis. Groups of ribosomes associated with the same molecule of mRNA are referred to as *polyribosomes* or *polysomes*. In the ribosomes the mRNA forms the template for producing a particular sequence of *amino acids*.

In the cytoplasm there is yet another form of RNA called *transfer* RNA or tRNA. For the incorporation of amino acids into a *polypeptide* chain, the amino acids must first be activated by reacting with ATP. Each activated amino acid then attaches itself to one end of a particular tRNA. The ribosome, with its associated ribosomal RNAs (rRNAs), moves along the mRNA in a zipper-like fashion,

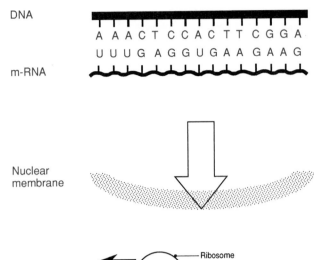

DNA

A A A C T C C A C T T C G G A

U U U G A G G U G A A G A A G

m-RNA

Nuclear
membrane

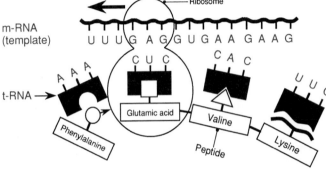

Ribosome

m-RNA
(template) U U U G A G G U G A A G A A G

CUC   CAC

AAA

t-RNA →

Glutamic acid   Valine   Lysine

UUC

Phenylalanine   Peptide

Fig. 2.8
Diagrammatic representation of the way in which genetic
information is translated into protein.

the amino acids linking up to form a polypeptide chain
(Fig. 2.8). When the completed polypeptide chain is
released, the ribosome reattaches itself to a new starting
point on a mRNA molecule.

Transcription involves extension of the RNA molecule
in the 5' to 3' direction. In any particular gene only one
DNA strand of the double helix acts as the so-called
template strand. The transcribed mRNA molecule is a
copy of the complementary coding or *sense* strand of the
DNA double helix. The particular strand of the DNA
double helix used for RNA synthesis appears to differ
throughout different regions of the genome. This transfer
of the genetic information from DNA to RNA to protein
has been called the *central dogma*.

THE GENETIC CODE

There are 20 different amino acids in protein. Since the
primary action of the gene is to synthesise protein, it
could be imagined that all genes could be reduced to 20
different combinations within the DNA molecule.

Genetic information is stored within the DNA molecule
in the form of a *triplet* code, that is, a sequence of three
bases determines one amino acid. The reason for believing

this is as follows. Only 20 different amino acids are
found in proteins and as the DNA molecule is composed
of four different nitrogenous bases, obviously a single
base cannot specify one amino acid, since this would
account for only four amino acids. If two bases were to
specify one amino acid there would only be 4^2 or 16
possible combinations. This is also not enough. If,
however, three bases specified one amino acid then the
possible number of combinations of the four bases would
be 4^3 or 64. This is more than enough to account for all
the 20 known amino acids and is known as the *genetic
code*.

THE TRIPLET BASIS

The first successful attempt to find the key to the genetic
code and so discover which triplet stands for which
amino acid was made by Nirenberg and Matthaei in
1961. These two investigators found that when they
added RNA containing only the nitrogenous base uracil
(U) to a mixture of amino acids, enzymes and ribosomes
a simple protein was synthesized containing only the
amino acid phenylalanine, even though all the other
amino acids were available in the mixture. In other
words, the triplet UUU codes for the amino acid
phenylalanine.

The next step was to introduce into the RNA molecule
containing only uracil (U) bases, an occasional adenine
(A), so that the nucleic acid consisted mainly of U but
with an occasional A occurring at random, e.g.
UUUAUUUAUUAUUU. ... In such a chain most of
the triplets would be UUU but a few would be UUA,
UAU or AUU, depending on where the chain was broken.
Using such a nucleic acid it was found that the resultant
protein was composed mainly of phenylalanine but a few
other amino acids had also been incorporated corresponding to the additional triplets containing adenine.
These other amino acids were leucine, isoleucine and
tyrosine. By similar experiments with various refinements,
triplet codes have been assigned to all 20 amino acids.
Some amino acids are coded for by more than one triplet
and so the code is said to be degenerate (Table 2.1). The
triplet of nucleotide bases in the mRNA which codes for a
particular amino acid is called a *codon* while the complementary triplet of the tRNA molecule which binds to it
with a particular amino acid is called an *anti-codon*.

NON-OVERLAPPING CODONS

There still remains the problem of whether the triplet
code is overlapping or not. If the sequence of bases in a
particular mRNA is UAAGCAUAGG, then the different
possible triplets are UAA, AAG, AGC, GCA, CAU,
AUA, UAG, and AGG. Obviously if the triplets overlap,

Table 2.1 Genetic code in terms of RNA triplets or codons (* chain termination)

1ST BASE	U	C	A	G	3RD BASE
			2ND BASE		
U	Phenylalanine	Serine	Tyrosine	Cysteine	U
	Phenylalanine	Serine	Tyrosine	Cysteine	C
	Leucine	Serine	*Ochre	*	A
	Leucine	Serine	*Amber	Tryptophan	G
C	Leucine	Proline	Histidine	Arginine	U
	Leucine	Proline	Histidine	Arginine	C
	Leucine	Proline	Glutamine	Arginine	A
	Leucine	Proline	Glutamine	Arginine	G
A	Isoleucine	Threonine	Asparagine	Serine	U
	Isoleucine	Threonine	Asparagine	Serine	C
	Isoleucine	Threonine	Lysine	Arginine	A
	Methionine	Threonine	Lysine	Arginine	G
G	Valine	Alanine	Aspartic acid	Glycine	U
	Valine	Alanine	Aspartic acid	Glycine	C
	Valine	Alanine	Glutamic acid	Glycine	A
	Valine	Alanine	Glutamic acid	Glycine	G

chaos would result if different tRNAs could attach themselves anywhere. In fact, tRNAs, with their respective amino acids, become attached in sequence along the mRNA starting at one end and gradually extending to the other. In the example given above one tRNA would become attached to UAA and when this was completed another would become attached to GCA and so on along the length of the mRNA. The order of the triplet codons in a gene is known as the *reading frame*.

In 1970, Khorana and colleagues succeeded in synthesising a gene de novo. They assembled the 77 base pairs of the gene which codes for the production of alanine tRNA in yeast. This artificial gene, while structurally correct, was non-functional both in cells and in the test tube mainly because it did not contain the *initiator* and *termination* signals that start and regulate the synthesis of tRNA. Subsequently Khorana and his associates succeeded in synthesising a wholly artificial gene which did function in a living cell.

It is of interest that the mitochondrial genetic code differs from the nuclear DNA code for 4 of the codons. Why this should be is a complete mystery. It is tempting to speculate that during evolution mitochondria, which are believed to have derived from some early independent organism, retained a genetic code which was subsequently abandoned by bacteria and all other organisms.

POST-TRANSCRIPTIONAL PROCESSING

Before the primary mRNA molecule leaves the nucleus, it undergoes a number of modifications or what is known as *processing*.

5' CAPPING

After transcription, the nascent mRNA is modified by the addition of a methylated guanine nucleotide to the 5' end of the molecule by an unusual 5' to 5' triphosphate linkage, the so-called *5' cap*.

POLYADENYLATION

The cleavage of the 3' end of the mRNA molecule from the DNA involves the addition of approximately 200 adenylate residues, the so-called *poly(A) tail*. The addition of the poly(A) tail is thought to make the mRNA more resistant to digestion by endogenous cellular nucleases.

mRNA SPLICING

After transcription, the intervening sequences or introns in the primary mRNA are excised, and the non-contiguous exons are *spliced* together to form the mature mRNA before its transportation to the ribosomes in the cytoplasm for translation (Fig. 2.9). The boundary between the introns and exons consists of a 5' donor GT dinucleotide and a 3' acceptor AG dinucleotide as well as surrounding short consensus sequences.

POST-TRANSLATIONAL PROCESSING

Many proteins, before they attain their normal structure or functional activity, undergo *post-translational modification* or *processing* which can involve either the addition of carbohydrate moieties or proteolytic cleavage, e.g. pro-insulin to insulin.

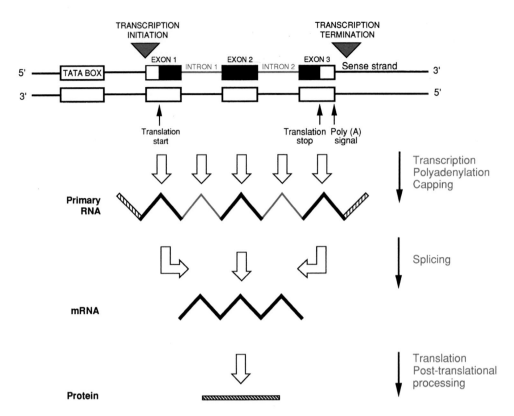

Fig. 2.9
Diagram of transcription, post-transcriptional processing, translation and post-translational processing.

RNA-DIRECTED DNA SYNTHESIS

It was initially believed that genetic information was only transferred from DNA to RNA and thence translated into protein. However, there is evidence, from the study of certain types of virus, retroviruses, that genetic information can occasionally flow in the reverse direction, i.e. from RNA to DNA (p. 165). This is referred to as RNA-directed DNA synthesis. It has been suggested that regions of DNA in normal cells serve as templates for the synthesis of RNA which in turn then acts as a template for the synthesis of DNA which later becomes integrated into the nuclear DNA of other cells. Homology between human and retroviral oncogene sequences could reflect this process (p. 166) which could be an important therapeutic approach in the treatment of inherited disease in humans (p. 279).

MUTATION

A *mutation* is defined as an alteration or change in the genetic material. Mutations are of two main kinds, either microscopically detectable gross structural chromosomal changes or sub-microscopic alterations involving one or more nucleotides (Table 2.2). However, when we speak about mutations in the present context usually we are talking about sub-microscopic changes at a *locus*, of which there are a number of different types.

Table 2.2 Types of mutation and possible consequences

Type of mutation	Consequence
Substitution (point mutation)	Silent – same amino acid Missense – altered amino acid, possible altered activity Nonsense – stop codon, premature termination of protein, possible loss of function/activity
Deletion/Insertion Multiple of 3 (codon)	Deletion/insertion of amino acid(s) in protein
Not multiple of 3	Altered reading frame or frameshift, altered amino acid sequence, often premature termination of protein through generation of termination codon with loss of function/activity
Dynamic/Unstable Triplet repeat	Altered gene expression, reduced transcription or translation, altered transcript?

TYPES OF MUTATION

Silent

Structural genes are responsible for the synthesis of protein, and a mutation of a base pair in a DNA molecule, or what is known as *point mutation*, can have various effects on the corresponding protein. The change can result in another triplet which codes for the same amino acid, a so-called *silent* mutation. In this case there will be no alteration to the properties of the resulting protein, an example of the degeneracy of the genetic code. Perhaps 20–25% of all possible single base changes are of this type.

Missense

In approximately 70–75% of cases, a single base mutation results in a different amino acid and the synthesis of an altered protein, a so-called *missense* mutation. This could affect the molecular structure of the protein so that there is a gross reduction, or even a complete loss, of biological activity. Alternatively the result could be a qualitative rather than a quantitative change in the protein such that it retains its normal biological activity (e.g. enzyme activity) but differs in characteristics such as its mobility on electrophoresis, its pH optimum, or its stability so that it is more rapidly broken down in vivo. Many of the abnormal haemoglobins (p. 118) are the result of missense mutations.

Nonsense

In approximately 2–4% of single base changes, the result is a so-called *nonsense* mutation which codes for one of the *stop codons*, ochre or amber, leading to termination of a *peptide* chain (Table 2.1). In most cases the shortened chain is unlikely to retain normal biological activity, particularly if the termination occurs, for example, before an important functional domain of the protein. A gene mutation can involve more than a single base in the DNA sequence, such as a rearrangement with an *insertion, deletion* or *duplication* of part of a gene or DNA sequence, with corresponding changes in biological activity.

Frame-shift

If any mutation involves the insertion or deletion of nucleotides which are not a multiple of three, it will disrupt the reading frame and constitute what is known as a *frame-shift mutation* in which the amino acid sequence subsequent to the mutation bears no resemblance to the normal sequence of that gene.

Dynamic

Recently, a new class of mutation has been identified which has emerged as an important and unexpected cause of mutation in inherited disease in humans. These have been called unstable or *dynamic* mutations and consist of triplet repeat sequences which, in affected persons, are of increased copy number when compared to the general population. Increase in the copy number of triplet repeat sequences, which is referred to as *triplet amplification* or *expansion*, has been identified as the mutational basis for a number of different single gene disorders including Huntington's disease (p. 86), Fragile X mental retardation (p. 224) and myotonic dystrophy (p. 249).

The mechanism by which amplification or expansion of the triplet repeat sequence occurs is not clear at present but it is postulated that it could involve two single stranded breaks within the repeat sequence with the DNA between the breakpoints 'sliding' as it is not anchored by a unique DNA sequence during DNA polymerization. Triplet expansions usually take place over a number of generations, providing an explanation for some unusual patterns of inheritance (p. 225) as well as possibly being the basis of the previously unexplained phenomenon of anticipation (p. 86).

EFFECTS OF MUTATIONS

If we consider conditions such as the inborn errors of metabolism (p. 127), the level of a particular enzyme can be reduced because it is not synthesised, or it can be synthesised but have reduced activity or stability. Rarely, a gene mutation can lead to the increased synthesis of an enzyme, resulting in increased activity, e.g. the Hektoen variant of G6PD (p. 145). The whole range of these different types of structural gene mutations is seen at the G6PD locus, where over 200 different mutants, with widely differing enzyme activities, have been recognised (p. 145).

In some genetic disorders, even though a specific protein is synthesised and its presence can be demonstrated by immunological methods, the protein is functionally inactive, as occurs in most patients with haemophilia (p. 82). This is known as *cross-reacting material*.

Mutations are usually harmful. It can be argued teleologically that evolutionary processes have resulted in a genetic make-up which is best adapted to the environment in which an organism lives, and any upset of such a balance would be detrimental. Sometimes, however, a new mutation is beneficial. Plant and animal breeders are continually looking for new mutations which could be of economic importance. Examples include strains of organisms or animals which are disease-resistant or have increased yield of a food product. In humans, however, a new mutation is much more likely to be recognised if its effects are detrimental, leading to a disorder or disease, rather than if it confers an increased resistance to infection or leads to a slightly longer survival time.

It is estimated that each individual carries about six *lethal* or semi-lethal recessive mutant alleles which in the homozygous state would have very serious effects. These are conservative estimates and the actual figure could be many times greater. Harmful alleles of all kinds constitute the so-called *genetic load* of the population.

MUTAGENS AND MUTAGENESIS

Naturally occurring mutations are referred to as *spontaneous mutations* and are thought to arise through chance errors in chromosomal division or DNA replication. Alternatively they can arise through exposure to environmental agents such as natural or artificial ionising radiation and chemical or physical mutagens.

IONISING RADIATION

Ionising radiation includes electromagnetic waves of very short wavelength (X-rays and gamma rays), and high energy particles (alpha particles, beta particles and neutrons). X-rays, gamma rays and neutrons have great penetrating power but alpha particles can penetrate soft tissues to a depth of only a fraction of a millimetre and beta particles only up to a few millimetres.

Measures of radiation

The amount of radiation received by irradiated tissues is often referred to as the 'dose' of radiation, which is measured in terms of *rads*. The rad (radiation absorbed dose) is a measure of the amount of any ionising radiation which is actually absorbed by the tissues. One rad is equivalent to 100 ergs of energy absorbed per gram of tissue. Many biological effects of ionising radiation depend on the volume of tissue exposed. In man, irradiation of the whole body with a dose of 300–500 rads is usually fatal, but in the treatment of malignant tumours as much as 10 000 rads can be given to a small volume of tissue without serious effects.

Humans can be exposed to a mixture of radiation and the *rem* (roentgen equivalent for man) is a convenient unit as it is a measure of any radiation in terms of X-rays. A rem of radiation is that absorbed dose which produces in a given tissue the same biological effect as one rad of X-rays. Expressing doses of radiation in term of rems permits us to compare the amounts of different types of radiation to which humans are exposed. A millirem (mrem) is one-thousandth of a rem. 100 rems is equivalent to 1 *sievert* (Sv), and 100 rads is equivalent to 1 *gray* (Gy) in SI units. For all practical purposes, sieverts and grays are approximately equal. In this discussion sieverts and millisieverts (mSv) will be used as the unit of measure.

Dosimetry

Dosimetry is the measurement of radiation. The dose of radiation is expressed in relation to the amount received by the gonads because it is the effects of radiation on *germ cells* rather than *somatic cells* which are important as far as transmission to future progeny is concerned. The *gonad dose* of radiation is often expressed as the amount received in 30 years. This period of time has been chosen because it corresponds roughly to the generation time in humans.

Sources of radiation

The various sources and average annual doses of the different types of natural and artificial ionising radiation are listed in Table 2.3. Natural sources of radiation include cosmic rays, external radiation from radioactive materials in certain rocks and internal radiation from radioactive materials in tissues. Artificial sources include diagnostic and therapeutic radiology, occupational exposure and fallout from nuclear explosions.

The average gonad dose of ionising radiation from radioactive fallout resulting from the testing of nuclear weapons is less than that from any of the sources of background radiation. However, the possibility of serious accidents involving nuclear reactors, as occurred at Three Mile Island in the United States in 1979 and at Chernobyl in the Soviet Union in 1986 with widespread effects, always has to be kept in mind.

Table 2.3 Approximate average doses of ionising radiation from various sources to the gonads of the general population (*including radon in dwellings) (data from Clarke R H, Southwood T R E 1989 Risks from ionizing radiation. Nature 338: 197–198)

Source of radiation	Average dose per year (mSv)	Average dose per 30 years (mSv)
Natural		
Cosmic radiation	0.25	7.5
External gamma radiation*	1.50	45.0
Internal gamma radiation	0.30	9.0
Artificial		
Medical radiology	0.30	9.0
Radioactive fallout	0.01	0.3
Occupational and miscellaneous	0.04	1.2
Total	2.40	72.0

Genetic effects

Experiments with animals and plants have shown that the number of mutations produced by irradiation is proportional to the dose; the larger the dose the more mutations produced. One important point is that there is no threshold below which irradiation has no effect. It is believed that even the smallest dose of radiation can produce a mutation. The genetic effects of ionising radiation are also cumulative so that each time a person is exposed to radiation the dose received has to be added to the amount of radiation already received. The total number of radiation-induced mutations is directly proportional to the total gonad dose.

Atomic radiation

Neel and Schull tackled the problem of trying to demonstrate the genetic effects of radiation by comparing the offspring of parents exposed to atomic radiation at the time Hiroshima and Nagasaki were bombed with those of parents who were not similarly exposed to this source of radiation. Analysis of several thousand births revealed no significant differences in the incidence of stillbirths, congenital malformations or neonatal deaths. This does not mean, however, that there are no genetic consequences of ionising radiation.

The genetic effects of radiation are not easy to assess for they are not manifest in the generation which is exposed to radiation but only in subsequent generations. If a dominant mutation is produced then it will be manifest in the next generation, but a recessive mutation will only be manifest if two heterozygotes with a mutation in the same gene have children. If a recessive mutant allele is very rare then the chance of this happening will be small. It was argued, however, that recessive mutations induced on the X chromosome would be immediately manifest in hemizygous (p. 82) male offspring of mothers who had been irradiated. If these mutants were lethal then the number of male births would be diminished; the *sex ratio* (number of male births divided by the number of female births) would be reduced. This is what would be expected if lethal recessive X-linked mutations were produced in the gonads of a woman who has been irradiated. If X-linked dominant lethal mutations were produced then there would be an equal chance of both male and female babies being eliminated and the sex ratio would remain unchanged. Recessive X-linked lethal mutations induced in the paternal gonads would have no effect on the sex ratio but dominant X-linked lethal mutations would lead to an excess of live male births with a resultant increase in the sex ratio. In other words, if a large enough sample was studied, one would expect that in the case of fathers exposed to radiation the sex ratio of their offspring would be increased whereas in the case of mothers exposed to radiation the sex ratio of their offspring would be decreased.

In the study of parents who had been exposed to atomic radiation in Japan, evidence was obtained by Neel and Schull of slight changes in the sex ratio which could be interpreted as being due to the production of X-linked mutations. In non-irradiated parents the sex-ratio was 0.5209 but in those parents who had received a dose of about 200 rads the sex-ratio was 0.5272 when the father had been irradiated and 0.5119 when the mother had been irradiated.

However, in an extension of this study published in 1966, it was not possible to confirm the effects of radiation on the sex-ratio. In fact, careful studies have revealed no higher incidence of abnormality among survivors' offspring than among the normal population and the practice of giving Green Cards to survivors' children, which gave certain medical and financial privileges, was abandoned in 1966.

The results of both these studies have to be considered with caution because many factors other than radiation can influence the sex ratio. For instance, the sex ratio is affected by paternal age and birth order, the proportion of males being highest in first births and decreasing with successive births.

Medical radiation

Similar results were obtained in studies looking at the offspring of parents who received pelvic radiotherapy. These showed a slight increase in the sex ratio when the father was the irradiated parent and a slight decrease when the mother was the irradiated parent.

Other attempts to detect genetic damage resulting from radiation have been made by comparing the incidence of abortions, stillbirths and congenital malformations in the offspring of radiologists and in the offspring of other medical specialists, the assumption being that radiologists are exposed to more radiation than other physicians. The results of these studies showed that there were slightly more abortions, stillbirths, and congenital malformations in the offspring of radiologists but the differences were not statistically significant.

Occupational radiation

A recent carefully controlled study of fathers working at the nuclear power plant at Sellafield in West Cumbria has revealed a significantly increased number of cases of leukaemia among their children. The results suggested that exposure to ionising radiation in some way led to leukaemia, possibly by inducing mutations in the germ cells of the fathers, though leukaemia is not strictly a genetic disorder. It will be instructive to see if in future there is any increase of genetic disorders in the offspring of such fathers, though so far there is no evidence of this.

Permissible dose

In summary, attempts to demonstrate that radiation causes genetic damage in humans have not been very convincing. This does not mean, however, that radiation does not cause genetic damage in humans. Experiments on other organisms have shown quite clearly that ionising radiation does cause mutations, the vast majority of which are harmful. The hazard from mutations induced in humans is not so much to ourselves as to our descendants. Unfortunately, in humans we do not have any easy way to demonstrate genetic damage caused by mutagens. Nevertheless the International Commission of Radiological Protection (ICRP), working in close liaison with various agencies of the United Nations (WHO, UNESCO, IAEA, etc.), has been mainly responsible for defining what is referred to as the maximum *permissible dose* of radiation. The maximum permissible *genetic dose* of radiation is an arbitrary safety limit and is probably very much less than that which would cause any significant effect on the frequency of harmful mutations within the population. It has been recommended that occupational exposure should not exceed 50 mSv in a year. However, there is currently much controversy over exactly what a permissible dose should be and some countries, such as the United States, set the upper limit significantly lower than many others. In the UK the National Radiological Protection Board advises that occupational exposure should not in fact exceed 15 mSv in a year. To put this into perspective, 1 mSv is roughly 50 times the dose received in a single chest X-ray and 100 times the dose incurred in flying from the UK to Spain in a jet aircraft!

There is no doubting the potential dangers, both somatic and genetic, of excessive exposure to ionising radiation. In the case of medical radiology the dose of radiation resulting from a particular procedure has to be weighed against the ultimate beneficial effect to the patient. In the case of occupational exposure to radiation, the answer lies in defining the risks and introducing and enforcing adequate legislation. With regard to the dangers from fallout from nuclear accidents and explosions the solution would seem obvious.

CHEMICAL AND PHYSICAL MUTAGENS

In humans, chemical mutagenesis could, in fact, be more important than radiation in producing genetic damage. Experiments have shown that certain chemicals such as mustard gas, formaldehyde, benzene, some basic dyes and even caffeine are mutagenic in animals. Many of these mutagenic substances are present in various agricultural, industrial and pharmaceutical chemicals in common use today. Consideration of animal data on the effects of chemicals on the induction of mutations makes it seem likely to be relevant in humans. High temperature is also known to increase the mutation rate in animals but again the relevance of this to humans is conjectural.

Concern over exposure to environmental chemicals with potential mutagenicity is receiving increasing attention although, again, formal proof of the consequences of such exposures is difficult to obtain.

ELEMENTS

1 Genetic information is stored in DNA (deoxyribonucleic acid) as a linear sequence of two types of nucleotides, the purines (adenine [A] and guanine [G]) and the pyrimidines (cytosine [C] and thymine [T]), linked by a sugar-phosphate backbone.

2 A molecule of DNA consists of two antiparallel strands held in a double helix by hydrogen bonds between the complementary G–C and A–T base pairs.

3 DNA replication has multiple sites of origin and is semi-conservative, each strand acting as a template for synthesis of a complementary strand.

4 Genes coding for proteins in higher organisms (eukaryotes) consist of coding (exons) and non-coding (introns) sections.

5 Transcription is the synthesis of a single stranded complemetary copy of one strand of the DNA of a gene which is known as the messenger RNA or mRNA. RNA (ribonucleic acid) differs from DNA in containing the sugar ribose and the base uracil in place of thymine.

6 mRNA is processed during transport from the nucleus to the cytoplasm, eliminating the non-coding sections. In the cytoplasm it becomes associated with the ribosomes where translation, i.e. protein synthesis, occurs.

7 The genetic code is 'universal' and consists of triplets (codons) of nucleotides, each of which codes for an amino acid or for termination of peptide chain synthesis. The code is degenerate, i.e. all but two amino acids are specified by more than one codon.

8 There are regulatory sequences in the 5' flanking regions of structural genes in eukaryotes. Many of the complex factors involved in the regulation and contol of expression of genes in humans will be revealed by research in the next decade or so.

FURTHER READING

Alberts B, Bray D, Lewis J et al 1994 Molecular biology of the cell, 3rd edn. Garland, London
Very accessible, well written and lavishly illustrated comprehensive text of molecular biology.

Beir V 1990 Health effects of exposure to low levels of ionizing radiation. National Academy Press, Washington
The fifth report of the National Research Council's Committee on the Biological Effects of Ionizing Radiations on the effects of low-dose radiation.

Darnell J, Lodish H, Baltimore D 1990 Molecular cellular biology. Freeman, New York
Published by Scientific American Books with very high quality illustrations.

Dawkins R 1989 The selfish gene, 2nd edn. Oxford University Press, Oxford
An interesting and controversial concept.

Jacob F, Monod J 1961 Genetic regulatory mechanisms in the synthesis of proteins. J Mol Biol 3: 318–356
A review article detailing the evidence for the hypothesis of regulatory genes.

Lewin B 1994 Genes V, 5th edn. Oxford University Press, Oxford
The fifth edition of this excellent textbook of molecular biology which has been further improved by simplification of the presentation along with excellent colour diagrams and figures.

Mettler F A, Moseley R D 1985 Medical effects of ionising radiation. Grune & Stratton, London
Good overview of all aspects of the medical consequences of ionising radiation.

Watson J D, Crick F H C 1953 Molecular structure of nucleic acids—a structure for deoxyribose nucleic acid. Nature 171: 737–738
The concepts in this paper, presented in just over one page, resulted in the authors receiving the Nobel Prize!

CHAPTER 3

Chromosomes

INTRODUCTION

Chromosomes are thread like structures located in the cell nucleus. The word chromosome is derived from the Greek chroma (= colour) and soma (= body). Very simply, chromosomes can be considered as being made up of genes. Their behaviour at somatic cell division in *mitosis* provides a means of ensuring that each daughter cell retains its own complete genetic complement. Similarly the behaviour of chromosomes during gamete formation in *meiosis* enables each mature ovum and sperm to contain a unique single set of parental genes. Chromosomes are quite literally the vehicles which facilitate reproduction and the maintenance of a species.

The study of chromosomes and cell division is referred to as *cytogenetics*. Prior to the 1950s it was believed, incorrectly, that each human cell contained 48 chromosomes and that human sex was determined by the number of X chromosomes present at conception. The field of cytogenetics developed rapidly following the development in 1956 of more reliable techniques for studying human chromosomes, which soon led to the realisation that abnormalities of chromosome structure and number could result in disturbance of growth and development.

CHROMOSOME STRUCTURE

Most of our knowledge of chromosome structure has been gained using light microscopy. Special stains selectively taken up by DNA have enabled each individual chromosome to be identified. These are best seen during cell division when the chromosomes are maximally contracted and the constituent genes can no longer be transcribed. Using this technique it can be seen that chromosomes are not uniform in width throughout their length, with each chromosome having a constriction which is referred to as a *centromere*. The exact structure of a centromere is unclear but it is known to be responsible for the movement of the chromosome at cell division.

The centromere divides the chromosome into short and long arms, designated p for 'petit' and q ('g' = grand) respectively. The tip of each end is referred to as a *telomere*.

Morphologically chromosomes are classified according to the position of the centromere. If this is located centrally, the chromosome is *metacentric*, if terminally it is *acrocentric*, and if the centromere is in an intermediate position the chromosome is *submetacentric* (Fig. 3.1). Acrocentric chromosomes can have stalk-like appendages called *satellites* which form the nucleolus of the resting interphase cell and contain multiple repeat copies of the genes for ribosomal RNA.

Individual chromosomes differ not only in the position of the centromere but also in their overall length. Based on the three parameters of length, position of the centromere and the presence or absence of satellites, early pioneers of cytogenetics were able to identify most individual chromosomes or at least subdivide them into groups labelled A–G on the basis of overall morphology (A = 1–3, B = 4–5, C = 6–12 + X, D = 13–15, E = 16–18, F = 19–20, G = 21–22 + Y). The advent of chromosome

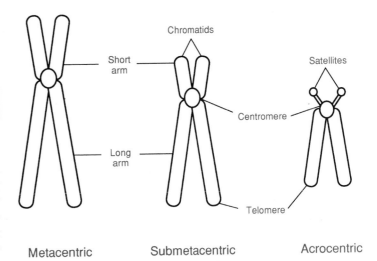

Fig. 3.1
Morphologically chromosomes are divided into metacentric, submetacentric and acrocentric depending on the position of the centromere.

banding (p. 25) has enabled very precise recognition of individual chromosomes and the detection of subtle chromosome abnormalities.

At the submicroscopic level, chromosomes are believed to consist of an extremely elaborate complex made up of supercoils of DNA, similar in overall structure to the tightly coiled network of wiring seen in a solenoid (p. 11). Under the electron microscope chromosomes can be seen to have a rounded, rather irregular morphology (Fig. 3.2).

Each somatic cell nucleus contains two sets of chromosomes, one of which has been inherited from each parent. Members of a pair of chromosomes are known as *homologues*. *Chromatin* is the name given to the material of which chromosomes are made, i.e. a combination of DNA and histone proteins. *Euchromatin* stains lightly and is believed to contain genes which are actively expressed. In contrast *heterochromatin* stains darkly and is believed to be made up largely of inactive unexpressed repetitive DNA.

CHROMOSOME NUMBER

In humans the normal cell nucleus contains 46 chromosomes, made up of 22 pairs of *autosomes* and a single pair of *sex chromosomes* – XX in the female and XY in the male.

One member of each of these pairs is derived from each parent. Somatic cells are said to have a *diploid* complement consisting of 46 chromosomes whereas gametes (ova and sperm) have a *haploid* complement of 23 chromosomes.

The total number of chromosomes in different organisms varies considerably but is constant for any particular species. In certain ferns there are as many as 500 chromosomes within a single nucleus and one small crustacean is estimated to have between 1500 and 1600 chromosomes per nucleus. At the other extreme, an intestinal worm is known in which the diploid number of chromosomes is only two.

A few years ago it was believed that the number of chromosomes could be of help in determining the relationship between various groups of primates. However investigations soon showed that the situation was much more complicated. Whereas the marmoset and certain monkeys resemble man in having 46 chromosomes, higher primates more closely related to humans, such as the chimpanzee, gorilla and orangutan, have 48 chromosomes. Amongst these primates the chromosomes of the chimpanzee most closely resemble those of humans. There is general agreement that the human number 2 chromosome is the product of the fusion of two chimpanzee chromosomes with many other

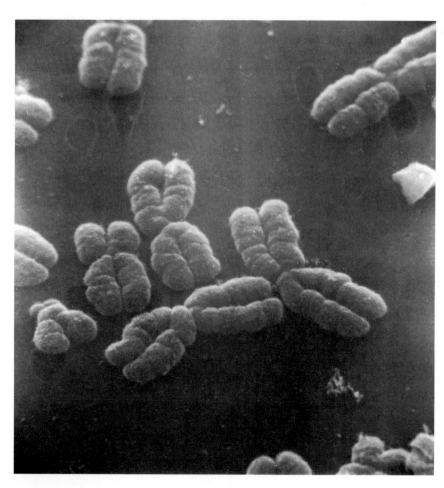

Fig. 3.2
Electron micrograph of human chromosomes showing the centromeres and well defined chromatids (courtesy of Dr Christine Harrison. Reproduced from Cytogenetics and Cell Genetics 1983, 35: 21–27 with permission of the publisher, S Karger AG, Basel).

differences between the chromosome complements in the two species being due to paracentric and pericentric inversions (p. 40). This observation has been exploited by molecular biologists to help map and clone genes in humans (p. 62).

THE SEX CHROMOSOMES

The X and Y chromosomes are known as the sex chromosomes because of their crucial role in sex determination. The X chromosome was originally labelled as such because of uncertainty as to its function when it was realised that in some insects this chromosome is present in some gametes but not in others. In these insects the male has only one sex chromosome (X) whereas the female has two (XX). In humans, and in most mammals, both the male and the female have two sex chromosomes – XX in the female and XY in the male. The Y chromosome is much smaller than the X and carries only a few genes of functional importance, most notably the testis determining factor (p. 71).

In the female each ovum carries an X chromosome, whereas in the male each sperm carries either an X or a Y chromosome. As there is a roughly equal chance of either an X-bearing sperm or a Y-bearing sperm fertilising an ovum, the numbers of male and female conceptions are approximately equal (Fig. 3.3). In fact more male babies are born than females, although during childhood and adult life the sex ratio evens out at 1:1.

The process of sex determination will be considered in detail later (p. 71).

METHODS OF CHROMOSOME ANALYSIS

Even before the beginning of the present century many investigators had attempted to determine the number of chromosomes in humans but their efforts were frustrated by technological limitations. It was generally believed that each cell contained 48 chromosomes until 1956 when Tjio and Levan correctly concluded on the basis of their studies that the normal human somatic cell contains only 46 chromosomes. The methods they used, with certain modifications, are now universally employed in all cytogenetic laboratories to analyse the chromosome constitution of an individual which is known as a *karyotype*. This term is also used to describe a photomicrograph of an individual's chromosomes, arranged in a standard manner.

CHROMOSOME PREPARATION

Any tissue with living nucleated cells which undergo division can be used for studying human chromosomes. Most commonly circulating lymphocytes from peripheral blood are used, although samples for chromosomal analysis can be prepared relatively easily using skin, bone-marrow, chorionic villi or cells from amniotic fluid (amniocytes).

In the case of peripheral (venous) blood, the lymphocytes are separated off and added to a small volume of nutrient medium containing phytohaemagglutinin, which stimulates T lymphocytes to divide. The cells are cultured under sterile conditions at 37°C for about 3 days, during which they divide and then colchicine is added to each culture. This drug has the extremely useful property of preventing formation of the spindle, thereby arresting cell division during metaphase, the time when the chromosomes are maximally condensed and therefore most easily visible. Hypotonic saline is then added which causes the cells to swell and release the chromosomes which are then fixed, mounted on a slide and stained ready for analysis (Fig. 3.4).

CHROMOSOME BANDING

Several different staining methods are used to enable the identification of individual chromosomes.

G (Giemsa) banding

This is the method most commonly used. The chromosomes are treated with trypsin which denatures their protein content and then with Giemsa stain which gives each chromosome a characteristic and reproducible pattern of light and dark bands (Fig. 3.5).

Q (Quinacrine) banding

This gives a banding pattern similar to that obtained with Giemsa, and requires examination of the chromosomes with a fluorescent microscope.

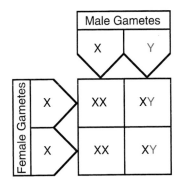

Fig. 3.3
Punnett's square showing sex chromosome combinations for male and female gametes.

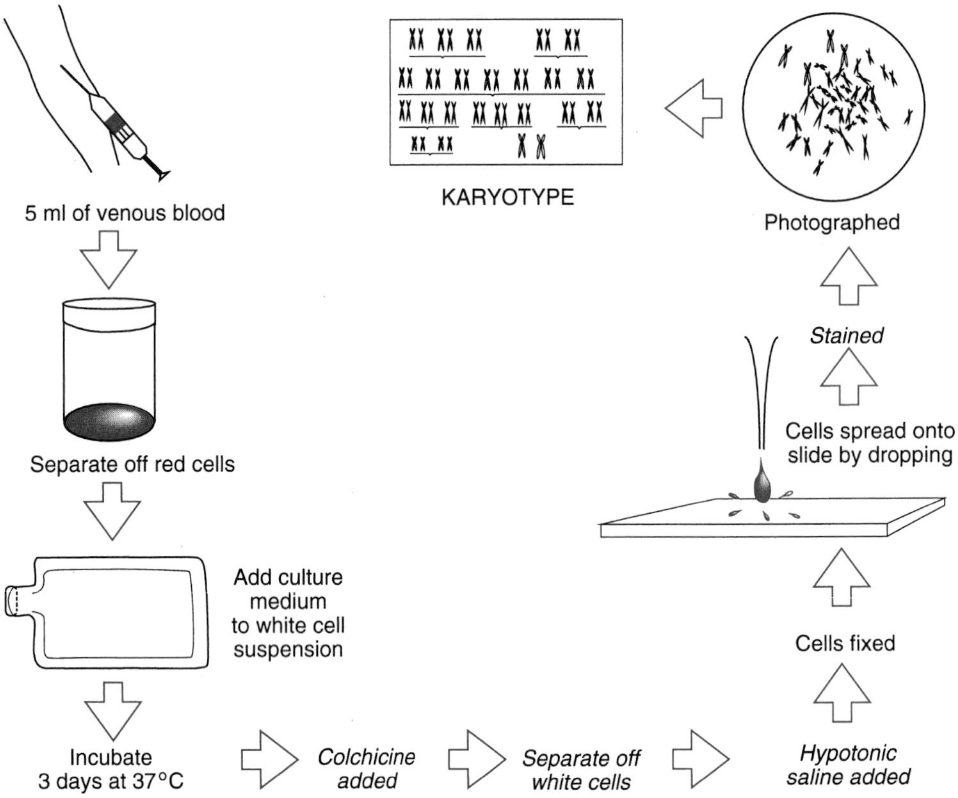

5 ml of venous blood

Separate off red cells

Add culture medium to white cell suspension

Incubate 3 days at 37°C

Colchicine added

Separate off white cells

Hypotonic saline added

Cells fixed

Cells spread onto slide by dropping

Stained

Photographed

KARYOTYPE

Fig. 3.4
Preparation of a karyotype.

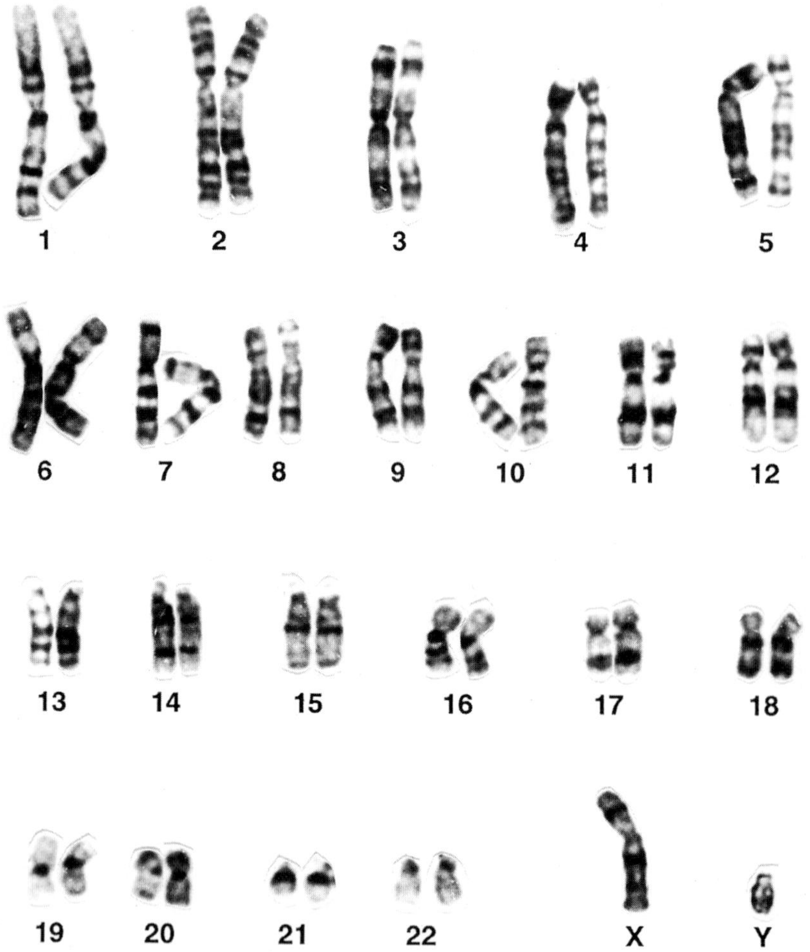

1	2	3	4	5
6	7	8	9	10	11	12
13	14	15	16	17	18
19	20	21	22	X	Y

Fig. 3.5
A normal G banded male karyotype.

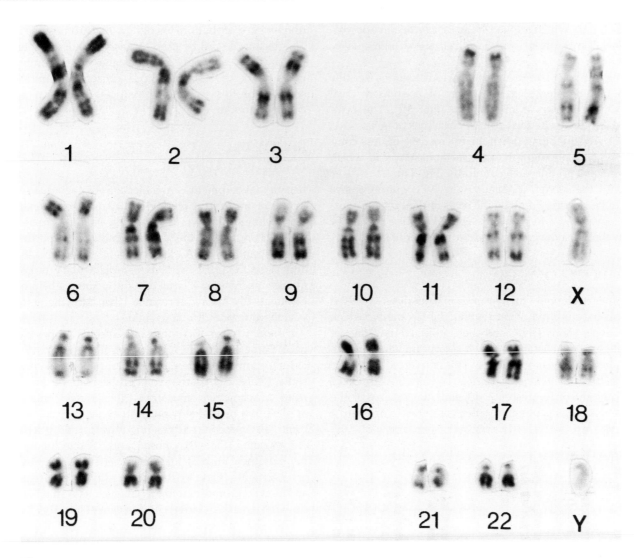

Fig. 3.6
A normal R banded male karyotype (courtesy of H.J. Evans).

R (Reverse) banding

If the chromosomes are heated before staining with Giemsa, the resulting light and dark bands are the reverse of those obtained using conventional G banding (Fig. 3.6).

C (Centromeric heterochromatin) banding

If the chromosomes are pre-treated with acid followed by alkali prior to G banding, the centromeres and other heterochromatic regions containing highly repetitive DNA sequences are preferentially stained.

G banding generally provides high quality chromosome analysis with approximately 400 bands per haploid genome. Each of these bands corresponds to approximately 8000 kilobases of DNA. High resolution banding of the chromosomes at an earlier stage of mitosis such as prophase or prometaphase provides greater sensitivity with up to 800 bands per haploid genome but is much more demanding technically. This involves first inhibit-

ing cell division with the folic acid antagonist, methotrexate. Folic acid is added to the culture medium which releases the cells into mitosis. Colchicine is then added at a specific time interval, when a higher proportion of cells will be in prometaphase and the chromosomes will not be fully contracted, giving a more detailed banding pattern.

CHROMOSOME ANALYSIS

Chromosome analysis involves first counting the number of chromosomes present in a specified number of cells or what are known as *metaphase spreads*, followed by careful analysis of the banding pattern of each individual chromosome in those cells. Usually the total chromosome count is determined in 10–15 cells, but if mosaicism is suspected then 30 or more cell counts will be undertaken. Detailed analysis of the banding pattern of the individual chromosomes is carried out on both members of each pair, which are known as *homologues*, in approximately 5 metaphase spreads which show high quality banding.

The banding pattern of each chromosome is specific and can be shown in the form of a stylised ideal karyotype known as an *idiogram* (Fig. 3.7). The cytogeneticist analyses each pair of *homologous chromosomes*, either whilst looking down the microscope or, less commonly, on a photograph of the metaphase spread which can now be produced electronically (Fig. 3.8).

Until the advent of banding in 1971, chromosomes could be classified only on the basis of their overall morphology. Now a formally presented *karyotype* will show each chromosome pair in descending order of size.

FLOW CYTOMETRY

Another technique for chromosome analysis involves cells being ruptured, stained with a fluorescent dye which selectively stains DNA, and then projected as a fine jet through a flow chamber across a laser beam which excites the chromosomes to fluoresce. This is referred to as *flow cytometry* or *fluorescent activated cell sorting* (FACS). Since the amount of fluorescence depends on the size of the chromosome, it is possible with a computer to draw up a

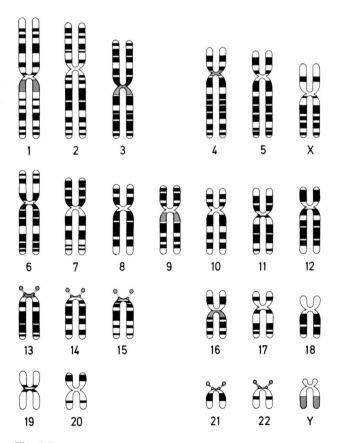

Fig. 3.7
An idiogram showing the banding patterns of individual chromosomes as revealed by fluorescent and Giemsa staining.

frequency distribution histogram of chromosome size. This technique can be used to analyse and separate out preparations of single chromosomes for recombinant DNA work (p. 45), but the expense and limited resolution of this technology reduces its clinical application at present.

FLUORESCENT IN SITU HYBRIDISATION

Recent developments in molecular biology have also made an impact on methods of chromosome analysis. The technique known as *fluorescent in situ hybridisation*, or FISH, relies on the unique ability of a portion of single-stranded DNA, known as a probe (p. 48), to anneal or hybridise with its complementary target sequence wherever it is located in the genome. The probe is conjugated with a fluorescent label allowing it to be visualised under ultraviolet light.

Different types of chromosome-specific probes can be used. Some are specific for the centromere of a particular chromosome (Plate 1) or a particular region of a chromosome (Plate 2). Alternatively probes can be prepared from a whole chromosome. When such probes are applied to a metaphase spread, they will hybridise to or *paint* all material originating from that particular chromosome (Plate 3). Consequently this technique can be extremely useful for characterising complex rearrangements (Plate 4) and for identifying the nature of additional chromosome material, such as a small supernumerary marker or ring chromosome (Plate 5).

FISH has a particular advantage in that it can be applied during interphase. This means that in theory it could be used to make a rapid diagnosis of a condition such as trisomy 21 in interphase nuclei from prenatal diagnostic samples, without the need for cell culture. At present this approach is not sufficiently reliable to justify its widespread introduction.

In the procedure known as *reverse painting*, an additional portion of unidentified chromosome material, such as a small *duplication* or marker chromosome, is extracted using a cell sorter. This is then amplified using the polymerase chain reaction (p. 48) and used as a probe for hybridisation to a normal metaphase spread. The origin of the unidentified chromosome segment or fragment is then revealed by identifying the chromosome to which it hybridises.

MITOSIS

At conception the human zygote consists of a single cell. This undergoes rapid division leading ultimately to the mature human adult, consisting of approximately 1×10^{14} cells in total. In most organs and tissues, such as bone

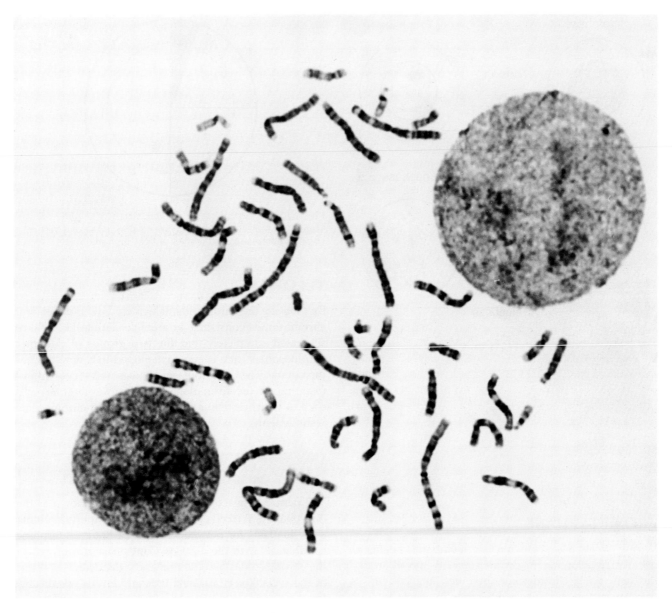

Fig. 3.8
A G banded metaphase spread (courtesy of Mr A. Wilkinson, Cytogenetics Unit, City Hospital, Nottingham).

marrow and skin, cells continue to divide throughout life. This process of somatic cell division during which the nucleus also divides is known as *mitosis*. During mitosis each chromosome divides into two daughter chromosomes one of which segregates into each daughter cell. Consequently the number of chromosomes per nucleus remains unchanged.

Prior to a cell entering mitosis, each chromosome will consist of two identical strands known as *chromatids* as a result of DNA replication having taken place during the S phase of the cell cycle (p. 30). Mitosis is the process whereby each of these pairs of chromatids separates and disperses into separate daughter cells.

Mitosis is a continuous process which usually lasts 1–2 hours, but for descriptive purposes it is convenient to distinguish five distinct stages. These are prophase, prometaphase, metaphase, anaphase and telophase (Fig. 3.9).

PROPHASE

During the initial stage of *prophase* the chromosomes condense and the mitotic spindle begins to form. Two *centrioles* form in each cell from which microtubules radiate as the centrioles move towards opposite poles of the cell.

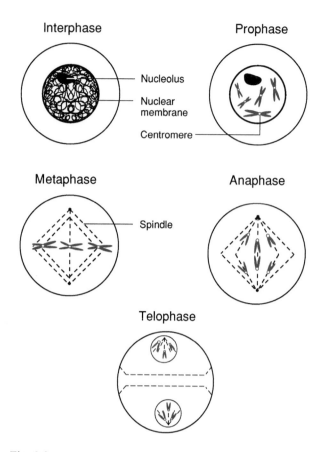

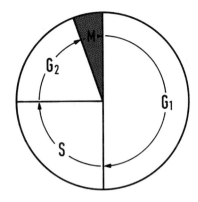

Fig. 3.10
Stages of the cell cycle. G_1 and G_2 are the first and second 'resting' stages of interphase. S is the stage of DNA replication.

Fig. 3.9
Stages of mitosis.

TELOPHASE

By *telophase* the chromatids, which are now independent chromosomes consisting of a single double helix, have separated completely and the two groups of daughter chromosomes each become enveloped in a new nuclear membrane. The cell cytoplasm also separates (cytokinesis) resulting in the formation of two new daughter cells each of which contains a complete diploid chromosome complement.

THE CELL CYCLE

The period between successive mitoses is known as the interphase of the cell cycle (Fig. 3.10). In rapidly dividing cells this lasts for between 16 and 24 hours. Interphase commences with the G_1 (G = Gap) phase during which the chromosomes become thin and extended. This phase of the cycle is very variable in length and is responsible for the variation in generation time within a cell population. Cells which have stopped dividing, such as neurones, usually arrest in this phase and are said to have entered a non-cyclic stage known as G_0.

The G_1 phase is followed by the S phase (S = synthesis), when DNA replication occurs and the chromatin of each chromosome is replicated. This results in the formation of two chromatids which give each chromosome their characteristic X-shaped configuration. The process of DNA replication commences at multiple points on a chromosome (p. 10).

Usually homologous pairs of chromosomes replicate in synchrony. However one of the X chromosomes is always late replicating. This is the inactive X chromosome (p. 72) which forms the *sex chromatin*, or the so-called *Barr body*, which can be visualised in interphase in female somatic cells. This used to be the basis of a rather unsatisfactory means of sex determination based on analysis of cells obtained by scraping the buccal mucosa – a 'buccal smear'.

PROMETAPHASE

During *prometaphase* the nuclear membrane begins to disintegrate allowing the chromosomes to spread around the cell. Each chromosome becomes attached at its centromere to a *microtubule* of the mitotic *spindle*.

METAPHASE

In *metaphase* the chromosomes become orientated along the equatorial plane or plate of the cell, where each chromosome is attached to the centriole by a microtubule forming the mature spindle. At this point the chromosomes are maximally contracted and therefore most easily visible. Each chromosome resembles the letter X in shape as the chromatids of each chromosome have separated longitudinally but remain attached at the centromere which has not yet undergone division.

ANAPHASE

In *anaphase* the centromere of each chromosome divides longitudinally and the two daughter chromatids separate to opposite poles of the cell.

Interphase is completed by a relatively short G_2 phase during which the chromosomes begin to condense in preparation for the next mitotic division.

MEIOSIS

Meiosis is the process of nuclear division which occurs during the final stage of gamete formation. Meiosis differs from mitosis in three fundamental ways:

1. Mitosis results in each daughter cell having a diploid chromosome complement (46). During meiosis the diploid count is halved so that each mature gamete receives a haploid complement of 23 chromosomes.
2. Mitosis takes place in somatic cells and during the early cell divisions in gamete formation. Meiosis occurs only at the final division of gamete maturation.
3. Mitosis occurs as a single one-step process. Meiosis can be considered as two cell divisions known as meiosis I and meiosis II, each of which can be considered as having prophase, metaphase, anaphase and telophase stages as in mitosis (Fig. 3.11).

MEIOSIS I

This is sometimes referred to as the stage of reduction division because during it the chromosome number is halved.

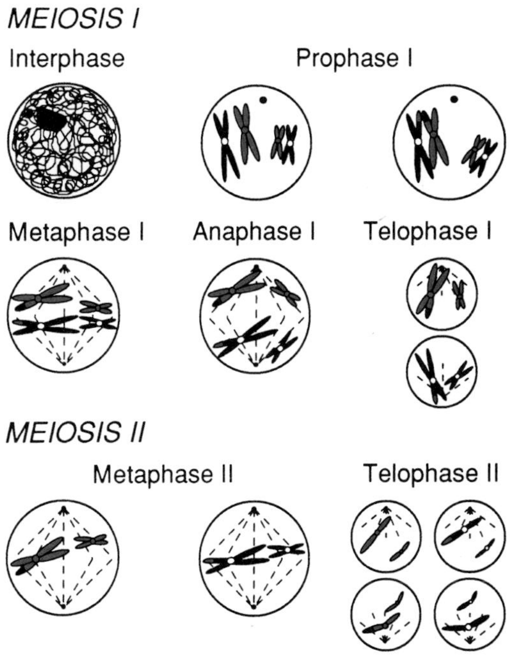

Fig. 3.11
Stages of meiosis.

Prophase I

Chromosomes enter this stage already split longitudinally into two chromatids joined at the centromere. Homologous chromosomes pair, and with the exception of the X and Y chromosomes in male meiosis, exchange of homologous segments occurs between non-sister chromatids, i.e. chromatids from each of the pair of homologous chromosomes. This exchange of homologous segments between chromatids occurs as a result of a process known as *crossing-over* or *recombination*. The importance of crossing-over in linkage analysis and risk calculation is considered later (pp. 100, 258).

During prophase I in the male, the X and Y chromosomes pair but do not exchange material. Pairing occurs between homologous segments at the tip of their short arms, with this portion of each chromosome being known as the *pseudoautosomal* region.

The prophase stage of meiosis I is relatively lengthy and can be subdivided into five stages.

Leptotene

The chromosomes become visible as they start to condense.

Zygotene

Homologous chromosomes align directly opposite each other, a process known as *synapsis*, and are held together at several points along their length by filamentous structures known as *synaptonemal complexes*.

Pachytene

Each pair of homologous chromosomes, known as a *bivalent*, becomes tightly coiled. Crossing-over occurs during which homologous regions of DNA are exchanged between chromatids.

Diplotene

The homologous recombinant chromosomes now begin to separate but remain attached at the points where crossing-over has occurred. These are known as *chiasmata*. On average small, medium and large chromosomes have 1, 2 and 3 chiasmata respectively, giving an overall total of approximately 50 recombination events per meiosis per gamete.

Diakinesis

Separation of the homologous chromosome pairs proceeds as the chromosomes become maximally condensed.

Metaphase I

The nuclear membrane disappears and the chromosomes become aligned on the equatorial plane of the cell where they have become attached to the spindle as in metaphase of mitosis.

Anaphase I

The chromosomes now separate to opposite poles of the cell as the spindle contracts.

Telophase I

Each set of haploid chromosomes has now separated completely to opposite ends of the cell which cleaves into two new daughter gametes, so-called *secondary spermatocytes* or *oocytes*.

MEIOSIS II

This is essentially similar to an ordinary mitotic division. Each chromosome, which exists as a pair of chromatids, becomes aligned along the equatorial plane and then splits longitudinally leading to the formation of two new daughter gametes, known as *spermatids* or *ova*.

THE CONSEQUENCES OF MEIOSIS

When considered in terms of reproduction and the maintenance of the species, meiosis achieves two major objectives. Firstly it facilitates halving of the diploid number of chromosomes so that each child receives half of its chromosome complement from each parent. Secondly it provides an extraordinary potential for generating genetic diversity. This is achieved in two ways:

1. When the bivalents separate during prophase of meiosis I, they do so independently of one another. This is consistent with Mendel's third law (p. 4). Consequently each gamete receives a selection of parental chromosomes. The likelihood that any two gametes will contain exactly the same chromosomes equals 1 in 2^{23}, i.e. approximately 1 in 8 million.
2. As a result of crossing-over, each chromatid will usually contain portions of DNA derived from both chromosomes of the parent. A large chromosome will typically consist of three or more segments of alternating parental origin. The ensuing probability that any two gametes will have an identical genome is therefore infinitesimally small.

This dispersion of DNA into different gametes is sometimes referred to as 'gene shuffling'.

GAMETOGENESIS

The process of gametogenesis shows fundamental differences in male and female (Table 3.1) which have quite distinct clinical consequences if errors occur.

OOGENESIS

Mature ova develop from oogonia by a complex series of intermediate steps. Oogonia themselves originate from primordial germ cells by a process involving 20–30 mitotic divisions which occur during the first few months of embryonic life. By the completion of embryogenesis at 3 months of intra-uterine life, the oogonia have begun to mature into primary oocytes which start to undergo meiosis. By birth all of the primary oocytes have entered a phase of maturation arrest, known as *dictyotene*, in which they remain suspended until meiosis I is completed at the time of ovulation when a single secondary oocyte is formed. This receives most of the cytoplasm. The other daughter cell from the first meiotic division consists largely of a nucleus and is known as a polar body. Meiosis II then commences during which fertilisation can occur. This second meiotic division results in the formation of a further polar body (Fig. 3.12).

It is proposed that the very lengthy interval between the onset of meiosis and its eventual completion, up to 50 years later, accounts for the well documented increase in chromosome abnormalities in the offspring of older mothers (p. 216). It is suggested that the accumulating effects of wear and tear on the primary oocyte during the dictyotene phase can damage the cell's spindle formation and repair mechanisms thereby predisposing to non-disjunction (p. 34).

SPERMATOGENESIS

In contrast, spermatogenesis is a relatively rapid process with an average duration of 60 to 65 days. At puberty spermatogonia, which will already have undergone approximately 30 mitotic divisions, begin to mature into

Table 3.1 Differences in gametogenesis in male and female

	Male	Female
Commences	Puberty	Early embryonic life
Duration	60–65 days	10–50 years
Number of mitoses in gamete formation	30–500	20–30
Gamete production per meiosis	4 spermatids	1 ovum + 3 polar bodies
Gamete production in adult life	100–200 million per ejaculate	1 ovum per menstrual cycle

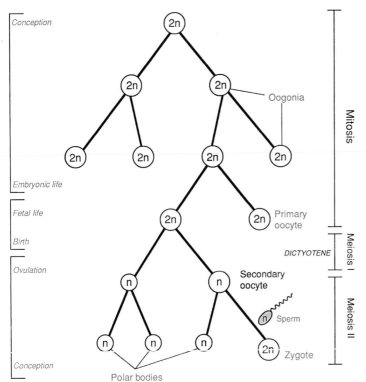

Fig. 3.12
Stages of oogenesis (n = the haploid number).

primary spermatocytes which enter meiosis I and emerge as haploid secondary spermatocytes. These then undergo the second meiotic division to form spermatids, which in turn develop without any subsequent cell division into mature spermatozoa, of which 100 to 200 million are present in each ejaculate.

Spermatogenesis is a continuous process involving many mitotic divisions, possibly as many as 20 to 25 per annum, so that mature spermatozoa produced by a man of 50 years or older could well have undergone several hundred mitotic divisions. The observed paternal age effect for new dominant mutations (p. 79) is consistent with the concept that many mutations arise as a consequence of DNA copy errors occurring during mitosis.

CHROMOSOME ABNORMALITIES

Specific disorders due to chromosome abnormalities are considered in Chapter 17. In this section discussion will be restricted to a review of the different types of abnormality which can occur. These can be divided into numerical and structural, with a third category consisting of different chromosome constitutions in two or more cell lines (Table 3.2).

NUMERICAL ABNORMALITIES

Numerical abnormalities involve the gain or loss of one or more chromosomes or what is known as *aneuploidy*, or the addition of one or more complete haploid complements or *polyploidy*. Loss of a single chromosome results in *monosomy*. Gain of one or two homologous chromosomes is referred to as *trisomy* and *tetrasomy* respectively.

Trisomy

The presence of an extra chromosome is referred to as trisomy. Most cases of Down's syndrome are due to the presence of an additional number 21 chromosome, hence Down's syndrome is often known as trisomy 21. Other autosomal trisomies which are compatible with survival

Table 3.2 Types of chromosome abnormality

Numerical	
Aneuploidy	—Monosomy
	—Trisomy
	—Tetrasomy
Polyploidy	—Triploidy
	—Tetraploidy
Structural	
Translocations	—Reciprocal
	—Robertsonian
Deletions	
Inversions	—Paracentric
	—Pericentric
Rings	
Isochromosomes	
Different cell lines	
Mosaicism	
Chimaerism	

to term are Patau's syndrome (trisomy 13) and Edwards' syndrome (trisomy 18). Most other autosomal trisomies result in early pregnancy loss with trisomy 16 being a particularly common finding in first trimester spontaneous miscarriages. The presence of an additional sex chromosome (X or Y) has only mild phenotypic effects (pp. 222–223).

Trisomy is usually caused by failure of separation of one of the pairs of homologous chromosomes during prophase of meiosis I. This failure of the bivalent to separate is called *non-disjunction*. Less often, trisomy can be caused by non-disjunction occurring during meiosis II when a pair of sister chromatids fail to separate. Either way the gamete receives two homologous chromosomes (*disomy*), and if subsequent fertilisation occurs a trisomic conceptus results (Fig. 3.13).

The origin of non-disjunction

The consequences of non-disjunction in meiosis I and meiosis II differ in the chromosomes found in the gamete. An error in meiosis I leads to the gamete containing both homologues of one chromosome pair. In contrast, non-disjunction in meiosis II results in the gamete receiving two copies of one of the homologues of the chromosome pair. Studies using centromeric DNA markers have shown that most children with an autosomal trisomy have inherited their additional chromosome as a result of non-disjunction occurring during one

Table 3.3 Parental origin of meiotic error leading to aneuploidy

Chromosome abnormality	Paternal (%)	Maternal (%)
Trisomy 13	15	85
Trisomy 18	5	95
Trisomy 21	5	95
45, X	80	20
47, XXX	5	95
47, XXY	55	45
47, XYY	100	0

of the maternal meiotic divisions (Table 3.3). Centromeric markers have to be used for these studies as the use of markers on either chromosome arm can give misleading results due to recombination.

Non-disjunction can also occur during an early mitotic division in the developing zygote. This would, however, result in the presence of two or more different cell lines, a phenomenon known as mosaicism (p. 41).

The causes of non-disjunction

The cause of non-disjunction is uncertain. The most favoured explanation is that of an ageing effect on the primary oocyte which can remain in a state of suspended inactivity for up to 50 years (p. 32). There is a well documented association between advancing maternal

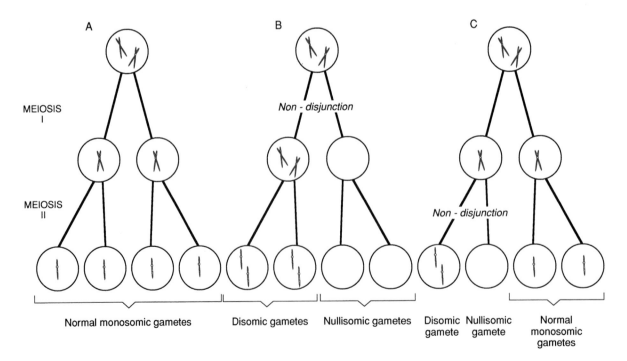

Fig. 3.13
Segregation at meiosis of a single pair of chromosomes in (A) normal meiosis, (B) non-disjunction in meiosis I and (C) non-disjunction in meiosis II.

age and increased incidence of Down's syndrome (Table 17.4). A maternal age effect has also been noted for trisomies 13 and 18.

An alternative explanation for the association of advancing maternal age with increased risk of autosomal trisomy is that survival of trisomic embryos could be the result of an age-related reduction in 'immunological' competence. Firm evidence for this theory is limited.

Other factors which have been implicated in causing non-disjunction include radiation and delayed fertilisation after ovulation. In animals it has been shown that an increased incidence of aneuploid embryos can result from lengthening of the interval between ovulation and fertilisation. It has been suggested that this could account for the relationship between maternal age and the incidence of Down's syndrome, as with increasing age intercourse is likely to occur less frequently, with delayed fertilisation therefore being more likely. The story is further complicated by the fact that in some species such as *Drosophila*, non-disjunction is under genetic control. This could account for those occasional families which seem to be prone to recurrent non-disjunction.

Monosomy

The absence of a single chromosome is referred to as monosomy. Monosomy for an autosome is almost always incompatible with survival to term, with the possible exception of a few very rare reported cases of monosomy 21. Absence of an X or a Y chromosome results in a 45,X karyotype which causes a condition known as Turner's syndrome (p. 222).

As with trisomy, monosomy can also result from non-disjunction in meiosis. If one gamete receives two copies of a homologous chromosome (disomy), the other corresponding daughter gamete will have no copy of the same chromosome (nullisomy). Monosomy can also be caused by loss of a chromosome as it moves to the pole of the cell during anaphase, an event known as *anaphase lag*.

Polyploidy

Polyploid cells contain multiples of the haploid number of chromosomes such as 69, *triploidy*, or 92, *tetraploidy*. In humans triploidy is found relatively often in material grown from spontaneous miscarriages but survival beyond mid-pregnancy is rare. Only a few triploid live births have been described and all have died soon after birth.

Triploidy can be caused by failure of a maturation meiotic division in ovum or sperm, leading, for example, to retention of a polar body, or by fertilisation of an ovum by two sperm, which is known as *dispermy*, or by a diploid sperm. When triploidy results from the presence of an additional set of paternal chromosomes, the placenta is usually swollen with what are known as hydatidiform changes (p. 70). In contrast when triploidy results from an additional set of maternal chromosomes, the placenta is usually small. Triploidy usually results in early spontaneous miscarriage (Fig. 3.14).

STRUCTURAL ABNORMALITIES

Structural chromosome rearrangements result from chromosome breakage with subsequent reunion in a different configuration. They can be balanced or unbalanced. In balanced rearrangements the chromosome complement is complete with no loss or gain of genetic material. Consequently, balanced rearrangements are generally harmless with the exception of rare cases in which one of the breakpoints damages an important functional gene. However, carriers of balanced rearrangements are often at risk of producing children with an unbalanced chromosomal complement.

When a chromosome rearrangement is unbalanced the chromosomal complement contains an incorrect amount of chromosome material and the clinical effects are usually very severe.

Translocations

A *translocation* refers to the transfer of genetic material from one chromosome to another. A *reciprocal translocation* is formed when a break occurs in each of two chromosomes with the segments being exchanged to form two new derivative chromosomes. A *Robertsonian translocation* is a particular type of reciprocal translocation in which the breakpoints are located at or close to the centromeres of two acrocentric chromosomes (Fig. 3.15).

Reciprocal translocations

A reciprocal translocation involves breakage of at least two non-homologous chromosomes with exchange of the fragments. Usually the chromosome number remains at 46, and if the exchanged fragments are of roughly equal size, a reciprocal translocation can often only be identified with detailed chromosomal banding studies. In general reciprocal translocations are unique to a particular family, although, for reasons which are unknown, balanced reciprocal translocations involving the long arms of chromosomes 11 and 22 are relatively common. The overall incidence in the general population of reciprocal translocations is approximately 1 in 500.

Segregation at meiosis
The importance of balanced reciprocal translocations lies in their behaviour at meiosis when they can segregate to

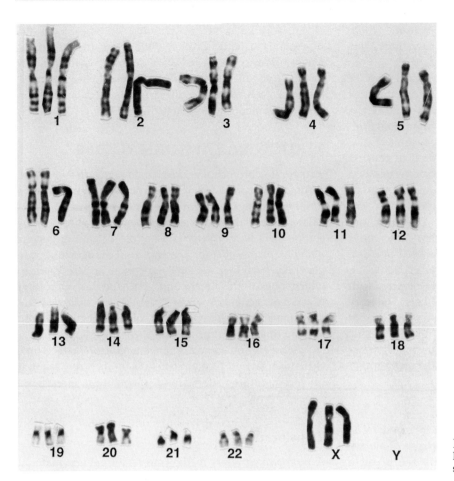

Fig. 3.14
Karyotype from products of conception of a
spontaneous miscarriage showing triploidy.

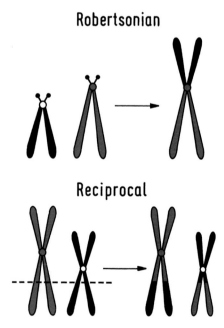

Fig. 3.15
Types of translocation.

generate significant chromosome imbalance. This can lead to early pregnancy loss or to the birth of an infant with multiple abnormalities. Problems can arise at meiosis because the chromosomes involved in the translocation cannot pair normally to form bivalents. Instead they form a cluster known as a *pachytene quadrivalent* (Fig. 3.16). The key point to note is that each chromosome aligns with homologous material in the quadrivalent.

2:2 segregation When the constituent chromosomes in the quadrivalent separate during the later stages of meiosis I they can do so in several different ways (Table 3.4). If alternate chromosomes segregate to each gamete, then the gamete will carry a balanced haploid complement (Fig. 3.17) and with fertilisation the embryo will either have normal chromosomes or carry the balanced rearrangement. If, however, adjacent chromosomes segregate together, this will invariably result in the gamete acquiring an unbalanced chromosome complement. For example, if the gamete inherits the normal number 11 chromosome and the derivative number 22 chromosome, then fertilisation will result in an embryo with monosomy for the distal long arm of chromosome 22 and trisomy for the distal long arm of chromosome 11.

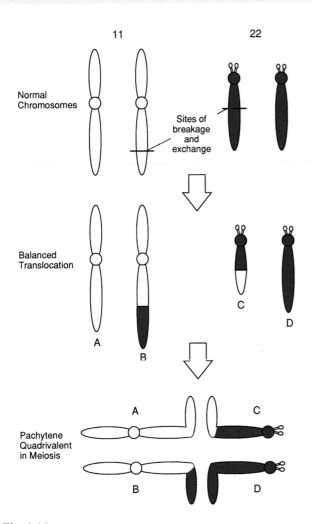

Fig. 3.16
Shows how a balanced reciprocal translocation involving chromosomes 11 and 22 leads to the formation of a quadrivalent at pachytene in meiosis I. The quadrivalent is formed to maintain homologous pairing.

Table 3.4 Patterns of segregation of a reciprocal translocation (see Figs 3.16 and 3.17)

Pattern of segregation	Segregating chromosomes	Chromosome constitution in gamete
2:2 Alternate	A + D	Normal
	B + C	Balanced translocation
Adjacent–1 (non-homologous centromeres segregate together)	A + C or B + D	Unbalanced leading to a combination of partial monosomy and partial trisomy
Adjacent–2 (homologous centromeres segregate together)	A + B or C + D	
3:1 Three chromosomes	A + B + C A + B + D A + C + D B + C + D	Unbalanced leading to trisomy in the zygote
One chromosome	A B C D	Unbalanced leading to monosomy in the zygote

3:1 segregation Another possibility is that three chromosomes segregate to one gamete with only one chromosome in the other gamete. If, for example, chromosomes 11, 22 and the derivative 22 segregate together to a gamete which is subsequently fertilised, this will result in the embryo being trisomic for the material present in the derivative 22 chromosome. This is sometimes referred to as *tertiary trisomy*. Experience has shown that with this particular reciprocal translocation, tertiary trisomy for the derivative 22 chromosome is the only viable unbalanced product. All other patterns of malsegregation lead to early pregnancy loss. Unfortunately tertiary trisomy for the derivative 22 chromosome is a very serious condition in which affected children show severe mental retardation and multiple abnormalities.

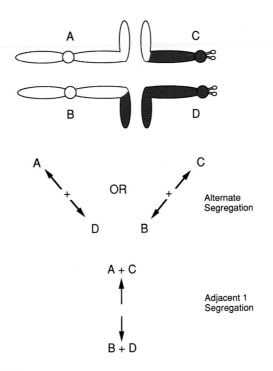

Fig. 3.17
Shows the different patterns of 2:2 segregation which can occur from the quadrivalent shown in Figure 3.16. See Table 3.4.

Risks in reciprocal translocations

When counselling a carrier of a balanced translocation it is necessary to consider the particular rearrangement to determine whether it could result in the birth of an abnormal baby. Usually this risk will lie somewhere between 1% and 10%. For carriers of the 11;22 translocation discussed, the risk has been shown to be 5%.

Robertsonian translocations

A Robertsonian translocation results from breakage of two acrocentric chromosomes (numbers 13, 14, 15, 21 and 22) at or close to their centromeres, with subsequent fusion of their long arms (Fig. 3.15). This is also referred to as *centric fusion*. The short arms of each chromosome are lost, this being of no clinical importance as they contain only genes for ribosomal RNA for which there are multiple copies on the various acrocentric chromosomes. The total chromosome number is reduced to 45 (Fig. 3.18). Since there is no loss or gain of important genetic material this is a functionally balanced rearrangement. The overall incidence of Robertsonian translocations in the general population is approximately 1 in 1000.

Segregation at meiosis

As with reciprocal translocations, the importance of Robertsonian translocations lies in their behaviour at meiosis. For example, a carrier of a 14q21q translocation can produce gametes with (Fig. 3.19):

1. A normal chromosome complement, i.e. a normal 14 and a normal 21.
2. A balanced chromosome complement, i.e. a 14q21q translocation chromosome.
3. An unbalanced chromosome complement possessing both the translocation chromosome and a normal 21. This will result in the fertilised embryo having Down's syndrome.
4. An unbalanced chromosome complement with a normal 14 and a missing 21.
5. An unbalanced chromosome complement with a normal 21 and a missing 14.
6. An unbalanced chromosome complement with the translocation chromosome and a normal 14 chromosome.

The last three combinations will result in zygotes with monosomy 21, monosomy 14 and trisomy 14 respectively. All of these combinations are incompatible with survival of the early conceptus.

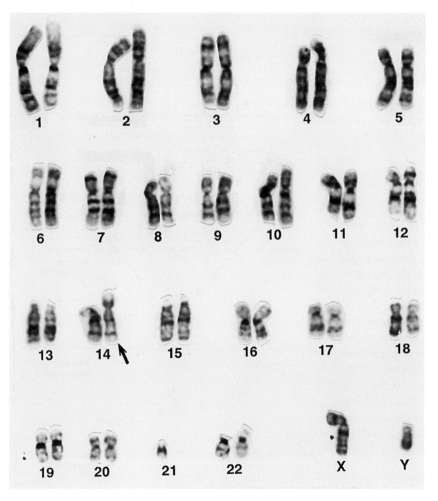

Fig. 3.18
Karyotype of a male carrier of a 14q21q Robertsonian translocation.

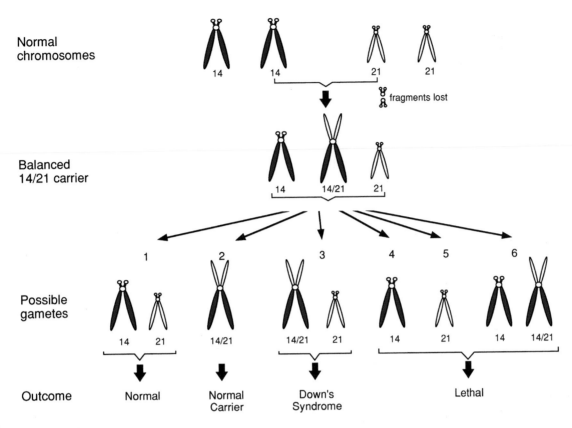

Normal
chromosomes

fragments lost

Balanced
14/21 carrier

Possible
gametes

1   2   3   4   5   6

14 21   14/21   14/21 21   14   21   14 14/21

Outcome   Normal   Normal   Down's   Lethal
Carrier   Syndrome

Fig. 3.19
Shows the formation of a 14q21q Robertsonian translocation and the possible gamete chromosome patterns which can be produced at meiosis.

Translocation Down's syndrome

The major practical importance of Robertsonian trans-locations is that they can predispose to the birth of babies with Down's syndrome as a result of the embryo inheriting two normal number 21 chromosomes (one from each parent) plus a translocation chromosome involving a number 21 chromosome. The clinical consequences are exactly the same as those seen in pure trisomy 21. However unlike trisomy 21, the parents of a child with translocation Down's syndrome have a relatively high risk of having further affected children if one of them carries the rearrangement in a balanced form.

Consequently the importance of performing a chromosome analysis in a child with Down's syndrome lies not only in confirmation of the diagnosis, but also in identification of those children with a translocation. In roughly two thirds of these latter children with Down's syndrome, the translocation will have occurred as a new ('de novo') event in the child, but in the remaining one third one parent will be a carrier. Other relatives can also be carriers. Consequently it is regarded as essential that efforts are made to identify all adult translocation carriers in a family so that they can be alerted to possible risks to future offspring. This is sometimes referred to as translocation tracing or 'chasing'.

Risks in Robertsonian translocations

Studies have shown that the female carrier of either a 13q21q or a 14q21q Robertsonian translocation runs a risk of approximately 10% for having a baby with Down's syndrome, whereas for male carriers the risk is 3–5%.

It is worth sparing a thought for the unfortunate carrier of a 21q21q Robertsonian translocation. All gametes will be either nullisomic or disomic for chromosome 21. Consequently all liveborn children will have Down's syndrome. This is one of the very rare situations in which offspring are at a risk of greater than 50% for having an abnormality. Other examples are the children of a mother with untreated phenylketonuria (p. 203) and parents who are both heterozygous for the same autosomal dominant disorder (p. 80).

Deletions

A *deletion* involves loss of part of a chromosome and results in monosomy of that segment of the chromosome. Usually a very large deletion will be incompatible with survival to term and as a general rule any deletion resulting in a loss of more than 2% of the total haploid genome will be lethal.

Deletions are now recognised as existing at two levels.

A microscopic or chromosomal deletion can be visualised under the microscope. Several deletion syndromes have been described such as the Wolf–Hirschhorn and cri-du-chat syndromes which involve loss of material from the short arms of chromosomes 4 and 5 respectively (p. 219). More recently *microdeletions* have been identified with the help of high resolution prometaphase cytogenetics augmented by fluorescent in situ hybridisation studies. For example it has been shown that several previously unexplained conditions such as the Prader–Willi and Angelman syndromes are due to microdeletions (p. 220).

Inversions

An *inversion* is a two-break rearrangement involving a single chromosome in which a segment is reversed in position, i.e. inverted. If the inversion segment involves the centromere it is termed a *pericentric inversion* (Fig. 3.20a). If it involves only one arm of the chromosome it is known as a *paracentric inversion* (Fig. 3.20b).

Inversions are balanced rearrangements which rarely cause problems in carriers unless one of the breakpoints has disrupted an important functional gene. A pericentric inversion involving chromosome number 9 occurs as a common structural variant or polymorphism, or what is known as a *heteromorphism*, and is not thought to be of any functional importance. However, other inversions, whilst not causing any clinical problems in balanced carriers, can lead to significant chromosome imbalance in offspring with important clinical consequences.

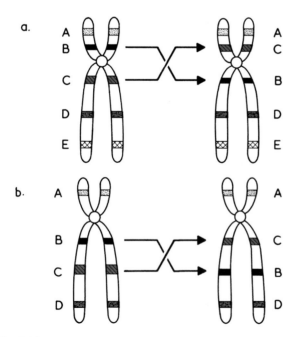

Fig. 3.20
Diagrammatic representation of (a) pericentric and (b) a paracentric inversion (courtesy of Dr J. Delhanty, Galton Laboratory, London).

Segregation at meiosis

Pericentric inversions

An individual who carries a pericentric inversion can produce unbalanced gametes if a cross-over occurs within the inversion segment during meiosis I, when an *inversion loop* forms as the chromosomes attempt to maintain homologous pairing at synapsis. For a pericentric inversion a cross-over within the loop will result in two complementary recombinant chromosomes, one with duplication of the distal non-inverted segment and deletion of the other end of the chromosome, and the other having the opposite arrangement (Fig. 3.21a).

The larger the segments involved in the duplication and deletion in the recombinant chromosome, the greater the degree of chromosome imbalance and the more likely the pregnancy will result in miscarriage. Therefore the smaller the size of the inversion, the greater will be the degree of imbalance and the more likely it becomes that all recombinant conceptions will miscarry.

The pooled results of several studies have shown that a carrier of a balanced pericentric inversion runs a risk of approximately 5–10% for having a child with viable imbalance if that inversion has already resulted in the birth of an abnormal baby. The risk is nearer 1% if the inversion has been ascertained because of a history of recurrent miscarriage.

Paracentric inversions

If a cross-over occurs in the inverted segment of a paracentric inversion this will result in recombinant chromosomes which are either acentric or dicentric (Fig. 3.21b). Acentric chromosomes, which strictly speaking should be known as *chromosomal fragments*, cannot undergo mitotic division so that survival of an embryo with such a rearrangement is extremely uncommon. Dicentric chromosomes are inherently unstable during cell division and are therefore also unlikely to be compatible with survival of the embryo. Overall the likelihood that a balanced parental paracentric inversion will result in the birth of an abnormal baby is extremely low.

Ring chromosomes

A *ring chromosome* is formed when a break occurs on each arm of a chromosome leaving two 'sticky' ends on the central position which reunites as a ring (Fig. 3.22). Inevitably the two distal chromosomal fragments are lost so that, if the involved chromosome is an autosome, the effects are usually very serious.

Ring chromosomes are often unable to complete mitotic division so that it is not unusual to find a ring chromosome in only a proportion of cells. The other cells in the individual are often monosomic due to absence of the ring chromosome.

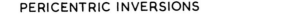

PERICENTRIC INVERSIONS

PARACENTRIC INVERSION

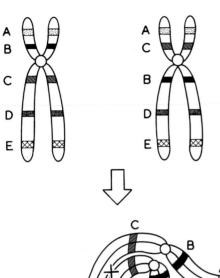
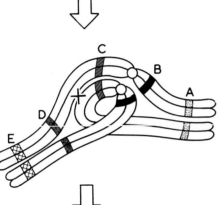
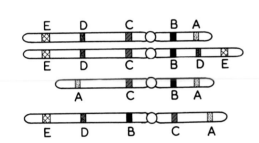
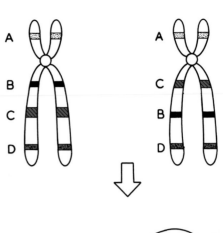
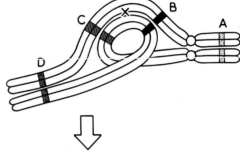
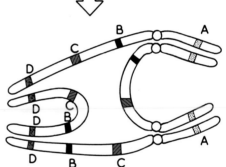

Fig. 3.21
Mechanism of production of recombinant unbalanced chromosomes from (a) a pericentric and (b) a paracentric inversion by crossing-over in an inversion loop (courtesy of Dr J. Delhanty, Galton Laboratory, London).

Isochromosomes

An *isochromosome* shows loss of one arm with duplication of the other. The most probable explanation for the formation of an isochromosome is that the centromere has divided transversely rather than longitudinally. The most commonly encountered isochromosome is that made up of two long arms of the X which accounts for approximately 20% of all cases of Turner's syndrome (p. 223).

MOSAICISM AND CHIMAERISM

Mosaicism

Mosaicism can be defined as the presence in an individual or in a tissue of two or more cell lines which differ in their genetic constitution but are derived from a single zygote. Chromosome mosaicism usually results from non-disjunction occurring in an early embryonic mitotic division with the persistence of more than one cell line. If, for example, the two chromatids of a number 21 chromosome failed to separate at the second mitotic division in a human zygote (Fig. 3.23) this would result in the 4 cell zygote having two cells with 46 chromosomes, one cell with 47 chromosomes (trisomy 21) and one cell with 45 chromosomes (monosomy 21). The ensuing cell line with 45 chromosomes would probably not survive so that the resulting embryo would be expected to show approximately 33% mosaicism for trisomy 21. Mosaicism accounts for 2–3% of all clinically recognised cases of Down's syndrome.

Mosaicism can also exist at a molecular level if a new

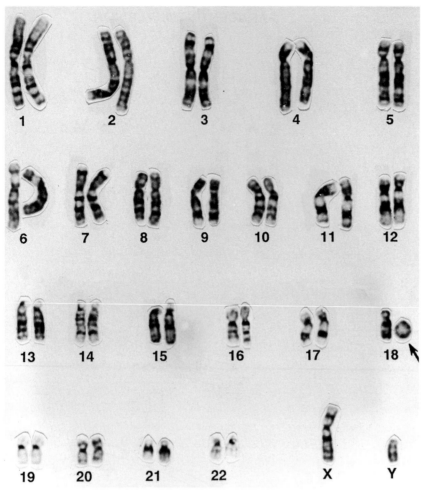

Fig. 3.22
Karyotype showing a ring chromosome 18 (arrowed).

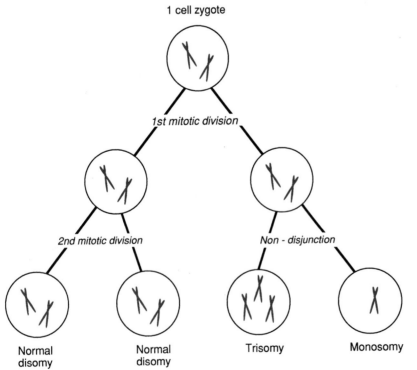

Fig. 3.23
Shows generation of somatic mosaicism due to mitotic non-disjunction.

mutation arises in a somatic or early germ-line cell division. The possibility of *germ-line* or *gonadal mosaicism* is a particular concern when counselling the parents of a child who is an isolated case of a condition such as Duchenne muscular dystrophy (p. 258).

Chimaerism

Chimaerism can be defined as the presence in an individual of two or more genetically distinct cell lines derived from more than one zygote. The word chimaera is derived from the mythological Greek monster which had the head of a lion, the body of a goat and the tail of a dragon.

In humans chimaeras are of two kinds: *dispermic chimaeras* and *blood chimaeras*.

Dispermic chimaeras

These are the result of double fertilisation whereby two genetically different sperm fertilise two ova and the resulting two zygotes fuse to form one embryo. If the two zygotes are of different sex, the chimaeric embryo can develop into an individual with true *hermaphroditism* (p. 226) and an XX/XY karyotype. Mouse chimaeras of this type can now be produced experimentally in the laboratory to facilitate the study of gene transfer.

Blood chimaeras

Blood chimaeras result from an exchange of cells, via the placenta, between non-identical twins in utero. For example, 90% of one twin's cells can have an XY karyotype with red blood cells showing predominantly blood group B, whereas the other twin can have 90% of cells showing an XX karyotype with red blood cells showing predominantly blood group A. It has long been recognised that when twin calves of opposite sex are born, the female can have ambiguous genitalia. It is now believed that this is due to gonadal chimaerism in the female calves which are known as freemartins.

CHROMOSOME NOMENCLATURE

A shorthand notation exists for chromosome abnormalities (Table 3.5). For example, a male with Down's syndrome due to trisomy 21 would be represented as 47,XY +21, whereas a female with 46 chromosomes and a deletion of the short arm of chromosome 5 (cri-du-chat syndrome) would be represented as 46,XX,5p- or 46,XX,del(5)(p).

By convention each arm of a chromosome is divided into regions and each region is subdivided into bands numbering always from the centromere outwards (Fig. 3.24). A given point on a chromosome is designated by the chromosome number, the arm (p or q), the region number and the band number. Therefore a chromosome report reading 46,XY,t(2;4)(p23;q25) would indicate a male with a reciprocal translocation involving the short arm of chromosome 2 at region 2 band 3 and the long arm of chromosome 4 at region 2 band 5.

Table 3.5 Symbols used in describing a karyotype

Term	Explanation
p	short arm
q	long arm
cen	centromere
del	deletion, e.g. 46, XX, del (1) (q21)
dup	duplication, e.g. 46, XY, dup (13) (q14)
i	isochromosome, e.g. 46, X, i (Xq)
inv	inversion, e.g. 46XX, inv (9) (p12q12)
r	ring, e.g. 46, XX, r (21)
t	translocation, e.g. 46, XY, t (2;4) (q21; q21)
ter	terminal or end, i.e. tip of arm e.g. pter or qter
/	mosaicism, e.g. 46, XY/47, XXY
+ or –	Before a chromosome: indicates gain or loss of that chromosome, e.g. 47, XY +21. After a chromosome: indicates gain or loss of part of that chromosome, e.g. 46, XX, 5p –

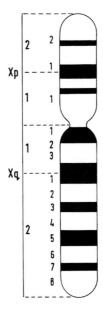

Fig. 3.24
An X chromosome showing the short and long arms each subdivided into regions and bands.

ELEMENTS

1 The normal human karyotype is made up of 46 chromosomes consisting of 22 pairs of autosomes and a pair of sex chromosomes, XX in the female and XY in the male.

2 Each chromosome consists of a short (p) and long (q) arm joined at the centromere. Chromosomes are analysed using cultured cells and specific banding patterns can be identified using special staining techniques.

3 During mitosis in somatic cell division, the two chromatids of each chromosome separate with one chromatid passing to each daughter cell. During meiosis, which occurs during the final stage of gametogenesis, homologous chromosomes pair, exchange segments, and then segregate independently to the mature daughter gametes.

4 Chromosome abnormalities can be structural or numerical. Numerical abnormalities include trisomy and polyploidy. In trisomy a single extra chromosome is present, usually as a result of nondisjunction in the first or second meiotic division. In polyploidy, three or more complete haploid sets are present instead of the usual diploid complement.

5 Structural abnormalities include translocations, inversions, rings and deletions. Translocations can be balanced or unbalanced. Carriers of balanced translocations are at risk of having children with unbalanced rearrangements who will usually be physically and mentally handicapped.

FURTHER READING

ISCN 1985 An international system for human cytogenetic nomenclatures. Karger, Basel
A report from an international committee giving full details of how chromosome abnormalities should be described.
Therman E 1986 Human chromosomes, 2nd edn. Springer-Verlag, New York
An easily read comprehensive introduction to human cytogenetics.
Tjio J H, Levan A 1956 The chromosome number of man. Hereditas 42: 1–6
A landmark paper which described a reliable method for studying human chromosomes and gave birth to the subject of clinical cytogenetics.
Vogel F, Motulsky A G 1986 Human genetics, problems and approaches, 2nd edn. Springer-Verlag, Berlin
An extremely comprehensive text-book of human genetics with a large section devoted to cytogenetics and cell division.

CHAPTER 4

Recombinant DNA technology

In the history of medical genetics, the 'chromosome breakthrough' in the mid–1950s was revolutionary. In the last two decades, *recombinant DNA* technology, equally revolutionary, has had a profound effect, not only in medical genetics (Fig. 4.1), but also in many other branches of medicine as well as in animal and plant breeding and diagnostic microbiology (Table 4.1).

In the early 1970s, the work of Davis and Mertz on restriction endonucleases, the development of the *plasmid* pSC101, named after its originator Stanley Cohen, and the introduction of the Southern blot technique, named after Ed Southern, must rank as seminal developments in the field.

PRINCIPLES OF RECOMBINANT DNA TECHNOLOGY

Recombinant DNA technology can be split into two main areas, DNA cloning and methods of DNA analysis.

Table 4.1 Applications of recombinant DNA technology

Gene structure/mapping/function

Population genetics
  relation to disease and population structure

Clinical genetics
  prenatal diagnosis
  presymptomatic diagnosis
  carrier detection

Diagnosis and pathogenesis of disease

Biosynthesis
  e.g. insulin, growth hormone, interferon

Treatment of genetic disease
  gene therapy

Agriculture
  e.g. nitrogen fixation

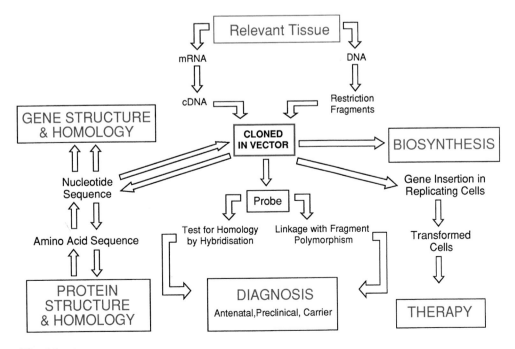

Fig. 4.1
Some of the applications of DNA technology in medical genetics.

DNA CLONING

There are six essential steps in the process of DNA cloning.

Generation of DNA fragments

Although fragments of DNA can be produced by mechanical shearing techniques, this is a very haphazard process producing fragments which vary in size. In the early 1970s it was recognised that certain microbes contained enzymes which cleave double stranded DNA in or near a particular sequence of nucleotides. These enzymes, called *restriction enzymes*, recognise a particular DNA sequence, usually 4 to 6 nucleotides in length, which is usually palindromic, i.e. with the same sequence of nucleotides on the two complementary strands of the DNA if read in one direction of polarity, e.g. 5' to 3' (Table 4.2). Well over 300 different restriction enzymes have been isolated from various bacterial organisms. Restriction endonucleases are named according to the organism from which they are derived, e.g. Eco RI is from *E. coli* and was the first restriction enzyme isolated from that organism.

The complementary pairing of bases in the DNA molecule, means that cleavage of double-stranded DNA by a restriction endonuclease always creates double-stranded breaks, and depending on which particular restriction enzyme is used, creates either a staggered or a blunt end (Fig. 4.2).

Digesting DNA from a specific source using a particular restriction enzyme will produce the same reproducible collection of DNA fragments each time the process is carried out.

Recombination of DNA fragments

DNA from any source, when digested with the same restriction enzyme, will produce DNA fragments with identical complementary ends, or termini. When DNA

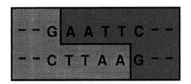

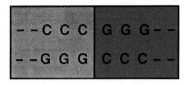

Fig. 4.2
Representation of the staggered and blunt ends generated by restriction digest of double-stranded DNA by Eco RI and Sma I.

has been cleaved by a restriction enzyme which produces staggered termini, these are referred to as being 'sticky' since they will unite under appropriate conditions with complementary sequences produced by the same enzyme on DNA of any source. The cohesive termini are initially held together by hydrogen bonding but are then sealed and stabilised with an enzyme called *DNA ligase*. *Ligation* of flush ended DNA fragments does not occur as readily and requires modification of the reaction conditions. The union of two DNA fragments produces what is referred to as a *recombinant DNA* molecule.

Vectors

A *vector* is the term for the carrier DNA molecule used in the cloning process which, through its own replication, will allow production of multiple copies of a particular DNA sequence of interest. There are four main types of vectors: plasmids, bacteriophages, cosmids and yeast artificial chromosomes (YACS). All replicate within a host organism.

Plasmids

Plasmids occur naturally in bacteria, to which they confer resistance to various antibiotics and heavy metals. They are inherited stably in an extrachromosomal state and consist of a circular duplex of DNA. Two of the original plasmids are pSC101 and pBR322, so designated after their originators, Stanley Cohen and Bolivar and Rodriguez (Fig. 4.3). Their advantage as vectors is that they possess a limited number of unique restriction sites and carry resistance to particular antibiotics, a characteristic which can be used to identify recombinant clones.

Bacteriophages

Bacteriophages, or *phages* for short, are *viruses* which infect bacteria, the DNA usually being in the form of a linear

Table 4.2 Some examples of restriction endonucleases with their nucleotide recognition sequence and cleavage sites

Enzyme	Organism	Cleavage site 5' 3'
Bam HI	*Bacillus amyloliquefaciens* H	G • G A T C C
Eco RI	*Escherichia coli* RY 13	G • A A T T C
Hae III	*Haemophilus aegyptius*	G G • C C
Hind III	*Haemophilus influenzae* Rd	A • A G C T T
Hpa I	*Haemophilus parainfluenzae*	G T T • A A C
Pst I	*Providencia stuartii*	C T G C A • G
Sma I	*Serratia marcescens*	C C C • G G G
Sal I	*Streptomyces albus* G	G • T C G A C

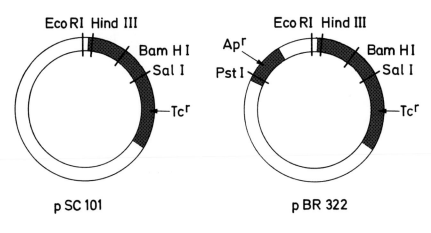

Fig. 4.3
Two plasmids used in recombinant DNA
technology showing drug resistance genes (Ap^r
= ampicillin resistance; Tc^r = tetracycline
resistance) and cleavage sites of restriction
endonucleases which cut the DNA only once.

duplex. The most extensively studied and utilised is the so-called lambda (λ) phage.

Cosmids

A *cosmid* is essentially a plasmid which has had all but the minimum vector DNA necessary for propagation removed to allow insertion of the largest possible foreign DNA fragment.

Plasmids can incorporate up to 10 kb (1 kb = 1 *kilobase* = 1000 bases) of 'foreign' DNA, lambda phage up to 20 kb, while cosmids can take inserts up to approximately 50 kb.

Yeast artificial chromosomes

A *yeast artificial chromosome*, YAC, consists of a plasmid which contains within it the minimum DNA sequences necessary for centromere formation, sequences that seed telomere formation and other DNA sequences known as autonomous replication sequences, all of which are necessary for accurate replication within yeast. YACs can incorporate DNA fragments up to 1000 kb in size.

The choice of vector used in cloning depends on a number of factors, such as the particular restriction enzyme being used and the size of the fragment to be inserted. The incorporation of a particular 'foreign' DNA sequence into a vector allows production of large amounts of that sequence (Fig. 4.4).

Transformation of the host organism

After introduction of the foreign DNA fragment into the vector, the recombinant vector can be introduced into the host cell by making its cell membrane permeable by a variety of different methods, which include exposing it, in the case of bacterial cells, to calcium salts. This technique is known as *transformation*. Only a small fraction of the host cells will be transformed and usually only by a single vector molecule.

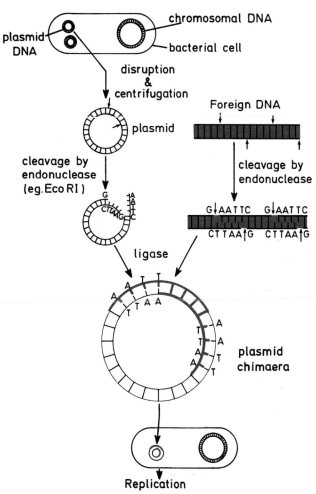

Fig. 4.4
Generation of a recombinant plasmid using Eco RI and
transformation of the host bacterial organism (from Emery A E H
1981 Lancet ii: 1406, with permission).

Cloning and screening for recombinant vectors

The next step is to grow the transformed host cells in culture medium to produce multiple identical copies of the various individual recombinant DNA molecules, i.e. *clones*.

In the case of the plasmid pBR322, if the restriction enzyme used to digest the vector DNA cuts within the drug resistance gene of the vector, then loss of antibiotic resistance of the host cells can be used as a screening procedure for recombinant plasmids. Thus, if the enzyme Pst I were used to generate DNA fragments and to cut the plasmid pBR322, any recombinant plasmids produced would make the bacterial host cells they transform sensitive to ampicillin, since this gene would no longer be functional, but they would remain resistant to tetracycline (Fig. 4.3).

Selection of specific clones

A number of techniques have been developed to detect the presence of clones with specific DNA sequence inserts. The most widely used method is by nucleic acid hybridisation. Colonies of transformed host bacteria are used to make replica plates which are then blotted on to a nitrocellulose filter to which nucleic acids bind. The DNA of the replica blots is then denatured to make the DNA single stranded which will allow it to hybridise with single-stranded radioactively-labelled DNA or RNA *probes* which can be detected by exposure to an X-ray film, a technique known as *autoradiography*. In this way a transformed host bacterial colony containing a sequence complementary to the probe can be detected and from its position on the replica plate, the colony containing that clone can be identified on the master plate, picked and cultured separately (Fig. 4.5).

DNA LIBRARIES

Different sources of DNA fragments can be used to make recombinant DNA molecules. DNA from nucleated cells is termed total or *genomic DNA*. DNA made by the action of the enzyme *reverse transcriptase* on mRNA is called *complementary DNA* or *cDNA*. It is possible to enrich for DNA sequences of particular interest by using a specific tissue as a source of mRNA; e.g. immature red blood cells which contain predominantly globin mRNA. The collection of recombinant DNA molecules generated from a specific source is referred to as a *DNA library*, e.g. a genomic or cDNA library. A DNA library using plasmids as a vector would need to consist of several hundred thousand clones to be large enough to contain the whole of the human genome. The use of YACs as cloning vectors with DNA digested by infrequently cutting restriction enzymes means that the whole of the human genome can be contained in a library of 13–14 000 clones.

DNA PROBES

DNA probes can come from a variety of sources which include random genomic DNA sequences, specific genes,

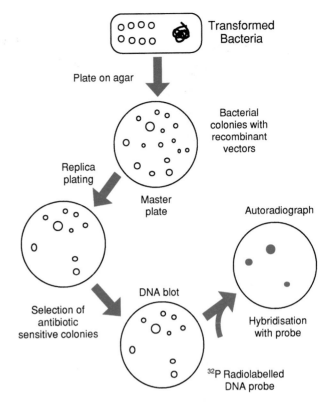

Fig. 4.5
Identification of recombinant DNA clones with specific DNA inserts by loss of antibiotic resistance, nucleic acid hybridisation and autoradiography.

cDNA sequences and DNA sequences produced synthetically based on knowledge of the protein amino acid sequence. A DNA probe can be radioactively labelled by a variety of processes, one of which is known as *nick translation*, whereby ³²P-labelled nucleotides are introduced into the DNA molecule. The sites where a radioactively labelled DNA probe hybridises with complementary DNA sequences on a nitrocellulose filter can be localised by autoradiography.

Non-autoradiographic labelling techniques can also be used to label DNA probes. Fluorescently labelled DNA probes are less sensitive than radiolabelled probes but are likely to replace their use because they avoid the use of radioactive isotopes.

THE POLYMERASE CHAIN REACTION

One of the most revolutionary developments in recombinant DNA is the technique which was originally called DNA sequence amplification but is now commonly known as the *polymerase chain reaction, PCR* (Fig. 4.6). PCR can be used to produce vast quantities of a DNA fragment provided that the base pair sequence of that region is known or can be inferred from the protein amino acid sequence.

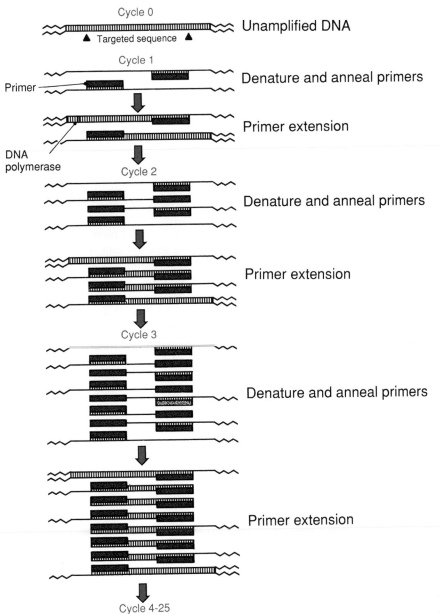

Fig. 4.6
Diagrammatic representation of the
polymerase chain reaction.

The technique involves synthesising two oligonucleotide primers of approximately 20 base pairs in length complementary to the DNA *flanking* a particular DNA sequence of interest. The primers are used to amplify that sequence by means of repeated cycles of denaturation through heating of the double-stranded source DNA, annealing of the primer sequences to the resulting single-stranded DNA, and extension of the primer DNA on the single-stranded DNA template using DNA polymerase to produce double-stranded copies of the DNA sequence of interest.

The successive cycles of DNA synthesis result in an exponential amplification of the target DNA sequence leading to a 10^5–10^6 fold increase in the amount of the DNA sequence of interest. This amplification results in sufficient quantities of DNA for direct visualisation by ultraviolet fluorescence after ethidium bromide staining, without the need to use indirect detection techniques such as radioactively or fluorescently labelled probes.

Use of PCR allows analysis of DNA from sources other than blood, such as buccal scrapings and pathological archival material. It is usually possible to start with quantities of DNA as small as that from a single cell! Great care has to be taken with PCR, however, as contaminating DNA from an extraneous source such as desquamated skin from a laboratory worker will also be amplified. This could give rise to false positive or negative results unless control studies to detect this possible source of error are carried out.

Another advantage of PCR is the rapid turn-round

time of samples for analysis. Initially the 20–25 cycles of amplification had to be carried out manually. In addition, the high temperatures required to denature the double-stranded DNA resulted in the inactivation of DNA polymerase I used for primer extension. This meant that further aliquots of that enzyme had to be added manually in each cycle of the amplification process. Man's ingenuity and nature combined to overcome these difficulties by automation of the temperature cycling, aided by the use of DNA polymerase isolated from the bacterium *Thermophilus aquaticus*, which grows naturally in hot springs and is heat-stable!

METHODS OF DNA ANALYSIS

SOUTHERN BLOTTING

DNA digested by a restriction enzyme is subjected to electrophoresis on an agarose gel. This separates the DNA or *restriction fragments* by size, the smaller fragments running faster than the larger ones. The DNA fragments in the gel are then denatured with alkali, making them single stranded and rendering them capable of hybridising with complementary DNA sequences. A 'permanent' copy of these single-stranded fragments is made by transferring them on to a nitrocellulose filter which binds the single-stranded DNA. In order to localise and visualise a particular DNA fragment of interest from the collection of fragments on the filter, a phosphorus-32, ^{32}P, radioactively labelled DNA probe which has been made single stranded is allowed to hybridise with DNA fragments in the *Southern blot* (Fig. 4.7).

RESTRICTION MAPPING

Hybridising a specific DNA probe to Southern blots of DNA from a particular source digested by a variety of different restriction enzymes, used in combination, allows a *restriction map* of a region of DNA to be constructed (Fig. 4.8).

DNA SEQUENCING

The cloning and amplification of a DNA fragment then allows its nucleotide sequence to be determined. The most commonly used approach is the dideoxy chain termination method. This involves making single-stranded DNA templates of the DNA fragment using a special phage vector and then adding an aliquot of this template DNA to 4 different reaction mixtures which include DNA polymerase, the 4 deoxynucleotides which have been radio-labelled and a short primer sequence. One of the 4 respective dideoxynucleotides is added to each of the 4 separate reaction mixtures. The dideoxynucleotides compete with their respective deoxynucleotide, inhibiting the DNA polymerase leading in each reaction mixture to DNA fragments of different length which terminate in their respective dideoxynucleotide. When the reaction products are run on a gel, a ladder of DNA sequences of differing lengths ending in the respective dideoxynucleotide is produced. The DNA sequence complementary to the single-stranded DNA template can be read directly from an autoradiograph of the gel (Fig. 4.9).

MUTATION SCREENING TECHNIQUES

Although sequencing a gene can be used to identify mutations within it, many genes in humans are several hundred thousand or even million base pairs in length making this an enormous task, especially if a single gene disorder is mutationally *heterogeneous*. Fortunately there are three techniques which can be used to screen for

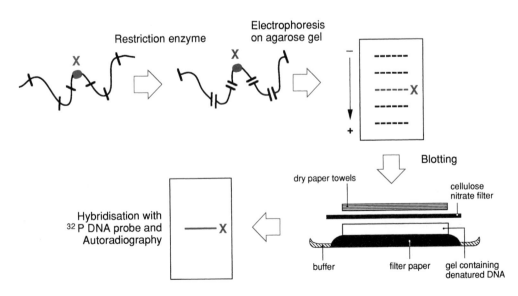

Fig. 4.7
Southern blot technique.

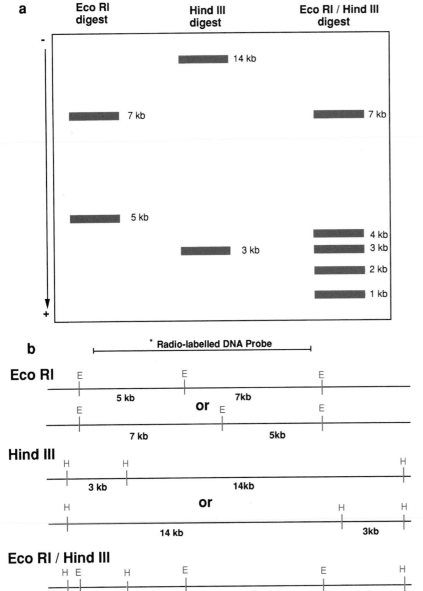

Fig. 4.8
a. Diagrammatic representation of a Southern blot of Eco RI and Hind III digests and Eco RI/Hind III double digests of a DNA fragment.
b. The possible Eco RI and Hind III restriction maps and the consequent combined Eco RI/Hind III double digest restriction map.

mutations. These differ in their ease of use and reliability.

Denaturing gradient gel electrophoresis

Denaturing gradient gel electrophoresis, DGGE, involves mixing a radiolabelled single-stranded DNA probe with the double-stranded DNA being screened, which is heated to make it single stranded. This mixture is electrophoresed on a denaturing gradient gel. DNA which is identical with the sequence of the DNA probe will form a homoduplex, which, under the denaturing conditions of the gel, will remain hybridised. Any mismatches of the DNA being screened with the DNA probe will result in the formation of a heteroduplex which, as it is run down the denaturing gradient of the gel, will become single stranded at a certain point resulting in a branched structure which has decreased mobility. This results in an altered position compared to the homoduplex which can be detected on an autoradiograph.

Single-stranded conformational polymorphism

Radiolabelled PCR products of double-stranded DNA, if made single stranded, fold up making a three dimensional structure. An alteration in the DNA sequence can result in a different conformation which, under appropriate gel conditions, results in a different electrophoretic mobility,

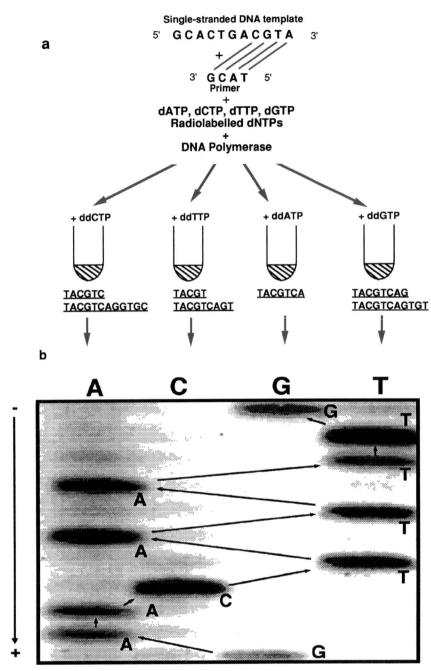

Fig. 4.9
a. Representation of the reagents added to a single-stranded DNA template and the resulting DNA sequences of different lengths ending in their respective dideoxynucleotides in the different reaction aliquots in the dideoxy method of DNA sequencing.
b. A portion of a sequencing gel from which the nucleotide sequence of the single-stranded DNA template can be read as arrowed (courtesy of Dr G. Taylor, DNA Laboratory, St James's Hospital, Leeds).

a so-called *single-stranded conformational polymorphism*, SSCP (Fig. 4.10).

Chemical cleavage mismatch

This method involves the addition of the chemicals hydroxylamine and osmium tetroxide which react with free cytosine and thymine nucleotides respectively. By denaturing the double-stranded DNA being screened and allowing it to hybridise with a single-stranded radiolabelled DNA probe, any mismatched cytosine or thymine nucleotides will be exposed and therefore be susceptible to reaction with the hydroxylamine and

osmium tetroxide. The addition of piperidine results in cleavage of the DNA being screened at any such sites, and this provides the basis of mutation identification through so-called *chemical cleavage mismatch*. The technique identifies mismatches on either strand and thereby indirectly detects adenine and guanine mismatches through their complementary nucleotides on the other strand.

NORTHERN BLOTTING

Messenger-RNA, although very unstable due to intrinsic cellular ribonucleases, can be isolated and, if run on an electrophoretic gel, can be transferred to a filter in a

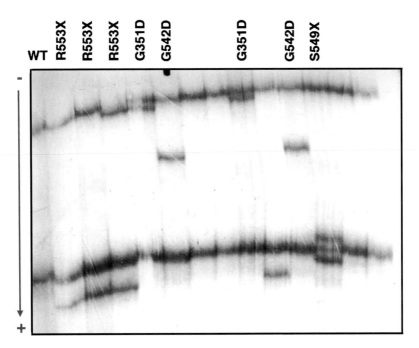

Fig. 4.10
An autoradiograph of a gel using single stranded conformational polymorphisms to detect known mutations in the cystic fibrosis gene (courtesy of Dr G. Taylor, Yorkshire Regional DNA Laboratory, St James's Hospital, Leeds).

process called *Northern blotting*. Hybridising the Northern blot with a radiolabelled probe allows determination of the size and quantity of the mRNA transcript. In single gene disorders in which no mutation has been identified in the coding sequences, an alteration in the size of the mRNA transcript suggests the possibility of a mutation in the non-coding regions of the gene such as the splice junction of the intron–exon border.

SITE DIRECTED MUTAGENESIS

It is possible to alter or modify DNA sequences in a directed fashion to produce 'tailor made' mutations. Techniques used include *homologous recombination*, in which one DNA sequence is replaced by another with close similarity but known specific differences, and insertional mutagenesis, where DNA sequences are disrupted by the insertion of foreign DNA. *Site directed mutagenesis* has been used to acquire a greater understanding of the relationship between structure and

function in protein and enzymes and has also enabled analysis of the controlling sequences in the flanking regions of eukaryotic structural genes as well as the production of transgenic animal models for inherited human disease (p. 282).

APPLICATIONS OF RECOMBINANT DNA TECHNOLOGY

ANALYSIS OF GENE STRUCTURE

Restriction mapping can reveal details of the structure of a gene and the adjacent region, as in the beta globin gene region which has allowed the ordering of the beta-like globin genes (Fig. 4.11). Each globin gene, including introns, is about 1.5 kb in length and the total length of the complex is about 50 kb including the intergenic DNA. Interestingly, the physical order of the beta-like globin genes corresponds to the order of expression of these genes during development (p. 115).

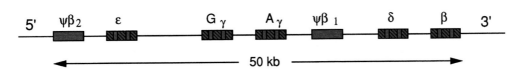

Fig. 4.11
Map of the human beta-globin gene region (ψ represents the position of pseudogenes).

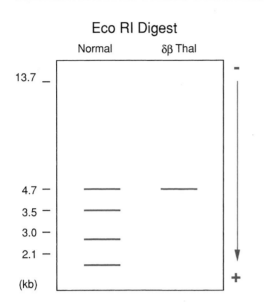

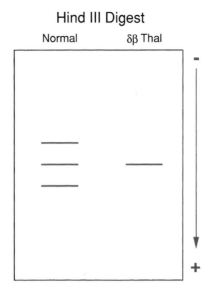

Fig. 4.12
Alteration in the Eco RI and Hind III restriction fragments in DNA from persons with delta-beta thalassaemia with a globin probe, compared with DNA from persons with two copies of the normal DNA sequence in the region of the delta and beta globin genes.

DNA ANALYSIS OF SINGLE GENE DISORDERS

Restriction mapping has been used in the analysis of the molecular basis of single gene disorders in humans. The approaches can be divided into direct and indirect methods.

Direct methods

Deletion detection

One of the first examples of the use of this approach was in the haemoglobinopathies. *Reticulocytes*, immature red blood cells, contain only globin mRNA, from which a radioactive complementary or cDNA probe for globin genes can be produced. This probe can then be used to identify and localise DNA fragments which contain the globin genes in an autoradiograph of a Southern blot. In the case of delta-beta thalassaemia (p. 125), the DNA probe complementary to the beta-globin gene does not hybridise with all the same DNA fragments as in normal persons, consistent with a deletion being the cause of this disorder (Fig. 4.12).

Mutation specific RFLPs

In some single gene disorders the mutation responsible eliminates a restriction enzyme recognition site. This direct approach has been used in sickle-cell disease using the restriction enzyme Mst II (Fig. 4.13). This approach is of limited use as it is relatively rare for mutations to occur within the recognition sequences of restriction endonucleases.

Allele specific oligonucleotides

If the mutational basis of a single gene disorder is a point mutation, it is possible to make short synthetic DNA sequences corresponding to the normal and mutant sequences. These are known as *oligonucleotide probes*. By using appropriate reaction conditions, the normal and

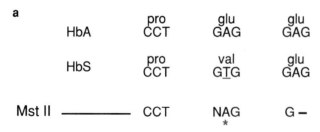

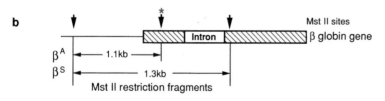

Fig. 4.13
a. The single base pair difference of thymine for adenine in the second nucleotide of the sixth codon of the beta globin gene between HbA and HbS, resulting in the substitution of valine for glutamic acid along with the recognition site nucleotide sequence of the restriction enzyme Mst II.
b. Representation of the two different sized DNA restriction fragments of 1.3 kb in persons with the sickle-cell allele (β^S) and 1.1 kb with the normal beta globin allele (β^A) consequent upon loss of the Mst II restriction site (*) due to A to T mutation in the first exon in persons with the sickle-cell allele.

a

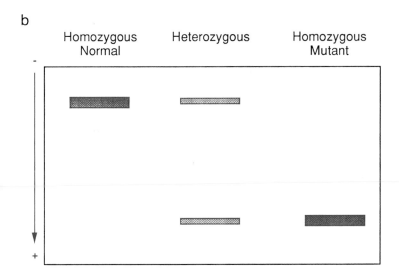

b

Fig. 4.14
a. Diagrammatic representation of the formation of homo- and heteroduplexes between target mutant and normal DNA sequences and allele specific oligonucleotides for the normal and mutant DNA sequences.
b. Diagrammatic representation of the resulting electrophoretic gel of homoduplexes and heteroduplexes of DNA from persons heterozygous and homozygous for the normal and mutant sequences with allele specific oligonucleotides for the normal and mutant beta globin sequence.

mutant DNA can be distinguished by demonstrating differential hybridisation of the normal and mutant oligonucleotide sequences to the normal and mutant DNA sequences (Fig. 4.14).

Indirect methods

DNA sequence polymorphisms

Techniques of DNA analysis have revealed that there is an enormous amount of DNA sequence variation in the human genome. This variation can be grouped into 2 main types, restriction fragment length polymorphisms and hypervariable DNA length polymorphisms.

Restriction fragment length polymorphisms
Variation in the nucleotide sequence of the human genome is common, occurring approximately once every 200 base pairs. These single base pair differences in DNA nucleotide sequences are inherited in a Mendelian codominant manner and are apparently without any phenotypic effects as they usually occur in intergenic DNA. If a difference in DNA sequence occurs within the recognition sequence of a restriction enzyme, the fragments produced by that restriction enzyme will be of different length in different people. This can be recognised by the altered mobility of the restriction fragments on gel electrophoresis, so-called *restriction fragment length polymorphisms, RFLPs*.

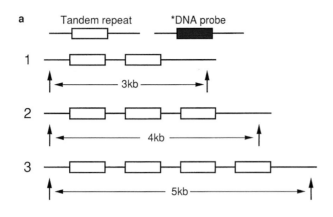

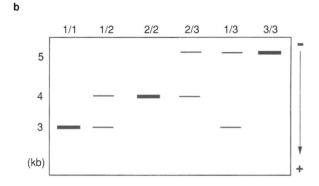

Fig. 4.15
a. Representation of the physical arrangement of different length DNA sequence variants due to variable number of tandem repeats.
b. Representation of an autoradiograph of electrophoretic gel of variable number tandem repeats hybridised to a probe to the tandem repeat sequence.

Hypervariable DNA length polymorphisms

Variable number tandem repeats DNA sequence polymorphisms have been demonstrated in human DNA which are *hypervariable*. This form of polymorphism has been shown to be inherited in a Mendelian codominant fashion and is due to the presence of variable numbers of tandem repeats of a short DNA sequence. These length differences are thought to have arisen by unequal exchanges either during recombination in meiosis (p. 241), sister chromatid exchange in mitosis (p. 227), or by errors in DNA replication of the repeat sequences. The resulting length variations are very highly polymorphic when compared to RFLPs and have the advantage that they can be demonstrated using any restriction enzyme provided it does not cleave within the DNA sequence of the repeat unit (Fig. 4.15).

The first two examples of this type of DNA sequence polymorphism demonstrated in humans were close to the human insulin gene on chromosome 11 and near the alpha globin locus on chromosome 16. The latter has proved to be useful clinically by demonstration of linkage to the major locus for adult onset polycystic kidney disease. This allows presymptomatic diagnosis in persons from

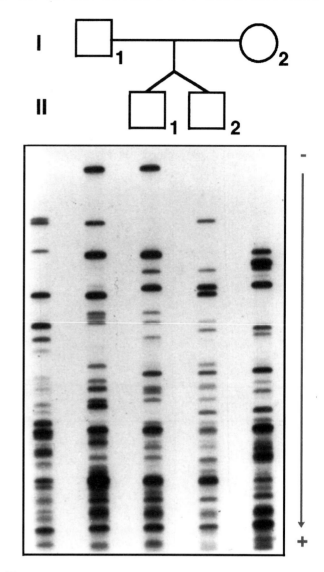

Fig. 4.16
An autoradiograph of a minisatellite DNA fingerprint of two parents, their two offspring and an unrelated individual. Each band in the two offspring is present in one of the two parents (courtesy of Professor A. Markham, St James's Hospital, Leeds).

families at risk for this late onset autosomal dominant disorder (p. 248).

Minisatellites Jeffreys identified a short 10–15 base-pair 'core' sequence with homology to many highly variable loci spread throughout the human genome. Using a probe containing tandem repeats of this core sequence, a pattern of hypervariable DNA fragments is identified which is sufficiently polymorphic to provide what has been called a *DNA fingerprint* which is unique and specific to an individual. The multiple variable size repeat sequences identified by the core sequence are known as *minisatellites* (Fig. 4.16).

It was hoped that minisatellite sequences would be useful in linkage studies of disease loci by enabling simultaneous analysis of many more loci than is possible using conventional RFLPs. Unfortunately, even if an individual family is large enough to demonstrate linkage of a specific disease locus to a particular hypervariable DNA fragment, the data from different families cannot be collated as the genomic localisation of each fragment is unknown. However, techniques are available for the identification of the unique DNA sequences immediately flanking the minisatellite. By using the entire minisatellite in high stringency hybridisation conditions it is possible to develop locus specific probes. These can then be used to add linkage data from further families as well as to allow assignment of the minisatellite to its location in the human genome.

Microsatellites   The human genome has been found to contain some 50–100 000 blocks of a variable number of tandem repeats of the dinucleotide CA:GT, so-called *CA repeats* or *microsatellites*. The difference in the number of CA repeats at any one site between individuals is very highly polymorphic and these have been shown to be inherited in a Mendelian codominant manner. Several thousand CA repeats which can be used in linkage

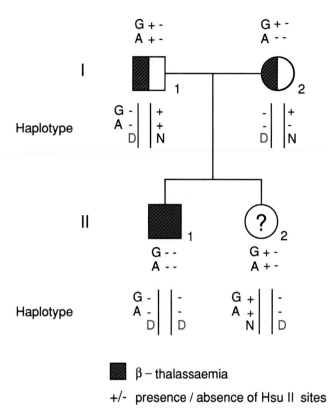

Fig. 4.18
The Hsu II linked RFLPs in the $^{G}\gamma$- and $^{A}\gamma$-globin structural genes confirm that the female sib (II$_2$) of the male with β thalassaemia is heterozygous for β thalassaemia, having inherited the β thalassaemia gene from her mother and the normal beta-globin gene from her father (N = normal, D = disease).

studies have been identified in the human genome so far (Fig. 4.17). More recently, highly polymorphic tri- and tetra-nucleotide repeats have also been identified, which can be used in a similar way.

CLINICAL APPLICATIONS

Locus linked DNA sequence variants

DNA sequence polymorphisms can be used in the analysis of inherited disease by application in linkage studies (p. 100). If the locus for a genetic disorder is shown to be linked to a DNA sequence polymorphism, this can be used for prenatal diagnosis (Fig. 4.18), to detect the presence of a gene in a person before the onset of symptoms (p. 250) and to identify female carriers of X-linked disorders (p. 247). The enormous advantage of the use of DNA sequence polymorphisms in these clinical situations is that it is not necessary to have knowledge of the basic biochemical defect or the nature of the mutation responsible, nor is it necessary to have access to a tissue in which the gene is expressed.

In order to be of use in the majority of families at risk for a particular single gene disorder, several different

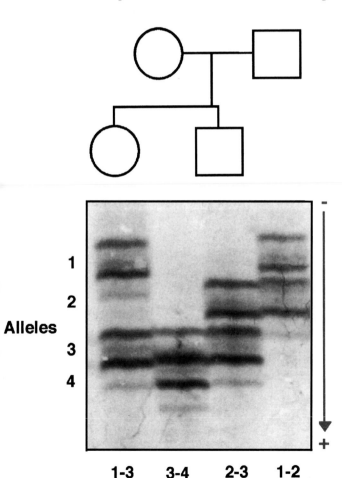

Fig. 4.17
An autoradiograph of a CA repeat microsatellite segregating in a family (courtesy of Dr G. Taylor, Yorkshire Regional DNA Laboratory, St James's Hospital, Leeds).

DNA sequence polymorphisms linked to the disease locus could need to be looked at as only a proportion of families will be informative for each specific DNA sequence polymorphism. Linked DNA sequence polymorphisms have been used clinically in a wide variety of single gene disorders which include beta thalassaemia, Duchenne muscular dystrophy, Huntington's disease and cystic fibrosis.

DNA sequence polymorphisms occur in mitochondrial as well as in nuclear DNA. In the former, the polymorphisms in the progeny are always of maternal origin as mitochondria are exclusively maternally inherited (pp. 12, 89).

Allele linked DNA sequence variants

Certain DNA sequence variants have been shown to occur in association with certain disease mutations more commonly than would be predicted by their individual frequencies in the population. In blacks of Afro-Caribbean origin with haemoglobin A, the normal beta globin gene usually occurs in a 7.6 or 7.0 kb DNA fragment of a Hpa I restriction enzyme digest and rarely in a 13.0 kb DNA fragment. On the other hand, the sickle-cell globin gene is found in the 13.0 kb Hpa I fragment nearly 90% of the time (Fig. 4.19). This particular type of RFLP can be termed allele-specific and is said to be in *linkage disequilibrium* with the mutation (p. 101).

DNA haplotypes

If a mutation-specific DNA sequence variant or deletion is not available for a particular disorder and closely linked DNA sequence polymorphisms are being used for

carrier testing, presymptomatic or prenatal diagnosis, there can be families in which the results of linkage studies will, despite the availability of these different types of DNA sequence polymorphisms, remain uninformative. In other words, the family does not possess the necessary variation at closely linked polymorphic sites to determine on which chromosome the disease allele is located. It is often possible, however, by looking at a number of different closely linked DNA sequence polymorphisms, for the family to be made informative by establishing what is known as a *haplotype*, i.e. the pattern of DNA sequence polymorphisms on the chromosomes with the disease allele and with the normal allele in that particular family.

This principle can be illustrated in an example (Fig. 4.20). In the pedigree shown the male child (II_1) is affected with the autosomal recessive disorder cystic fibrosis. If the DNA sequence polymorphisms A and B are closely linked *markers* flanking the cystic fibrosis locus, then in each parent marker allele 2 must be in coupling with the cystic fibrosis mutation. One can then infer that the normal cystic fibrosis gene is flanked by marker allele 1 at both sites in each parent. Analysis of the marker alleles in the affected child's sister (II_2) would predict her to be homozygous for the normal gene at that locus.

In some diseases certain DNA haplotypes occur more frequently with particular mutations than would be predicted by their individual frequency in the population, i.e. they are in linkage disequilibrium with the mutation (p. 101). This phenomenon can be utilised clinically in carrier detection, presymptomatic and prenatal diagnosis.

Molecular pathology

There are now more than 6000 recognised Mendelian characteristics in humans, many of which are associated with disease. In excess of 2000 genes in humans have been cloned and in a rapidly increasing number the mutational basis has been identified (Table 4.3). Where no identifiable protein or enzyme abnormality has as yet been detected, the finding of linked DNA sequence polymorphisms will lead to the isolation and cloning of the structural gene, allowing recognition of its protein product. This process has been called *reverse genetics*.

Diagnosis in non-genetic disease

The polymerase chain reaction can be used to detect the presence of DNA sequences specific to a particular infectious organism before conventional evidence such as an antibody response or the results of cultures are available. An example is the screening of blood products for the presence of DNA sequences from the *human immunodeficiency virus* (HIV) to ensure their safety, e.g.

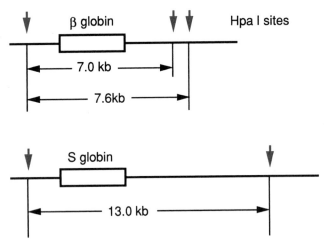

Fig. 4.19
The Hpa I restriction site polymorphism to the 3' side of the beta globin gene has been shown to be in linkage disequilibrium with the sickle-cell mutation, producing a 13.0 kb fragment with the HbS allele rather than a 7.0 or 7.6 fragment with DNA from persons with a normal beta globin gene.

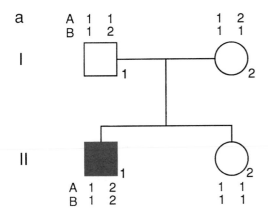

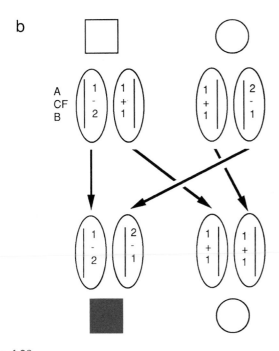

Fig. 4.20
a. A two generation family with a child affected with the autosomal recessive disorder, cystic fibrosis, with DNA sequence polymorphisms at flanking loci A and B. Neither marker on its own is fully informative. Together they produce a haplotype which is fully informative.
b. Inferred DNA sequence haplotype at the cystic fibrosis and flanking loci which allows one to infer II$_2$ is homozygous normal for the cystic fibrosis gene.

Table 4.3 Single gene diseases in humans with their molecular basis (HGPRT = hypoxanthine-guanine phosphoribosyl transferase)

Disorder	Nature of molecular defect
Autosomal dominant	
Antithrombin III deficiency	Deletions, point mutations, insertions
Familial hypercholesterolaemia	Deletions, point mutations, duplication, insertion (Alu repeat)
Huntington's disease	CAG triplet repeat expansion
Myotonic dystrophy	CTG triplet repeat expansion
Neurofibromatosis Type I (von Recklinghausen's disease)	Deletions (Alu repeat), point mutations, insertions
Osteogenesis imperfecta	Deletions, point mutations
Autosomal recessive	
α$_1$-antitrypsin deficiency	Point mutations, deletions, insertions, duplications
Congenital adrenal hyperplasia due to 21-hydroxylase deficiency	Point mutations, deletions
Cystic fibrosis	Deletions, point mutations, insertions
Growth hormone deficiency (rare familial form)	Deletions
Phenylketonuria	Point mutations, deletions, insertions
Tay–Sachs disease	Deletions, point mutations
X-linked	
Chronic granulomatous disease	Deletions, point mutations
Duchenne/Becker muscular dystrophy	Deletions, duplications, point mutations
Fragile X mental retardation	CGG triplet repeat expansion
Haemophilia A (Factor VIII deficiency)	Point mutations, deletions, insertions, duplications, inversions
Haemophilia B (Factor IX deficiency)	Point mutations, deletions, insertions
Lesch—Nyhan syndrome (HGPRT deficiency)	Deletions, point mutations, insertions, duplications
Ornithine transcarbamylase deficiency	Deletions, point mutations

The extreme sensitivity of PCR also means it has potential applications in malignancy for detecting residual disease or recurrence after treatment for disorders such as leukaemia. This is vital to the timing, continuation, duration and reinstitution of chemotherapy.

GENE MAPPING

This can be divided into two main types. The first involves techniques used to assign a gene or DNA sequence to a specific chromosome or a particular region of a chromosome, i.e. *chromosome mapping*. The second, finer, level of analysis provides detailed mapping information at the DNA level, which includes physical relationships to flanking DNA sequence polymorphisms, and the detailed structure of the gene, i.e. *DNA mapping*.

screening pooled Factor VIII concentrate for use in males with haemophilia A. Another example is the identification of DNA sequences specific to bacterial or viral organisms responsible for acute overwhelming infections, where early diagnosis allows prompt institution of the correct antibiotic or antiviral agent with the prospect of reducing morbidity and mortality.

CHROMOSOME MAPPING TECHNIQUES

Gene dosage

The study of persons with chromosome abnormalities looking for increased amounts of a particular protein in trisomic individuals (p. 33), and decreased amounts in individuals with deletions (p. 39), can allow assignment of structural genes to a particular chromosome. The genes for the enzymes superoxide dismutase and red cell acid phosphatase were provisionally assigned to chromosomes 21 and 2 respectively by this means.

Somatic cell hybridisation

Somatic cell genetics has been invaluable in gene mapping studies. This technique involves taking cells from two different species and fusing them, a process facilitated by the presence of the Sendai virus or by the use of the chemical polyethyleneglycol. The chromosome constitution of the resulting *somatic cell hybrid* shows a preferential loss of the human chromosomes from the cells (Fig. 4.21). By staining the chromosomes present

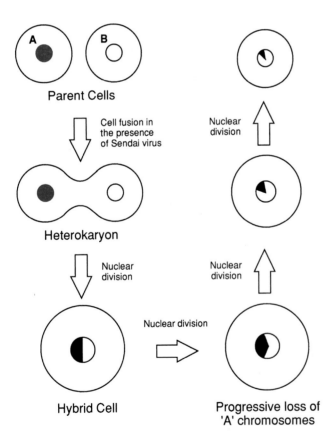

Parent Cells

Cell fusion in the presence of Sendai virus

Heterokaryon

Nuclear division

Nuclear division

Nuclear division

Nuclear division

Hybrid Cell

Progressive loss of 'A' chromosomes

Fig. 4.21
Diagrammatic representation of the hybridisation of human and mouse cells and subsequent selective loss of chromosomes from the hybrid cells.

and analysing the human biochemical markers expressed, it is possible to determine which human chromosomes have been retained and select interspecific hybrids which contain different human chromosome(s). A panel of somatic cell hybrid clones which retain different human chromosomes can be selected which will enable assignment of any expressed enzyme or protein to a particular human chromosome.

It is also possible to isolate somatic cell hybrids with a particular human chromosome or gene by choosing genes which can be selected for in the culture medium. The presence of aminopterin in the medium, which inhibits purine and pyrimidine synthesis necessary for nuclear and therefore cell division, will stop growth of cells in culture. If, however, thymidine kinase activity is present, which allows synthesis of nucleotides from thymidine, cells will be able to grow. Rodent cells do not possess the enzyme thymidine kinase. If, therefore, they are fused with human cells, after several generations of cell division only somatic cell hybrids with chromosome 17 are found to survive. This led to the identification that the gene for this particular enzyme is located on chromosome 17 in humans.

Cells from humans with structural chromosome abnormalities such as translocations (p. 35), deletions (p. 39) and inversions (p. 40) can be used to allow more specific chromosomal mapping of a particular gene or DNA sequence. The use of recombinant DNA technology in somatic cell hybrids allows detection and mapping of DNA sequences without the need for gene expression, thereby extending the usefulness of this approach in gene mapping. The development of the technique known as *chromosome-mediated gene-transfer* allows establishment of somatic cell hybrids with particular DNA sequences or specific genes, allowing more detailed gene mapping.

In situ hybridisation

In this technique single stranded radiolabelled DNA sequences are incubated under special conditions with standard chromosome preparations so that they will hybridise with homologous DNA sequence(s) in the genome. This allows mapping of single copy genes or DNA sequences on the chromosomes by exposure of the preparation to an X-ray film, a technique known as *in situ hybridisation*. The availability of non-radioactive labelling techniques, has allowed development of *fluorescent in situ hybridisation* which has found widespread clinical and research use (p. 28).

DNA MAPPING TECHNIQUES

In single-gene disorders which have been mapped by genetic linkage to a particular region of a chromosome, even with closely linked markers, the gene of interest can be in a region several million base pairs in length. There are a number of techniques which are useful in gene mapping at this intermediate level of analysis.

Pulsed field gel electrophoresis

Conventional agarose gel electrophoresis can resolve DNA fragments up to approximately 20 000 base-pairs in size. Use of *pulsed field gel electrophoresis*, PFGE, in which DNA fragments are subjected alternately to two approximately perpendicular fields in the electrophoretic gel, enables separation of DNA fragments of up to 2 000 000 base-pairs in size. Digestion of DNA with restriction enzymes such as Not I and Pvu I results in relatively larger DNA fragments, since these enzymes have 6–8 base pair nucleotide recognition sequences which occur less frequently in DNA. Analysis of restriction digests of genomic DNA using these infrequently cutting restriction enzymes allows construction of physical maps of relatively large stretches of DNA not amenable to resolution by conventional restriction mapping studies.

Chromosome jumping/linking

Circularisation of DNA fragments produced by restriction enzyme digestion in the presence of a plasmid sequence cut with the same restriction enzyme, followed by digestion with a second restriction enzyme, which does not cleave within the plasmid sequence, allows deletion of the 'internal' DNA from these fragments (Fig. 4.22). The plasmid sequence acts as an identifying 'tag' and allows cloning of the ends of the original DNA fragments which, with complementary libraries, can be used to map markers directionally which are hundreds of kilobases apart. This has been called *chromosome jumping* or *linking*.

Yeast artificial chromosome contigs

A number of genes such as the cystic fibrosis, dystrophin and neurofibromatosis genes are up to 2 000 000–3 000 000 base-pairs in length. Detailed mapping of such genes and their flanking regions using conventional vectors requires a large number of overlapping clones. The development of yeast artificial chromosomes (p. 47) has allowed the cloning of large segments of genomic DNA. Cloning of DNA fragments of this size into YACs facilitates analysis of major genomic rearrangements as found in the immunoglobulin genes. This technique has also found widespread use in long range physical mapping for gene cloning by the production of overlapping YAC clones or *contigs*, allowing 'chromosome walking' when flanking linked markers have been identified.

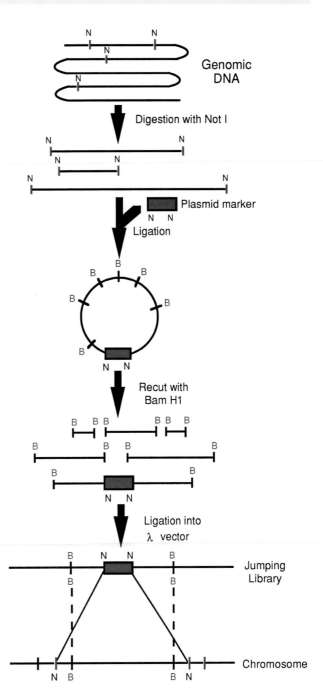

Fig. 4.22
Representation of the production of linking or jumping clones. N and B refer to restriction enzyme cleavage sites for Not I and BamH I.

POSITIONAL CLONING

Despite lack of knowledge of the product of a gene, a variety of techniques can be used to localise a gene to a particular region of a chromosome and lead to its cloning. This approach is known as *positional cloning*.

Zoo blots

The structure and relative position of many genes have been highly conserved during evolution so that in closely related species there are large areas of homology consistent with evolutionary divergence from a common ancestor. If a particular DNA sequence or gene is isolated from another species it can be relatively easily mapped to the human genome by a combination of approaches such as somatic cell hybridisation and FISH. Southern blots of DNA from a variety of species demonstrating the presence of homologous sequences for such a gene comprise what is known as *zoo blots*. If a gene is found to be highly conserved throughout evolution then it is thought likely to represent an important functional gene.

HTF islands

A number of the infrequently cutting restriction enzymes, such as Hpa II, contain one or more CpG dinucleotides within the nucleotide recognition sequence necessary for DNA cleavage. Methylation of the cytosine residue of this dinucleotide pair prevents cleavage of the DNA by these restriction enzymes. It has been found that CpG dinucleotides occur with one-quarter of the frequency which would be predicted from the base composition of genomic DNA and that they are non-randomly distributed within the genome. Clusters of undermethylated CpG dinucleotides have been found near transcription initiation sites at the 5′ end of many genes and are called methylation-free *Hpa II tiny fragments* or *HTF islands*. Therefore cleavage at one of these sites identifies a methylation-free region and can be used to identify the likely location of genes within a stretch of DNA. Not all genes, however, are associated with HTF islands, particularly those which show tissue-specific expression. Conversely not all HTF islands are found in association with genes.

Persons with single gene disorders and chromosome abnormalities

Occasionally individuals are recognised with single gene disorders who are also found to have chromosome abnormalities. The first clue that the gene responsible for Duchenne muscular dystrophy, DMD (p. 238), was located on the short arm of the X chromosome was the identification of a number of females with DMD who were also found to have a chromosomal rearrangement between an autosome and a particular portion of the short arm of one of their X chromosomes. Isolation of DNA clones spanning the region of the X chromosome involved in the rearrangement led in one such female to more detailed gene mapping information as well as to the eventual cloning of the DMD or dystrophin gene (p. 240).

At the same time as these observations, a male was reported with three X-linked disorders, Duchenne muscular dystrophy, chronic granulomatous disease and retinitis pigmentosa. He also had an unusual X-linked red cell group known as the McLeod phenotype. It was suggested that he could have a deletion of the short arm of his X chromosome in the proposed region of the Duchenne muscular dystrophy gene. Detailed prometaphase chromosome analysis revealed this to be the case. DNA from this individual was used in vast excess to hybridise in competitive reassociation, under special conditions, with DNA from persons with multiple X chromosomes to enrich for DNA sequences which he lacked, the so-called *phenol enhanced reassociation technique*, hence pERT, which allowed isolation of DNA clones containing portions of the DMD gene.

Individuals with a chromosome abnormality and a single gene disorder are rare, but their recognition is important as they have provided the vital first clue for linkage analysis and gene mapping studies in the cloning of several important disease genes in humans. Polyposis coli (p. 173) is another disorder in which the gene responsible was cloned through the observation of an individual with the disease and an abnormality involving the long arm of one of his number 5 chromosomes.

Identification of expressed sequences

Once a gene has been mapped to a particular region of the human genome, techniques can be used to identify genes in the region concerned. One, known as *exon trapping*, involves using a recombinant plasmid vector with splice site sequences which, with intact splice sites in the cloned DNA, results in normal RNA processing. The resulting RNA can be amplified by PCR to identify coding sequences which can be screened for mutations.

Candidate genes

Genes which are located in the region of the human genome to which a single gene disorder maps constitute what are known as *candidate genes*. This term, however, is usually reserved for genes whose function, taking into account knowledge of the disease process, suggests that they are likely to be responsible. An example in which this latter approach has led to the recognition of a locus responsible for a genetic disorder without the need for exhaustive physical mapping and cloning, is the identification of mutations in the gene for the photosensitive retinal protein rhodopsin in some patients with autosomal dominant retinitis pigmentosa (p. 81).

THE HUMAN GENE MAP

The rate at which DNA sequences and genes are being mapped is increasing exponentially, producing what has been called the 'anatomy of the human genome' (Fig. 4.23). As a consequence, any human gene map (Fig. 4.24) is out of date almost as soon as it has been collated! This is likely to be especially so, given the resources being directed into the human genome project over the next decade (p. 284).

POSSIBLE BIOLOGICAL HAZARDS OF RECOMBINANT DNA TECHNOLOGY

Recombinant DNA technology has a very great deal to offer to medicine but there has been concern that potentially serious hazards of this technology should not be ignored. These same techniques are being used to improve animal and plant stocks for food production, and recombinant microbial strains are being engineered to deal with environmental waste products. Certain factions suggest that insufficient consideration is being given to the serious potential consequences which could follow introduction of the use of these techniques. For example, it is claimed that the engineered microbial strains, if released into the environment, could cause far more problems than they solve. These concerns, in many instances, are likely to be more theoretical than practical.

The main concern surrounding DNA technology is the danger of producing organisms which could contain genes for cancer susceptibility or be immune to all known antibiotics. After all, one of the host organisms which is commonly used in such experiments is *E. coli*, which is ubiquitous being a normal commensal of the bowel. These are matters which have been of considerable public concern and were the subject of the famous Asilomar Conferences in California in the mid-1970s.

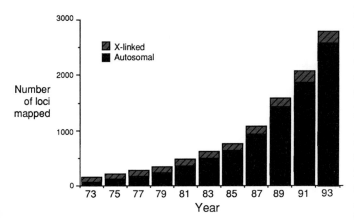

Fig. 4.23
The number of DNA sequences mapped to the human genome over the last 20 years (from McKusick).

The consensus of scientific opinion now, however, seems to be that these dangers have been very much exaggerated. Various authorities, such as the Genetic Manipulation Advisory Group (GMAG) in Britain and the National Institutes of Health in the United States, have laid down very careful guidelines for research in this field.

TECHNIQUES TO MINIMISE BIOHAZARD

There have been two main approaches to limiting potential hazards of DNA technology. These can be separated into physical and biological containment methods.

Physical containment

Here the object is to make sure that any microorganisms of potential danger are contained within the laboratory. Laboratories are graded, according to the type of experiments being conducted, from C I (minimum containment), which involves little more than the use of careful techniques, to C IV (maximum containment), where containment is of an exceptionally high order. This high level of containment is used in laboratories involved in biological warfare such as Porton Down in Britain and Camp Detrick in the United States. Even with specially designed laboratories having special ventilator systems and where every care is taken to maintain containment, infections can occur.

Biological containment

Host organisms used in recombinant DNA work have been attenuated, or 'crippled', so that they cannot survive outside the confines of laboratory culture conditions. This is achieved by careful selection of particular mutants which led, for example, to the production of the *E. coli* K12 strain 1776 (after the year of American independence!) which requires many complex growth factors if it is to survive outside the laboratory. At the same time, complementary work has produced safer vectors. The combination of physical containment and the use of attenuated organisms should reduce the risk of any possible hazard.

From the evidence available to date, it seems that the hazards of genetic engineering have, perhaps, been overemphasised in the past and that the risks are more imagined than possible. Accordingly, the guidelines set out by the GMAG on which types of procedure can be carried out at the various levels of containment have been relaxed. Nevertheless, great care will continue to have to be exercised in this field, if for no other reason than to allay the fears of the general public.

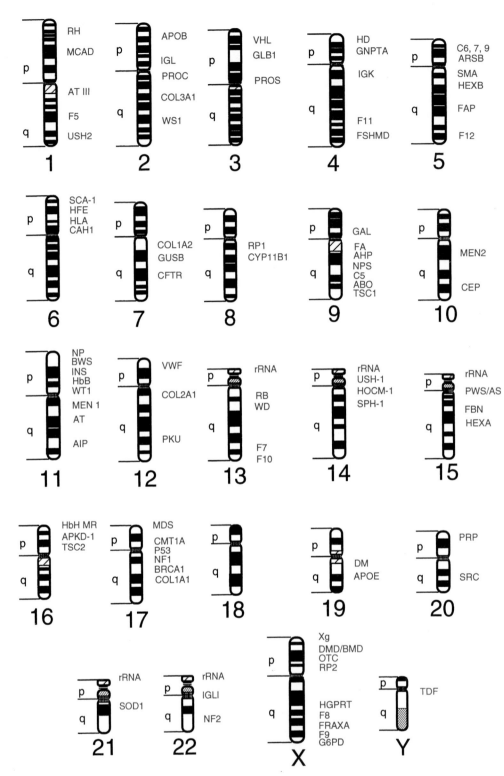

Fig. 4.24
A gene map of the human genome with examples of some of the more common or important single genes and disorders (from McKusick).

Key to Fig. 4.24

ABO—ABO blood group
AHP—Acute hepatic porphyria
AIP—Acute intermittent porphyria
APKD–1—Adult polycystic kidney disease—locus 1
APOB—Apolipoprotein B
APOE—Apolipoprotein E
ARSB—Mucopolysaccharidosis type VI, Maroteaux–Lamy syndrome
AS—Angelman syndrome
AT—Ataxia telangiectasia
AT III—Antithrombin III
BRCA1—Familial breast/ovarian cancer locus-1
BWS—Beckwith–Wiedemann syndrome
C5—Complement factor 5
C6—Complement factor 6
C7—Complement factor 7
C9—Complement factor 9
CAH1—Congenital adrenal hyperplasia, 21-hydroxylase
CEP—Congenital erythropoietic porphyria
CFTR—Cystic fibrosis transmembrane conductance regulator
CMT1A—Charcot–Marie–Tooth disease type 1a
COL1A1—Collagen type 1, alpha-1 chain, osteogenesis imperfecta
COL1A2—Collagen type 1, alpha-2 chain, osteogenesis imperfecta
COL2A1—Collagen type 2, Stickler syndrome
COL3A1—Collagen type 3, alpha-1 chain, Ehlers–Danlos syndrome type IV
CYP11B1—Congenital adrenal hyperplasia, 11-beta hydroxylase
DM—Myotonic dystrophy
DMD/BMD—Dystrophin, Duchenne and Becker muscular dystrophy
F5—Coagulation protein V
F7—Coagulation protein VII
F8—Coagulation protein VIII, Haemophilia A
F9—Coagulation protein IX, Christmas disease, Haemophilia B
F10—Coagulation protein X
F11—Coagulation factor XI
F12—Coagulation factor XII
FA—Friedreich's ataxia
FAP—Familial adenomatous polyposis, polyposis coli, Gardner syndrome
FBN—Fibrillin, Marfan syndrome
FraxA—Fragile X mental retardation
FSHMD—Facio–scapulo–humeral muscular dystrophy
GAL—Galactosaemia
GLB1—GM1 gangliosidosis
G6PD—Glucose-6-phosphate dehydrogenase
GNPTA—Mucopolysaccharidosis type I, Hurler syndrome
GUSB—Mucopolysaccharidosis type VII, Sly syndrome
HbB—Beta globin gene

HbH MR—Alpha-thalassaemia mental retardation
HD—Huntington's disease
HEXA—Hexosaminidase A, Tay–Sachs disease
HEXB—Hexosaminidase B, Sandhoff disease
HFE—Haemochromatosis
HGPRT—Hypoxanthine guanine phosphoribosyl transferase, Lesch–Nyhan syndrome
HLA—Major histocompatibility locus
HOCM-1—Hypertrophic obstructive cardiomyopathy type 1
IGK—Immunoglobulin kappa light chain
IGL—Immunoglobulin lambda light chains, κ on chromosome 2, λ on chromosome 22
INS—Insulin
MCAD—Acyl Co-A dehydrogenase, medium chain
MDS—Miller–Dieker syndrome
MEN1—Multiple endocrine neoplasia syndrome type 1
MEN2—Multiple endocrine neoplasia syndrome type 2
NF1—Neurofibromatosis type 1, von Recklinghausen's disease
NF2—Neurofibromatosis type 2, bilateral acoustic neuroma
NP—Niemann–Pick disease
NPS—Nail–patella syndrome
OTC—Ornithine transcarbamylase
p53—p53 protein, Li–Fraumeni syndrome
PKU—Phenylketonuria
PROC—Protein C, coagulopathy disorder
PROS—Protein S, coagulopathy disorder
PRP—Prion disease protein
PWS—Prader–Willi syndrome
RB—Retinoblastoma
RH—Rhesus null disease, Rhesus blood group
RP1—Retinitis pigmentosa locus 1
RP2—Retinitis pigmentosa locus 2, X-linked
rRNA—Ribosomal RNA
SCA1—Spinocerebellar ataxia locus 1
SPH1—Spherocytosis type 1
SMA—Spinal muscular atrophy
SOD1—Superoxide dismutase, familial motor neurone disease
SRC—Proto-oncogene, Rous sarcoma virus
TDF—Testis determining factor
TSC1—Tuberous sclerosis, locus 1
TSC2—Tuberous sclerosis, locus 2
USH1—Usher syndrome type 1
USH2—Usher syndrome type 2
VHL—von Hippel–Lindau syndrome
VWF—von Willebrand disease
WD—Wilson's disease
WS1—Waardenburg syndrome, type 1
WT1—Wilms' tumour 1 gene
Xg—Xg blood group

ELEMENTS

1 Restriction enzymes allow DNA from any source to be cleaved into reproducible fragments based on their specific nucleotide recognition sequences. These fragments can be made to re-combine enabling their incorporation into a suitable vector, with subsequent transformation of a host organism by the vector leading to the production of clones containing a particular DNA sequence.

2 Techniques including Southern blotting, the use of allele-specific oligonucleotide probes, the polymerase chain reaction, mutation screening and DNA sequencing can be used to identify or analyse in detail specific DNA sequences of interest.

3 These techniques can be used for analysing normal gene structure and function and revealing the molecular pathology of inherited disease. This provides a means for presymptomatic diagnosis, carrier detection and prenatal diagnosis either by direct mutational analysis or indirectly through linkage studies in families.

4 Gene mapping techniques which include somatic cell hybridisation, in situ hybridisation, pulsed field gel electrophoresis, the use of yeast artificial chromosome contigs and positional cloning techniques are beginning to reveal the 'anatomy of the human genome'.

5 Recombinant DNA technology is potentially biologically hazardous but these risks can be minimised by physical and biological containment methods.

FURTHER READING

Botstein D, White R L, Skolnick M, Davis R W 1980 Construction of a genetic linkage map in man using restriction fragment length polymorphisms. Am J Hum Genet 32: 314–331
One of the original papers describing the concept of linked RFLPs.
McKusick V A 1994 Mendelian inheritance in man, 11th edn. Johns Hopkins University Press, London
A computerised catalogue of the dominant, recessive and X-linked Mendelian traits and disorders in humans with a brief clinical commentary and details of the mutational basis if known. Also available on-line, up-dated weekly!
Sambrook J, Fritsch E F, Maniatis T 1989 Molecular cloning–a laboratory manual, 2nd edn. Cold Spring Harbor Laboratories Press, Cold Spring Harbor
The standard beginner's laboratory manual of basic recombinant DNA techniques.
Strachan T 1992 The human genome. βios Scientific Publishers, Oxford
A brief outline of the approaches to and discoveries from study of the molecular biology of the human genome.
Weatherall D J 1991 The new genetics and clinical practice, 3rd edn. Oxford University Press, Oxford
A lucid overview of the application of DNA techniques in clinical medicine.

Developmental genetics

INTRODUCTION

The formation and subsequent development of a human being are extremely complex processes which are still only poorly understood. Both genetic and environmental factors play important roles. Given a suitable environment, genes inherited from both parents determine how a small cluster of undifferentiated cells derived from the fertilised egg or zygote develop over a period of approximately 12 weeks into a recognisably human fetus. The physiological processes which take place within these first 12 weeks following conception fall within the realm of embryology. In this chapter we are not concerned so much with the mechanics of these structural changes as with the way these processes are under genetic control. It is this aspect of biology which constitutes the field of *developmental genetics*.

Prenatal life can be divided into three main stages – pre-embryonic, embryonic and fetal (Table 5.1). During the pre-embryonic stage a small collection of cells becomes distinguishable, firstly as a double-layered or *bilaminar disc*, and then as a triple-layered or *trilaminar disc* which is destined to develop into the human infant. During the embryonic stage, cranio-caudal and dorso-ventral axes are established, as cellular aggregation and differentiation lead to tissue and organ formation. The final fetal stage is characterised by rapid growth and development as the embryo, now known as a *fetus*, matures into a viable human infant.

On average this extraordinary process lasts approximately 38 weeks. By convention pregnancy is usually dated from the first day of the last menstrual period (LMP) preceding conception, so that the normal length of gestation is often stated incorrectly as lasting for 40 weeks.

FERTILISATION AND GASTRULATION

Fertilisation, the process by which the male and female gametes fuse, occurs in the Fallopian tube. Of the 100–

Table 5.1 Main events in the development of a human infant

Stage	Time from conception	Length of embryo/fetus
Pre–embryonic		
First cell division	30 hours	
Zygote reaches uterine cavity	4 days	
Implantation	5–6 days	
Formation of bilaminar disc	12 days	0.2 mm
Lyonisation in female	16 days	
Formation of trilaminar disc and primitive streak	19 days	1 mm
Embryonic stage		
Organogenesis	4–8 weeks	
Brain and spinal cord are forming	4 weeks	4 mm
First signs of heart and limb buds		
Brain, eyes, heart and limbs developing rapidly	6 weeks	17 mm
Bowel and lungs beginning to develop		
Digits have appeared. Ears, kidneys, liver and muscle are developing	8 weeks	4 cm
Palate closes and joints form	10 weeks	6 cm
Sexual differentiation almost complete	12 weeks	9 cm
Fetal stage		
Fetal movements felt	16–18 weeks	20 cm
Eyelids open. Fetus is now viable with specialised care	24–26 weeks	35 cm
Rapid weight gain due to	28 weeks	40 cm
growth and accumulation of	↓	↓
fat as lungs mature	38 weeks	50 cm

200 million spermatozoa deposited in the female genital tract only a few hundred reach the site of fertilisation. Of these only a single spermatozoon succeeds in penetrating first the *corona radiata*, then the *zona pellucida* and finally the oocyte cell membrane, whereupon the oocyte completes its second meiotic division (Fig. 3.12, p. 33).

After the sperm has penetrated the oocyte and the meiotic process has been completed, the two nuclei, now known as *pronuclei*, fuse thereby restoring the diploid number of 46 chromosomes. The fertilised ovum or zygote then undergoes a series of mitotic divisions to consist of 2 cells by 30 hours, 4 cells by 40 hours and 12–16 cells by 3 days when it is known as a *morula*.

Further cell division leads to formation of a *blastocyst* which consists of an inner cell mass or *embryoblast*, which is destined to form the embryo, and an outer cell mass or *trophoblast*, which gives rise to the placenta. The process of converting the inner cell mass into firstly a bilaminar and then a trilaminar disc is known as *gastrulation*, and takes place between the beginning of the second and the end of the third weeks.

Between 4 and 8 weeks body form is established beginning with the formation of the primitive streak at the caudal end of the embryo. The germinal layers of the trilaminar disc give rise to ectodermal, mesodermal and endodermal structures (Table 5.2). The neural tube is formed and neural crest cells migrate to form sensory ganglia, the sympathetic nervous system, pigment cells, and both bone and cartilage in parts of the face and branchial arches. Disorders involving cells of neural crest origin, such as neurofibromatosis (p. 233), are sometimes referred to as neurocristopathies. This period between 4 and 8 weeks is referred to as the period of organogenesis as it is during this interval that all of the major organs are formed as regional specialisation proceeds in a cranio-caudal direction down the axis of the embryo.

MOLECULAR ASPECTS OF DEVELOPMENT

Information about the genetic factors which initiate, maintain and direct embryogenesis is limited. However, genetic studies of the fruit fly, *Drosophila melanogaster*, have identified several genes and gene families which play important roles in the early developmental processes. Most of these genes produce proteins called *transcription*

Table 5.2 Organ and tissue origins

Ectodermal
Central nervous system
Peripheral nervous system
Epidermis including hair and nails
Subcutaneous glands
Dental enamel

Mesodermal
Connective tissue
Cartilage and bone
Smooth and striated muscle
Cardiovascular system
Urogenital system

Endodermal
Thymus and thyroid
Gastro-intestinal system
Liver and pancreas

factors. These control RNA transcription from the DNA template by binding to specific regulatory DNA sequences forming complexes which initiate transcription by RNA polymerase.

Transcription factors can switch genes on and off by activating or repressing gene expression. It is likely that important transcription factors control many other genes in a coordinated sequential cascade involving the regulation of fundamental embryological processes such as segmentation, induction, migration, differentiation and programmed cell death or what is known as *apoptosis*. It is believed that these processes are mediated by growth factors, cell receptors and chemicals known as *morphogens*. These are thought to stimulate cell receptors and to show a concentration gradient across a structure such as a limb bud, thereby determining axial development and tissue specificity. Examples of growth factors identified in developing chick limb buds include fibroblast growth factor and bone morphogenetic protein, which is related to transforming growth factor. There is also evidence that in limb buds the main morphogen involved in digit formation and differentiation is retinoic acid.

DEVELOPMENTAL GENES IN VERTEBRATES

Three gene families have been identified in vertebrates which show strong sequence homology with developmental regulatory genes in *Drosophila*. These are the homeotic genes, the paired box genes and genes which encode transcription factors containing zinc fingers.

HOMEOBOX (HOX) GENES

In *Drosophila* a class of genes known as the *homeotic* genes have been shown to determine segment identity. Mutations in these genes result in major structural abnormalities such as the development of a leg instead of an antenna. Homeotic genes contain a conserved 180 base pair sequence know as the *homeobox* which is believed to be characteristic of genes involved in spatial pattern control and development. Proteins from homeobox containing, or what are known as Hox, genes are therefore important transcription factors which specify cell fate and establish a regional axis.

Four homeobox gene clusters have been identified in humans (Table 5.3). Each cluster contains a series of closely linked genes. In vertebrates such as mice it has been shown that these genes are expressed in segmental units in the hindbrain and in the somites formed from axial mesoderm. In each Hox cluster there is a direct linear correlation between the position of the gene and its temporal and spatial expression, an observation which

Table 5.3 Homeobox gene clusters in humans

Cluster	Number of genes	Chromosome location
Hox 1 (=Hoxa)	11	7p
Hox 2 (=Hoxb)	9	17q
Hox 3 (=Hoxc)	9	12q
Hox 4 (=Hoxd)	9	2q

points to these genes playing a crucial role in early morphogenesis.

No homeobox mutations have been identified in humans and it is likely that any such mutation would be so devastating that the embryo would not survive. Transgenic mice with mutations in certain Hox genes have been found to have multiple severe abnormalities often involving development of the face and skull.

PAIRED-BOX (PAX) GENES

The *paired-box* is a highly conserved DNA sequence which encodes approximately 130 amino acids. Genes which contain a paired-box are known as Pax genes and were first identified in *Drosophila*. They encode DNA-binding proteins, which are almost certainly transcription control factors, and play an important role in development right across the animal kingdom.

Eight Pax genes have been identified in mice and humans through their homology with the *Drosophila* paired-box sequence. In mice, mutations in Pax 1, Pax 3 and Pax 6 cause vertebral malformations, pigmentary abnormalities and small eyes respectively. In humans, mutations which disrupt the DNA binding domain of Pax 3 cause Waardenburg's syndrome, an autosomal dominant disorder characterised by deafness, white forelock and iris heterochromia (Plate 6). Mutations in Pax 6 cause absence of the iris, i.e. aniridia. Curiously, rearrangements in Pax 3 have been identified in a rare childhood tumour known as alveolar rhabdomyosarcoma. These rearrangements are generated by a translocation which interrupts the Pax locus and leads to formation of a novel hybrid transcript. Thus different mutations or rearrangements involving Pax 3 can cause quite different and unrelated human disorders.

ZINC FINGER GENES

The term *zinc finger* is used to describe the finger like projection formed by amino acids positioned between two separated cysteine residues which form a complex with a zinc ion. Many DNA binding proteins contain zinc fingers indicating that the genes which encode these proteins play important developmental regulatory roles.

It has recently been shown that interruption of a multiple zinc finger gene known as GLI3 on chromosome 7 causes a malformation syndrome known as Greig cephalopolysyndactyly. This autosomal dominant disorder is characterised by cranial and hand abnormalities which can take the form of additional and/or webbed digits (Fig. 5.1). Mutations in the Wilms' tumour (WT1) gene on the short arm of chromosome 11 (p. 220), in addition to leading to a risk of developing the renal malignancy, can also lead to a characteristic syndrome with abnormal sexual differentiation and disordered renal development known as the Denys–Drash syndrome.

MOLECULAR GENETICS AND MULTIPLE MALFORMATIONS

The identification of mutations in transcription control genes provides an attractive explanation for the presence of apparently unrelated abnormalities in multiple malformation syndromes. Thus developmental gene mutations provide one explanation for the phenomenon of pleiotropy whereby a single gene exerts multiple and widespread effects (p. 78). In morphogenesis the concept of the *developmental field* has been suggested to account for a set of apparently unrelated embryonic primordia which react together to a single underlying insult which can be genetic or environmental. It is possible that many developmental field defects and multiple congenital abnormality syndromes will be shown to be due to mutations in transcription control genes.

The concept of the developmental field can be extended to include all organs or tissues which share a common embryological origin. Thus in the ectodermal dysplasias, which are usually caused by single gene mutations, abnormalities occur in tissues of ectodermal origin such as hair, teeth, nails and sweat glands (Table 5.2). Similarly in axial mesodermal dysplasia, which usually occurs as a *sporadic* event in a family, organs of mesodermal origin such as the heart, kidneys and vertebrae show abnormal development. Several other conditions such as the VATER association (p. 198) also involve mainly organs of mesodermal origin. Most if not all of the abnormalities in Waardenburg's syndrome can be explained by an abnormality in cells derived from the neural crest. These observations show how a knowledge of embryology, molecular genetics and dysmorphology can help provide a rational explanation for the findings in congenital multiple malformation syndromes.

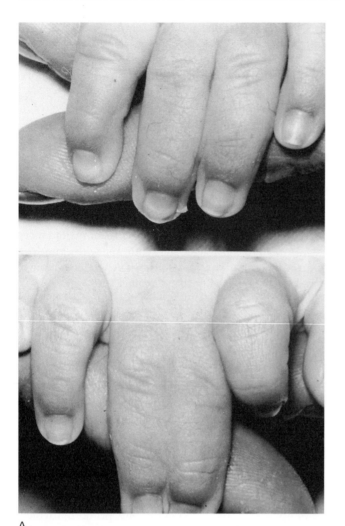

A

HYDATIDIFORM MOLES

Occasionally conception results in an abnormal pregnancy in which the placenta consists of a proliferating disorganised mass known as a *hydatidiform mole*. These changes can be either partial or complete (Table 5.4).

PARTIAL HYDATIDIFORM MOLE

Chromosome analysis of tissue from partial moles reveals the presence of 69 chromosomes, i.e. triploidy (p. 35). Using DNA polymorphisms it has been shown that 46 of these chromosomes are always derived from the father with the remaining 23 being maternal in origin. This doubling of the normal haploid paternal contribution of 23 chromosomes can be due to either fertilisation by two sperm, which is known as *dispermy*, or to duplication of a haploid sperm chromosome set by a process known as *endoreduplication*.

In these pregnancies the fetus rarely if ever survives to term. Triploid conceptions only survive to term if the additional chromosome complement is maternally derived, in which cases partial hydatidiform changes do not occur. Even in these situations it is extremely uncommon for a triploid infant to survive for more than a few hours or days after birth.

Fig. 5.1
(A) Hands and (B) feet of a child with Greig cephalopolysyndactyly syndrome. There is evidence of both polydactyly (extra digits) and syndactyly (webbed digits).

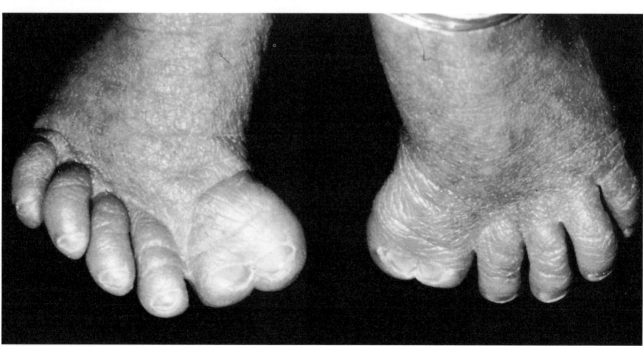

B

Table 5.4 Characteristics of partial and complete hydatidiform moles

	Partial	Complete
Number of chromosomes	69	46
Parental origin of chromosomes	23 – maternal 46 – paternal	all 46 paternal
Fetus present	Yes – but not viable	No
Malignant potential	Very low	High

COMPLETE HYDATIDIFORM MOLE

Complete moles have only 46 chromosomes, but these are exclusively paternal in origin. A complete mole is caused by fertilisation of an empty ovum by either two sperm or by a single sperm which undergoes endoreduplication. The opposite situation of an egg undergoing development without being fertilised by a sperm, a process known as *parthenogenesis*, occurs in lower animals such as arthropods but has never been reported in humans!

The main importance of complete moles lies in their potential to undergo malignant change into invasive choriocarcinoma. This can usually be treated very successfully by chemotherapy, but if untreated the outcome can be fatal. Malignant change is seen only very rarely with partial moles.

DIFFERENT EXPRESSION OF PARENTAL CHROMOSOMES IN TROPHOBLAST AND EMBRYOBLAST

Studies in mice have shown that when all nuclear genes in a zygote are derived from the father, the embryo fails to develop, whereas trophoblast development proceeds relatively unimpaired. In contrast, if all of the nuclear genes are maternal in origin, the embryo develops normally but extra-embryonic development is very poor. The observations outlined above on partial and complete moles indicate that a comparable situation exists in humans with paternally derived genes being essential for trophoblast development and maternally derived genes being necessary for early embryonic development. These phenomena are relevant to the concept of genomic imprinting (p. 88).

SEXUAL DIFFERENTIATION AND DETERMINATION

The sex of an individual is determined by the X and Y chromosomes (p. 25). The presence of a Y chromosome leads to maleness regardless of the number of X chromosomes present. Absence of a Y chromosome results in female development.

Although the sex chromosomes are present from conception, differentiation into male or female does not commence until approximately 6 weeks. Up to this point both the Müllerian and Wolffian duct systems are present and the embryonic gonads, although consisting of cortex and medulla, are still undifferentiated. From 6 weeks onwards the embryo develops into a female unless the testis determining factor initiates a sequence of events which prompt the undifferentiated gonads to develop into testes.

In 1990 it was shown that the testis determining factor or gene is located on the short arm of the Y chromosome close to the pseudoautosomal region (p. 31). This gene is now referred to as being located in the *sex-determining region of the Y* chromosome (SRY). It encodes a sequence of amino acids which show homology to a DNA-binding motif indicating that it is likely to be a transcription regulator.

Evidence that the SRY gene is the primary factor which determines maleness comes from several observations:

1. SRY sequences are present in XX males. These are infertile phenotypic males who appear to have a normal 46,XX karyotype.
2. Mutations or deletions in the SRY sequences are found in many XY females. These are infertile phenotypic females who are found to have a 46,XY karyotype.
3. In mice the SRY gene is expressed only in the male gonadal ridge as the testes are developing in the embryo.
4. Transgenic XX mice which have a tiny portion of the Y chromosome containing the SRY region develop into males with testes.

Considered from the evolutionary point of view and for the maintenance of the species, it would clearly be impossible for the SRY gene to be involved in crossing-over with the X chromosome during meiosis I. Hence the SRY gene has to lie outside the pseudoautosomal region. There has to be pairing of the X and Y chromosomes, however, as otherwise they would segregate on average into the same gamete during meiosis 50% of the time. Nature's compromise has been to ensure that only a small portion of the X and Y chromosomes are homologous and therefore pair during meiosis I. Unfortunately the close proximity of the SRY gene to the pseudoautosomal region means that, occasionally, it can get caught up in a recombinational event. This almost certainly accounts for the majority of XX males, in whom molecular and FISH studies show evidence of Y chromosome sequences at the distal end of one X chromosome short arm (Plate 2).

Once the SRY gene is expressed, the medulla of the undifferentiated gonad develops into a testis in which

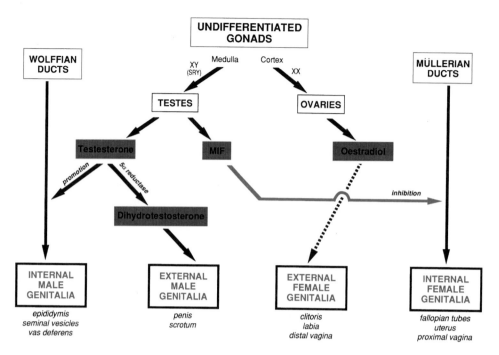

Fig. 5.2
Summary of the main events involved in sex determination (SRY = sex determining region of the Y chromosome, MIF = Müllerian inhibitory factor).

the Leydig cells begin to produce testosterone (Fig. 5.2). This leads to stimulation of the Wolffian ducts, which form the male internal genitalia, and also to masculinisation of the external genitalia. This latter step is mediated by dihydrotestosterone which is produced from testosterone by the action of 5 alpha-reductase (p. 226). The Sertoli cells in the testes produce a hormone known as Müllerian inhibitory factor which causes the Müllerian duct system to regress.

In the absence of normal SRY expression, the cortex of the undifferentiated gonad develops into an ovary. The Müllerian duct forms the internal genitalia. The external genitalia fail to fuse and grow as in the male and instead evolve into normal female external genitalia. Without the stimulating effects of testosterone, the Wolffian duct system regresses.

Normally sexual differentiation is complete by 12 to 14 weeks gestation, although the testes do not migrate into the scrotum until late pregnancy. Abnormalities of sexual differentiation are uncommon but they are important causes of infertility and sexual ambiguity and are considered further in Chapter 17.

X CHROMOSOME INACTIVATION

As techniques were developed for studying chromosomes it was noted that in female mice one of the X chromosomes often differed from all other chromosomes in the extent to which it was condensed. In 1961 Dr Mary Lyon proposed that this *heteropyknotic* X chromosome was

inactivated, citing as evidence her observations on the mosaic pattern of skin colouration seen in mice known to be heterozygous for X-linked genes which influence coat colour. Subsequent events have confirmed the validity of Dr Lyon's hypothesis, and in recognition of her foresight the process of *X-inactivation* is often referred to as *Lyonisation*.

The process of X-inactivation occurs early in development at around 15–16 days gestation when the embryo consists of approximately 5000 cells. Normally either of the two X chromosomes can be inactivated in any particular cell. Thereafter the same X chromosome is inactivated in all daughter cells (Fig. 5.3). This differs from marsupials in which the paternally derived X chromosome is consistently inactivated.

The inactive X chromosome exists in a condensed form during interphase when it appears as a darkly staining mass of chromatin known as the *sex-chromatin* or *Barr body*. During mitosis the inactive X chromosome is late replicating. Laboratory techniques have been developed for distinguishing which X chromosome is late replicating in each cell. This can be useful for confirming that one of the X chromosomes is structurally abnormal, as usually an abnormal X chromosome will be preferentially inactivated, or more precisely only those haematopoietic stem cells in which the normal X chromosome was active will have survived. Apparent non-random inactivation also occurs if one of the X chromosomes is involved in a translocation with an autosome (p. 240).

The process of X-inactivation is achieved by methylation

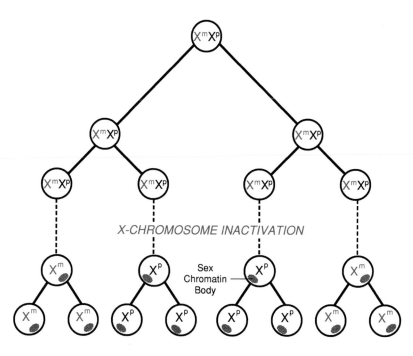

X-CHROMOSOME INACTIVATION

Sex
Chromatin
Body

Fig. 5.3
X chromosome inactivation during development.
The maternally and paternally derived X
chromosomes are represented as X^m and X^p
respectively.

and is initiated by a locus close to the centromere on the long arm known as the *X-inactivation centre*. This hypermethylation of the inactive X chromosome has been utilised in carrier detection studies for X-linked immunodeficiency diseases using methylation sensitive restriction enzymes (p. 156). Not all of the X chromosome is inactivated. Genes in the pseudoautosomal region at the tip of the short arm remain active as do other loci elsewhere on the short and long arms such as the X inactivation centre. If all loci on the X chromosome were inactivated then all women would have the clinical features of Turner's syndrome and the presence of more than one X chromosome in a male, e.g. 47,XXY or two in a female, e.g. 47,XXX, would have no phenotypic effects. There are, in fact, quite characteristic clinical features in these disorders (p. 222).

X chromosome inactivation provides a satisfactory explanation for several observations:

1. Barr bodies – In men and women with more than one X chromosome, the number of Barr bodies visible at interphase is always one less than the total number of X chromosomes. For example men with a 47,XXY karyotype have a single Barr body whereas women with a 47,XXX karyotype have two Barr bodies.
2. Dosage compensation – Women with two normal X chromosomes have the same blood levels of X chromosome protein products, such as factor VIII, as normal men who of course have only one X chromosome. An exception to this phenomenon of *dosage compensation* is the level of steroid sulphatase in blood which is increased in women as compared with men. Not surprisingly it has been shown that the locus for steroid

sulphatase, deficiency of which causes a skin disorder known as ichthyosis, is in the pseudoautosomal region.

3. Mosaicism – Mice which are heterozygous for X-linked genes affecting coat colour show mosaicism with alternating patches of different colour rather than a homogeneous pattern. This is consistent with patches of skin being clonal in origin in that they are derived from a single stem cell in which one or other of the X chromosomes is expressed but not both. Thus, each patch reflects which of the X chromosomes was active in the original stem cell. Similar effects are seen in tissues of clonal origin in women who are heterozygous for X-linked mutations such as ocular albinism (Plate 7, p. 83). Other evidence confirming that X-inactivation leads to mosaicism in females comes from studies of the expression of the enzyme glucose-6-phosphate dehydrogenase (p. 145) in clones of cultured fibroblasts from women heterozygous for variants of this gene. Each clone is derived from a single cell and expresses one of the variants but never both. The clonal origin of tumours can be confirmed in women who are heterozygous for such variants by demonstration of expression of only one of the variants in the tumour.
4. Problems of carrier detection – Carrier detection for X-linked recessive disorders based only on examination of clinical features or on indirect assay of gene function is notoriously difficult and unreliable. Cells in which the X chromosome with the normal gene is active can have a selective advantage or can correct the defect in closely adjacent cells in which the X chromosome with the abnormal gene is active. For example, only a proportion of carriers of Duchenne

muscular dystrophy show evidence of muscle damage as indicated by measurement of creatine kinase in serum (p. 246). Fortunately the development of molecular methods for carrier detection in X-linked disorders can bypass these problems as techniques such as Southern blotting are not influenced by methylation unless methylation sensitive restriction enzymes are used.

5. Manifesting heterozygotes – Occasionally a woman is encountered who shows mild or even full expression of an X-linked recessive disorder. One possible explanation is that she is a *manifesting heterozygote* in whom, by chance, the X chromosome bearing the normal gene has been inactivated in significantly more than 50% of relevant cells. This is referred to as *skewed X-inactivation* (p. 84). There is some evidence that X chromosome inactivation can itself be under genetic control as families with several manifesting carriers of disorders such as Duchenne muscular dystrophy and Fabry's disease have been reported.

TWINNING

Twinning occurs frequently in humans although the incidence in early pregnancy as diagnosed by ultrasonography is greater than at delivery, presumably as a result of death and subsequent resorption of one of the twins in a proportion of twin pregnancies. The overall incidence of twinning in the United Kingdom is approximately 1 in 80 of all pregnancies, so that approximately 1 in 40 (i.e. 2 out of 80) of all individuals is a twin.

Twins can be *identical* or *non-identical* – *monozygotic* (MZ) or *dizygotic* (DZ) – depending on whether they originate from a single conception or from two separate conceptions (Table 5.5). Comparison of the incidence of

Table 5.5 Summary of differences between monozygotic and dizygotic twins

	Monozygotic	Dizygotic
Origin	Single egg fertilised by a single sperm	Two eggs each fertilised by a single sperm
Incidence	1 in 300 pregnancies	Varies from 1 in 100 to 1 in 500 pregnancies
Proportion of genes in common	100%	50%
Fetal membranes	70% monochorionic and diamniotic 30% dichorionic and diamniotic rarely monochorionic and monoamniotic.	Always dichorionic and diamniotic

disease in identical and non-identical twins reared apart and together can provide information about the relative contributions of genetics and environment to the cause of many of the common diseases of adult life as discussed in Chapter 14.

MONOZYGOTIC TWINS

Monozygotic twinning occurs in about 1 in 300 births in all populations which have been studied. MZ twins originate from a single egg which has been fertilised by a single sperm. A very early division, occurring in the zygote before separation of the cells which make the chorion, results in dichorionic twins. Division during the blastocyst stage from days 3 to 7 results in monochorionic diamniotic twins. Division after the first week leads to monoamniotic twins.

MZ twins are genetically identical although rarely they can be discordant for a single gene trait or chromosome abnormality because of a post-zygotic somatic mutation or non-disjunction respectively. Curiously, MZ female twins can show quite striking discrepancy in X chromosome inactivation. There are several reports of female MZ twin pairs only one of whom is affected with an X-linked recessive condition such as Duchenne muscular dystrophy or haemophilia. In these rare examples both twins have the mutation and both show non-random X inactivation but in opposite directions.

Very late division occurring more than 2 weeks after conception can result in conjoined twins. This occurs in less than 1 in 50 000 pregnancies. Conjoined twins are sometimes referred to as *Siamese*, in memory of Chang and Eng who were born in 1811 in Thailand, then Siam, joined at the upper abdomen. Chang and Eng made a successful living out of showing themselves at travelling shows in the United States, where they settled and married. Somehow they both managed to have large numbers of children despite remaining conjoined until they died within a few hours of each other at the age of 61 years.

DIZYGOTIC TWINS

The incidence of DZ twinning varies from approximately 1 in 100 deliveries in Afro-Caribbean populations to 1 in 500 deliveries in Asia and Japan. In Western European Caucasians the incidence is approximately 1 in 120 deliveries. Other factors which convey an increased risk for DZ twinning are increased maternal age, a positive family history and the use of ovulatory inducing drugs such as clomiphene.

DZ twins result from the fertilisation of two ova by two sperm and are no more closely related genetically than brothers and sisters. Hence they are sometimes referred to as *fraternal twins*. DZ twins are dichorionic and diamniotic although they can have a single fused placenta if implantation occurs at closely adjacent sites.

DETERMINATION OF ZYGOSITY

This used to be established by study of the placenta and membranes and also by analysis of polymorphic systems such as the blood groups, the HLA antigens and other biochemical markers. Now zygosity is most easily determined using highly polymorphic molecular markers such as those identified by DNA fingerprinting (pp. 56, 212).

ELEMENTS

1 Three developmental gene families known as Hox, Pax and zinc finger containing genes have been identified in vertebrates. These are believed to act as transcription control factors which initiate and regulate sequential developmental processes.

2 For normal development a haploid chromosome set must be inherited from each parent. A paternal diploid complement results in a complete hydatidiform mole if there is no maternal contribution and in triploidy with a partial hydatidiform mole if there is a haploid maternal contribution.

3 A testis determining factor on the Y chromosome, known as SRY, stimulates the undifferentiated gonads to develop into testes. This, in turn, sets off a series of events leading to male development. In the absence of SRY expression the human embryo develops into a female.

4 In females one of the X chromosomes is inactivated in each cell in early embryogenesis. This can be either the maternally derived or the paternally derived X chromosome. Thereafter in all daughter cells the same X chromosome is inactivated. This process, known as Lyonisation, explains the presence of the Barr body in female nuclei and achieves dosage compensation of X chromosome gene products in males and females.

5 Twins can be monozygotic (identical) or dizygotic (fraternal). Monozygotic twins originate from a single zygote which divides into two during the first 2 weeks after conception. Monozygotic twins are genetically identical. Dizygotic twins originate from two separate zygotes and are no more genetically alike than brothers and sisters.

FURTHER READING

Brueton L A, Winter R M 1993 Molecular aspects of morphogenesis. Baillière's Clinical Paediatrics: The New Genetics. Baillière Tindall, London 1: 2 345–373
A clear account of known developmental genes and molecular aspects of limb development.

Lindor N M, Ney J A, Gaffey T A et al 1992 A genetic review of complete and partial hydatidiform moles and nonmolar triploidy. Mayo Clinic Proceedings 67: 791–799
A comprehensive review of the mechanisms involved in the formation of hydatidiform moles.

Lyon M F 1961 Gene action in the X-chromosome of the mouse (*Mus musculus L.*). Nature 190: 372–373
The original proposal of X inactivation. Very short and easily understood.

Pritchard D J 1986 Foundations of developmental genetics. Taylor & Francis, London
A text-book covering all aspects of developmental genetics including the general principles of embryology and genetics.

Sinclair A H, Berta P, Palmer M S et al 1990 A gene from the human sex-determining region encodes a protein with homology to a conserved DNA-binding motif. Nature 346: 240–244
Report of the identification of the testis determining factor gene known as SRY.

Slack J M W 1991 From egg to embryo, 2nd edn. Cambridge University Press, Cambridge
A comprehensive review of the knowledge of regional specification of early development in a number of vertebrate and non-vertebrate organisms.

CHAPTER 6

Patterns of inheritance

FAMILY STUDIES

If we wish to investigate the genetics of a particular trait or disorder in humans, we usually have to rely either on observation of the way in which it is transmitted from one generation to another, or on study of its frequency among relatives.

An important reason for studying the pattern of inheritance of disorders within families is to enable advice to be given to members of a family regarding the likelihood of their developing it or passing it on to their children, i.e. *genetic counselling* (p. 207). Taking a family history can, in itself, provide a diagnosis. For example, a child could come to the attention of a doctor having a fracture after a seemingly trivial injury. A family history of relatives with a similar tendency to fracture and blue

sclerae (Plate 8), would suggest the diagnosis of brittle bone disease, also known as osteogenesis imperfecta (p. 197). In the absence of a positive family history then other diagnoses would have to be considered.

PEDIGREE DRAWING AND TERMINOLOGY

A family tree is a short hand system of recording the pertinent information about a family. It usually begins with the person through whom the family came to the attention of the investigator. This person is referred to as the *index case*, *proband* or *propositus*, or if female, the *proposita*. The position of the proband in the family tree is indicated by an arrow. Information about the health of the rest of the family is obtained by asking about brothers, sisters, parents and maternal and paternal

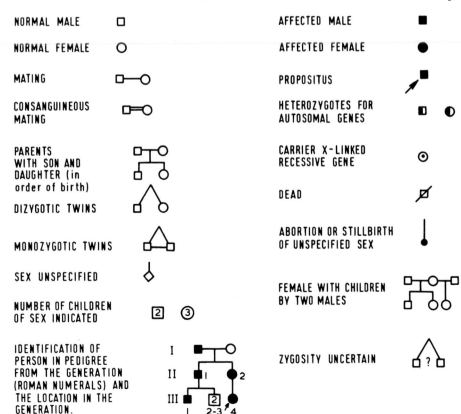

NORMAL MALE

NORMAL FEMALE

MATING

CONSANGUINEOUS MATING

PARENTS WITH SON AND DAUGHTER (in order of birth)

DIZYGOTIC TWINS

MONOZYGOTIC TWINS

SEX UNSPECIFIED

NUMBER OF CHILDREN OF SEX INDICATED

IDENTIFICATION OF PERSON IN PEDIGREE FROM THE GENERATION (ROMAN NUMERALS) AND THE LOCATION IN THE GENERATION. PROPOSITA IS III₄

AFFECTED MALE

AFFECTED FEMALE

PROPOSITUS

HETEROZYGOTES FOR AUTOSOMAL GENES

CARRIER X-LINKED RECESSIVE GENE

DEAD

ABORTION OR STILLBIRTH OF UNSPECIFIED SEX

FEMALE WITH CHILDREN BY TWO MALES

ZYGOSITY UNCERTAIN

Fig. 6.1
Symbols used in family trees.

relatives with the relevant information being carefully recorded in the pedigree chart (Fig. 6.1).

MENDELIAN INHERITANCE

Over 6000 traits or disorders in humans exhibit simple single gene *unifactorial* or *Mendelian inheritance*. However, characteristics such as height, and many common familial disorders, do not usually follow a simple pattern of inheritance (p. 105).

A trait or disorder which is determined by a gene on an autosome is said to show *autosomal inheritance*, whereas a trait or disorder determined by a gene on one of the sex chromosomes is said to show *sex-linked inheritance*.

AUTOSOMAL DOMINANT INHERITANCE

A dominant trait is one which manifests in a *heterozygote*, i.e. a person possessing both the abnormal or *mutant* allele and the normal allele. It is often possible to trace a dominantly inherited trait or disorder through many generations of a family (Fig. 6.2). In South Africa the vast majority of cases of porphyria variegata can be traced back to one couple in the late 17th century. This is a metabolic disorder characterised by skin blistering due to increased sensitivity to sunlight and the excretion of urine which becomes 'port-wine' coloured on standing due to the presence of porphyrins (p. 138) (Fig. 6.3). This pattern of inheritance is sometimes referred to as 'vertical' transmission.

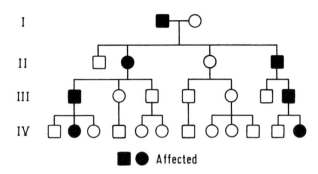

Fig. 6.2
Family tree of an autosomal dominant trait.

Genetic risks

Each gamete from an individual with a dominant trait or disorder will contain either the normal allele or the mutant allele. If we represent the dominant mutant allele as 'A' and the recessive normal allele as 'a', then the various possible combinations of the gametes can be represented in a Punnett's square (Fig. 6.4). Any child born to a person affected with a dominant trait or disorder has a 1 in 2 (50%) chance of inheriting it and being similarly affected.

Pleiotropy

Autosomal dominant traits can involve only one organ or part of the body. A common example is polydactyly. However, many autosomal dominant disorders in humans can manifest in a number of different systems of the body in a variety of ways, so-called *pleiotropy*. An example is tuberous sclerosis (p. 249), in which affected

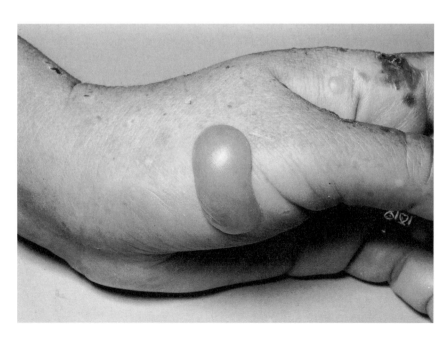

Fig. 6.3
Blistering skin lesions on the hand in porphyria variegata.

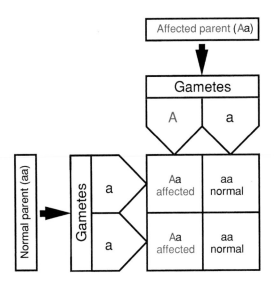

Fig. 6.4
Punnett's square showing possible gamete combinations for an autosomal dominant allele.

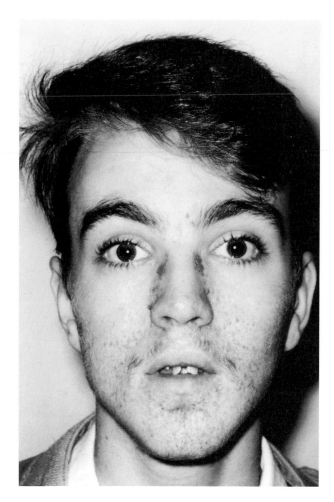

Fig. 6.5
Facial rash of angiokeratoma in a male with tuberous sclerosis.

individuals can present with learning difficulties, epilepsy and a classical facial rash known as adenoma sebaceum which can be confused with acne but is histologically angiokeratomous, being composed of blood vessels and fibrous tissue (Fig. 6.5).

Variable expressivity

The clinical features can show striking variation from person to person in autosomal dominant disorders. This difference in involvement between individuals is referred to as *variable expressivity*.

Reduced penetrance

Some autosomal dominant traits or disorders exhibit a wide range of severity between individuals even within a family in which the same mutation is responsible. In osteogenesis imperfecta some individuals can be so mildly affected that the condition hardly affects their everyday life, while others can have repeated fractures from fairly trivial injuries. In some individuals the presence of the mutation can go undetected, so-called *non-penetrance* or in lay terms 'skipping a generation'. This variation in the expression of a mutant allele is thought to be the result of the modifying effects of other genes, as well as due to interactions with environmental factors.

Reduced penetrance and the variable expressivity of the pleiotropic effects of a mutant allele need to be taken into account when giving genetic counselling to individuals at risk for autosomal dominantly inherited disorders (p. 254).

New mutations

In autosomal dominant disorders an affected person will usually have an affected parent. Sometimes, however, a trait can appear in an individual in one generation when no one else in previous generations has been affected. An example is achondroplasia, a form of short-limbed dwarfism (Fig. 6.6), in which the parents are usually of normal stature. The sudden unexpected appearance of a condition arising as a result of a mistake occurring in the transmission of a gene is called a *new mutation*. In this instance the dominant mode of inheritance of achondroplasia could only be confirmed by persons with achondroplasia having in equal proportions offspring with achondroplasia and normal stature.

There are other possible explanations for a disorder appearing to arise as a new dominant mutation. It is possible that one of the parents can, in fact, be heterozygous for the mutant allele but be so mildly affected that it has not previously been detected, i.e. reduced or non-penetrance. The variable expressivity of the

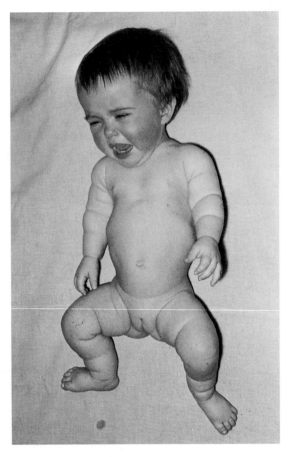

Fig. 6.6
Child with short-limbed dwarfism due to achondroplasia.

pleiotropic manifestations of a mutant allele also needs to be considered as a possible explanation. Another possibility for the appearance of an apparent new mutation is that the stated father is not the child's true father, i.e. *non-paternity* (p. 212).

New dominant mutations, in certain instances, have been associated with an increased age of the father. It is believed that this is due to the large number of mitotic divisions which male gamete stem cells undergo during a reproductive lifetime (p. 32).

Codominance

Codominance is the term used for two traits which are both expressed in the heterozygote. In persons with blood group AB it is possible to demonstrate both A and B blood group substances on the red blood cells so that the A and B blood groups are therefore codominant (p. 86).

Homozygosity for autosomal dominant traits

The rarity of most autosomal dominant disorders and diseases means that they usually only occur in the heterozygous state. There are, however, reports of

children born to couples where both parents are heterozygous for a dominantly inherited disorder. Offspring of such couples are, therefore, at risk of being homozygous. In the limited number of such observations, affected individuals appear to be either more severely affected, as has been reported with achondroplasia, or have an earlier age of onset, as in familial hypercholesterolaemia (p. 134). The heterozygote having a phenotype intermediate between the homozygotes for the normal and mutant alleles is consistent with what is known as *intermediate inheritance*.

Conversely, with other dominantly inherited disorders, such as Huntington's disease, homozygous affected individuals seem to have the same age of onset and severity as heterozygotes. There is also an intriguing report of individuals who have been shown by DNA analysis to be homozygous for myotonic dystrophy but are clinically unaffected, as if the two different mutations have cancelled each other out!

AUTOSOMAL RECESSIVE INHERITANCE

Recessive traits and disorders are only manifest when the allele is present in a double dose, i.e. homozygosity for a mutant allele. Both the parents and the offspring of persons homozygous for a recessive mutant allele are obligate heterozygotes and by definition are perfectly healthy with no features to show that they are carriers. The family tree for recessive traits differs considerably from that found in autosomal dominant traits (Fig. 6.7). It is not possible to trace an autosomal recessive trait or disorder through the family, i.e. all the affected individuals in a family are usually in a single sibship, that is, they are brothers and sisters. This is sometimes referred to as 'horizontal' inheritance.

Consanguinity

Enquiry into the family history of individuals affected with rare recessive traits or disorders, reveals their

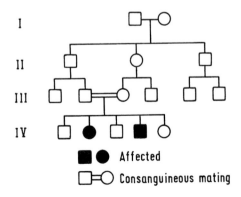

Fig. 6.7
Family tree of an autosomal recessive trait.

parents to be related more often than parents in the general population. Generally speaking, the rarer a recessive trait or disorder, the greater the frequency of consanguinity among the parents of affected individuals. In cystic fibrosis, the commonest autosomal recessive disorder in persons of Western European origin (p. 235), the frequency of parental consanguinity is little greater than in the general population. In oculocutaneous albinism (p. 130) the parents of roughly 1 in 20 affected children are first cousins. In alkaptonuria, one of the original inborn errors of metabolism (pp. 3, 130), which is an exceedingly rare condition, a quarter or more of the parents are first cousins. Bateson and Garrod, in 1902, reasoned that rare alleles for disorders such as alkaptonuria are more likely to 'meet up' in the offspring of cousins than in the offspring of parents who are unrelated.

Genetic risks

If we represent the normal dominant allele as 'A' and the recessive mutant allele as 'a', then each parental gamete carries either the mutant or the normal allele (Fig. 6.8). The various possible combinations of gametes mean that the offspring of two heterozygotes have a 1 in 4 (25%) chance of being homozygous affected, a 1 in 2 (50%) chance of being heterozygous unaffected and a 1 in 4 (25%) chance of being homozygous unaffected.

Pseudodominance

If an individual who is homozygous for an autosomal recessive disorder marries a carrier of the same disorder, their children have a 1 in 2 (50%) chance of being affected. Such a pedigree is said to exhibit *pseudodominance* (Fig. 6.9).

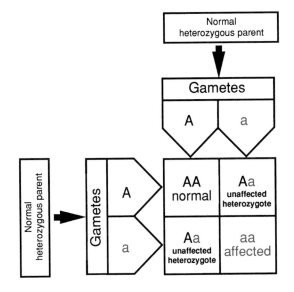

Fig. 6.8
Punnett's square showing possible gametic combinations for heterozygous carrier parents of an autosomal recessive allele.

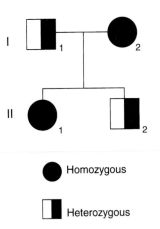

Homozygous

Heterozygous

Fig. 6.9
A pedigree with a woman (I_2) homozygous for an autosomal recessive disorder whose husband is heterozygous for the same disorder. They have a homozygous affected daughter so that the pedigree shows pseudodominant inheritance.

Genetic heterogeneity

It is known that many disorders can be inherited in various ways due to a number of different genes. An example is retinitis pigmentosa which can be inherited in a dominant, recessive and X-linked manner. This is known as *genetic heterogeneity*.

In addition, a disorder inherited in the same manner can be due to mutations in more than one gene. For example, it is recognised that sensorineural deafness often shows autosomal recessive inheritance. Deaf persons, by virtue of their schooling and involvement in the deaf community, often choose to have children with another deaf person. It would be expected that if two deaf persons were homozygous for the same recessive gene, all of their children would be similarly affected. Families have been described in which all the children born to deaf parents have had perfectly normal hearing. The explanation for this must be that the parents were not homozygous for a mutant allele at the same locus and that different genes can cause sensorineural deafness. This phenomenon is referred to as *locus heterogeneity*, i.e. two or more genes can show the same phenotype but are in fact genetically distinct.

The offspring of parents homozygous at different loci are *double heterozygotes*. In addition, disorders with the same phenotype due to different genetic loci are known as *genocopies*, while the same phenotype being due to environmental causes is known as a *phenocopy*.

Compound heterozygotes

Heterogeneity can also occur at a genotypic or allelic level. In the majority of single gene disorders, for example in beta thalassaemia, a large number of different mutations have been identified (p. 124). Individuals have been identified who have two different allelic mutations at the same locus. These are known as *compound heterozygotes*. Most individuals affected with an autosomal recessive disorder are probably, in fact, compound heterozygotes rather than true homozygotes, unless their parents are related when they are likely to be homozygous by descent.

SEX-LINKED INHERITANCE

Sex-linked inheritance refers to the pattern of inheritance shown by genes carried on either of the sex chromosomes. Genes carried on the X chromosome are referred to as being *X-linked*. Genes carried on the Y chromosomes are referred to as being *Y-linked* or *holandric*.

X-linked recessive inheritance

An X-linked recessive trait is one determined by a gene carried on the X chromosome and usually only manifests in males. A male with a mutant allele on his single X chromosome is said to be *hemizygous* for that allele. Diseases inherited in an X-linked manner are transmitted by healthy heterozygous female carriers to affected males, as well as by affected males to their *obligate carrier* daughters with a consequent risk to male grandchildren through these daughters (Fig. 6.10). This type of pedigree is sometimes said to show 'diagonal' or a 'knight's move' pattern of inheritance.

The mode of inheritance whereby only males are affected by a disease which is transmitted by normal females was appreciated by the Jews nearly 2000 years ago. They excused from circumcision the sons of all the sisters of a mother who had sons with the 'bleeding disease', i.e. haemophilia. The sons of the father's sibs were not excused. Queen Victoria was a carrier of haemophilia and her carrier daughters, who were perfectly healthy, introduced the gene into the Russian

and Spanish Royal families. Fortunately for the British Royal family, Queen Victoria's son, Edward VII, did not inherit the gene, and so could not transmit it to his descendants.

Genetic risks

A male transmits his X chromosome to each of his daughters and his Y chromosome to each of his sons. If a male affected with haemophilia has children with a normal female, then all his daughters will be carriers but none of his sons will be affected (Fig. 6.11). A male cannot transmit an X-linked trait to his son, with the very rare exception of uniparental heterodisomy (p. 88).

For a carrier female of an X-linked recessive disorder having children with a normal male, each son has a 1 in 2 (50%) chance of being affected and each daughter has a 1 in 2 (50%) chance of being a carrier (Fig. 6.12).

Some X-linked disorders are not compatible with survival to the reproductive age and are not, therefore, transmitted by affected males. Duchenne muscular dystrophy is the commonest form of muscular dystrophy and is a severe disease, with an onset in early childhood. The first signs in an affected male are a waddling gait, difficulty in climbing stairs unaided and a tendency to fall over easily. By about the age of 10 years affected boys can no longer walk and have to use a wheelchair. The muscle weakness gradually progresses and affected males ultimately become confined to bed and usually die before reaching the age of 20 years (Fig. 6.13). Since affected boys do not usually survive to reproduce, the disease is transmitted entirely by healthy female carriers

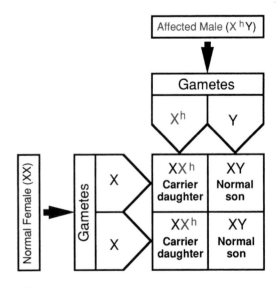

Fig. 6.11
Punnett's square showing possible gamete combinations for the offspring of a male affected by an X-linked recessive disorder (X^h represents a mutation for an X-linked gene).

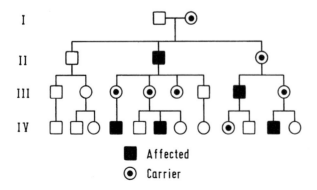

Fig. 6.10
Family tree of an X-linked recessive trait in which affected males reproduce.

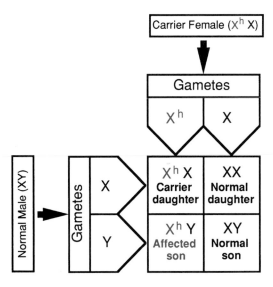

Fig. 6.12
Punnett's square showing possible gamete combinations for the offspring of a female carrier of an X-linked recessive disorder (X^h represents a mutation for an X-linked gene).

(Fig. 6.14). Often the case is the only one in the family having occurred as the result of a new mutation (p. 16).

Variable expression in heterozygous females

In humans, several X-linked disorders are known in which heterozygous females have a mosaic phenotype with a mixture of features of the normal and mutant alleles. In ocular albinism the iris and ocular fundus of affected males are completely lacking in pigment. Careful examination of the ocular fundus in females heterozygous for ocular albinism reveals a mosaic pattern of pigmentation (Plate 7). This mosaic pattern of involvement can be explained through the random process of X-inactivation. In the pigmented areas the normal gene is on the active X chromosome while in the depigmented areas the mutant allele is on the active X chromosome.

Females affected with X-linked recessive disorders

Very rarely a woman can exhibit an X-linked recessive trait. There are several explanations for how this can happen.

Homozygosity for X-linked recessive disorders
Another example of an X-linked recessive trait is red–green colour blindness, the inability to distinguish between the colours red and green. About 8% of males are red–green colour blind and although it is unusual, about 1 in 150 women is red–green colour blind. Therefore a female can be affected with an X-linked recessive

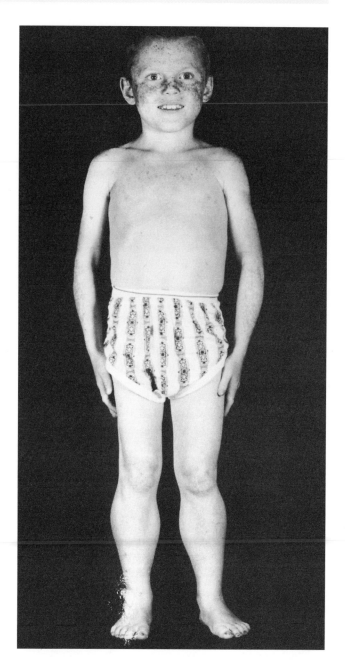

Fig. 6.13
Boy with Duchenne muscular dystrophy; note the enlarged calves and wasting of the thigh muscles.

trait due to homozygosity, although this is uncommon due to the rarity of most X-linked conditions. A female could be a homozygote because her mother was a carrier and her father was affected. Although extremely unlikely, a female could also be homozygous if her father was affected and her mother was normal but a mutation occurred on the X chromosome transmitted to the daughter, or her mother was a carrier and her father was normal but a mutation occurred on the X chromosome he transmitted to his daughter.

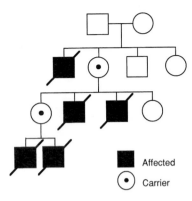

Fig. 6.14
Family tree of Duchenne muscular dystrophy with the disorder being transmitted by carrier females and affecting males who do not survive to transmit the disorder.

Skewed X-inactivation

The process of X-inactivation occurs randomly, there being an equal chance of either of the two X chromosomes in a heterozygous female being inactivated in any one cell. By chance, however, in an occasional heterozygous carrier female, the active X chromosome in most of her cells could be the one bearing the mutant allele. If this happens, a carrier female would exhibit some of the symptoms and signs of the disease and be a so-called *manifesting heterozygote* or *carrier*. This has been reported in a number of X-linked disorders including Duchenne muscular dystrophy and haemophilia A (p. 74). In addition, there is evidence that the expression of certain X-linked genes could be under some sort of genetic control because of the occasional occurrence of several manifesting carriers in the same family.

Numerical X chromosome abnormalities

A female could manifest an X-linked recessive disorder through being a carrier and having only a single X chromosome, i.e. Turner's syndrome (p. 222). Women with Turner's syndrome who have also had haemophilia or Duchenne muscular dystrophy have been reported.

X-autosome translocations

Females with a translocation involving one of the X chromosomes and an autosome can be affected with an X-linked recessive disorder. The X chromosome involved in the translocation remains preferentially active in order to maintain the activity of the autosomal part of the derivative chromosome. If the break point of the translocation disrupts a gene on the X chromosome, then a female can be affected with an X-linked recessive disorder as the X chromosome involved in the translocation remains preferentially active. The observation of females affected with Duchenne muscular dystrophy with X-autosome translocations involving the same region of the short arm of the X chromosome helped to map the

Duchenne muscular dystrophy gene (p. 239). This is a technique which has been used in positional cloning of a number of genes in humans (p. 62).

X-linked dominant inheritance

Although uncommon, just as there are dominant and recessive autosomal traits, there are *X-linked dominant* as well as recessive X-linked traits. An X-linked dominant trait is manifest in the heterozygous female as well as in the male who has the mutant allele on his single X chromosome (Fig. 6.15). This pattern of inheritance superficially resembles that of an autosomal dominant trait because both daughters and sons of an affected female have a 1 in 2 (50%) chance of being affected. There is, however, an important difference. With an X-linked dominant trait an affected male transmits the trait to all his daughters but to none of his sons. Therefore in families with an X-linked dominant disorder there is an excess of affected females and direct male to male transmission cannot occur.

An example of an X-linked dominant trait is vitamin D-resistant rickets. Rickets can be due to a dietary deficiency of vitamin D, but in vitamin D-resistant rickets, the disorder occurs even when there is an adequate intake of vitamin D. Affected persons are refractory to normal doses of vitamin D. In the X-linked dominant form of vitamin D-resistant rickets both males and females are affected, though the females usually have less severe skeletal changes than the males.

Another example of an X-linked dominant trait is the Xg blood group. Persons whose blood reacts with a specific antiserum to Xg blood group substance are said to be Xg (a+). Those persons who do not react are said to be Xg (a–). Xg (a+) is dominant to Xg (a–) and heterozygous females are therefore always Xg (a+). Approximately 90% of females and 60% of males are Xg (a+).

A similar mosaic pattern of involvement can be demonstrated in females heterozygous for an X-linked dominant gene. An example is the mosaic pattern of

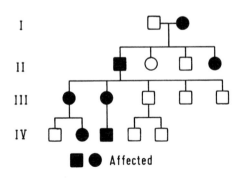

Fig. 6.15
Family tree of an X-linked dominant trait.

abnormal pigmentation of the skin which follows developmental lines (p. 221) seen in females heterozygous for the X-linked dominant disorder incontinentia pigmenti (Plate 9).

Y-linked inheritance

Y-linked or *holandric inheritance* implies that only males are affected and that an affected male transmits the trait to all his sons but to none of his daughters. In the past it has been suggested that such bizarre-sounding conditions as porcupine skin, hairy ears and webbed toes are Y-linked traits. With the possible exception of hairy ears, these claims of holandric inheritance have not stood up to more careful study. Recent evidence clearly indicates, however, that the H–Y histocompatibility antigen (p. 160) and genes involved in spermatogenesis are carried on the Y chromosome and therefore manifest holandric inheritance. The family surname also shows this pattern of inheritance!

Partial sex-linkage

Another term which is occasionally used is that of *partial sex-linkage*. This refers to genes carried on what is believed to be the homologous portions of the X and Y chromosomes. During meiosis pairing occurs between the homologous distal parts of the short arms of the X and Y chromosomes, the so-called *pseudoautosomal region*. As a result of a cross-over, a gene could be transferred from the X to the Y chromosome or vice versa. There is some evidence for partial sex-linkage in certain animals, but in humans the evidence is far less compelling. Partial sex-linkage has been proposed as a possible explanation for certain diseases which appear to be X-linked in some families, Y-linked in others and show a confused pattern of inheritance in yet others. Diseases which have been thought to exhibit partial sex-linkage include total colour-blindness, which results in a complete inability to recognise colours, and certain rare skin disorders. It is, however, extremely difficult in human pedigree data to distinguish between partial sex-linkage and autosomal inheritance. In humans, partial sex-linkage is an interesting possibility for which there is, as yet, no conclusive evidence.

Sex influence

Some autosomal traits are expressed more frequently in one sex than another, so-called *sex influence*. Gout and presenile baldness are examples of sex-influenced autosomal dominant traits, males being predominantly affected in both cases. The influence of sex in these two examples is probably through the effect of male hormones. Gout, for example, is very rare in women before the menopause but the frequency increases in later life. Hippocrates is credited with having been among the first to note that 'eunuchs neither get gout nor grow bald'.

Sex limitation

Sex limitation refers to the appearance of certain features in individuals of only one sex. Examples include virilization of female infants affected with the autosomal recessive endocrine disorder, congenital adrenal hyperplasia (p. 134) and hydrometrocolpos in females affected with certain autosomal recessive syndromes (p. 198).

ESTABLISHING THE MODE OF INHERITANCE OF A GENETIC DISORDER

In experimental animals it is possible to arrange specific types of mating but in humans the geneticist approaches the problem indirectly by fitting likely models of inheritance to the observed outcome in the offspring. In human disorders which are newly recognised, family studies can usually allow the mode of inheritance to be established. Certain features are necessary to support a particular mode of inheritance.

Autosomal dominant inheritance

In order to determine whether a trait or disorder is inherited in an autosomal dominant manner, there are 3 specific features which need to be observed. The first is that it affects both males and females in equal proportions. The second is that it is transmitted from one generation to the next. The third is that all forms of transmission between the sexes are observed, i.e. male to male, female to female, male to female and the converse. The former two exclude the possibility of the gene being on one of the sex chromosomes. In the case of sporadically occurring disorders, increased paternal age is suggestive of a new autosomal dominant mutation.

Autosomal recessive inheritance

There are 3 features in a family which suggest the possibility of autosomal recessive inheritance. The first is that the disorder affects males and females in equal proportions. The second is that it usually only affects individuals in one generation in a single sibship, i.e. brothers and sisters, and does not occur in previous and subsequent generations. Lastly, consanguinity in the parents provides further support for autosomal recessive inheritance.

X-linked recessive inheritance

There are 3 main features necessary to establish X-linked recessive inheritance. The first is that the trait or disorder should affect males almost exclusively. The second is that X-linked recessive disorders are transmitted through carrier females to their sons. Affected males, if they survive to reproduce, can have affected grandsons through their daughters who are obligate carriers. The third is that affected males cannot transmit the disorder to their sons.

X-linked dominant inheritance

There are 3 features necessary to establish X-linked dominant inheritance. The first is that males and females are affected but affected females occur more frequently than affected males. Secondly, females are usually less severely affected than males. Thirdly, while affected females can transmit the disorder to male and female children, affected males can only transmit the disorder to their daughters, all of whom will be affected.

Multiple alleles

So far, each of the traits we have considered has involved only two alleles, the normal and the mutant. Some genes have more than two allelic forms, i.e. *multiple alleles*. Multiple alleles are the result of a normal gene having mutated to produce various different alleles, some of which can be dominant and others recessive to the normal allele. In the case of the ABO blood group system (p. 158), there are at least four alleles (A1, A2, B and O). An individual can possess any two of these alleles which can be the same or different (AO, A_2B, OO, and so on). Alleles are carried on homologous chromosomes and therefore a person transmits only one allele for a certain trait to any particular offspring. For example, if a person has the genotype AB, he will transmit to any particular offspring either the A allele or the B allele but never both or neither (Table 6.1).

The preceding remarks concerning the inheritance of multiple alleles relate only to genes located on the autosomes. If a series of alleles were carried on the X chromosome then a woman would have two, either of which she could transmit to a particular offspring, whereas a man would only have one allele to transmit. An example of multiple allelism on the X chromosome is provided by the alleles at the G6PD locus (p. 145).

NON-MENDELIAN INHERITANCE

A number of disorders are known which do not follow classical patterns of Mendelian inheritance. In recent

Table 6.1 Possible genotypes, phenotypes and gametes formed from the four alleles A_1, A_2, B and O at the ABO locus

Genotype	Phenotype	Gametes
A_1A_1	A_1	A_1
A_2A_2	A_2	A_2
BB	B	B
OO	O	O
A_1A_2	A_1	A_1 or A_2
A_1B	A_1B	A_1 or B
A_1O	A_1	A_1 or O
A_2B	A_2B	A_2 or B
A_2O	A_2	A_2 or O
BO	B	B or O

years several different mechanisms have been recognised which can account for this.

ANTICIPATION

In some autosomal dominant traits or disorders, such as myotonic dystrophy, the onset of the disease occurs at an earlier age in the offspring than in the parents, or the disease occurs with increasing severity in subsequent generations. This phenomenon is called *anticipation*. It used to be argued that this effect was due to a *bias of ascertainment* as a result of the way in which cases were collected, with persons in whom the disease begins earlier or is more severe being more likely to be ascertained. Secondly, only those individuals who are less severely affected tend to have children and finally, because the observer is in the same generation as the affected presenting probands, many individuals who at present are unaffected would, by necessity, if they developed the disease, do so later in life.

Despite these reservations, however, recent studies have shown that in a number of disorders, including Huntington's disease and myotonic dystrophy (p. 249), anticipation is, in fact, a real biological phenomenon occurring as a result of the expansion of unstable triplet repeat sequences (p. 17). An expansion of the CTG triplet repeat in the 3' untranslated end of the myotonic dystrophy gene occurring predominantly in maternal meiosis appears to be the explanation for the severe neonatal form of myotonic dystrophy which usually only occurs when the gene is transmitted by the mother (Fig. 6.16). A similar expansion in the CAG expansion in the 5' untranslated end of the Huntington's disease gene (Fig. 6.17) in the paternal meiosis appears to account for the increased risk of juvenile Huntington's disease when the gene is transmitted by the father.

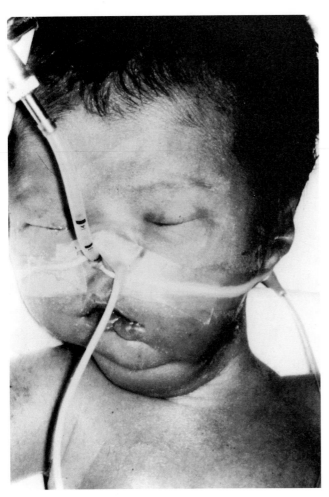

Fig. 6.16
Newborn baby with severe hypotonia requiring ventilation due to having inherited myotonic dystrophy from his mother.

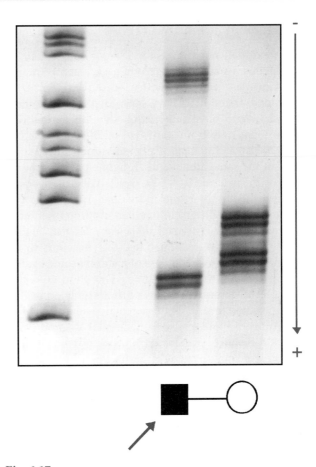

Fig. 6.17
Silver staining of a 5% denaturing gel of the PCR products of the CAG triplet in the 5' untranslated end of the Huntington's disease gene from an affected male and his wife showing her to have two similar size repeats in the normal range (20 and 24 copies) and him to have one normal sized triplet repeat (18 copies) and an expanded triplet repeat (44 copies). The bands in the left lane are standard markers to allow sizing of the CAG repeat (courtesy of Alan Dodge, Regional DNA Laboratory, St Mary's Hospital, Manchester).

MOSAICISM

An individual, or a particular tissue of the body, can consist of more than one cell type or line, through an error occurring during mitosis at any stage after conception. Mosaicism of either somatic or germ cells can account for some instances of unusual patterns of inheritance.

Somatic mosaicism

The possibility of somatic mosaicism is suggested by the features of a single gene disorder being less severe in an individual than usual or by their being confined to a particular part of the body in a so-called *segmental* distribution. Depending on when a mutation arises in development, it can be transmitted to the next generation with full expression if the mutation is also present in a proportion of germ-line cells. This is referred to as *germ-line* or *gonadal mosaicism*.

Gonadal mosaicism

There have been many reports of families with various autosomal dominant disorders, such as achondroplasia and osteogenesis imperfecta, and X-linked recessive disorders, such as Duchenne muscular dystrophy and haemophilia, in which the parents are phenotypically and genetically normal by all known tests, but in which more than one of their children have been affected. The most favoured explanation for these observations is gonadal mosaicism in one of the parents, i.e. a proportion of the gonadal cells have the mutation. Direct evidence of this has been provided by the demonstration of a mutation in the collagen gene responsible for osteogenesis imperfecta in a proportion of individual sperm from a clinically normal father who had two affected infants with different partners. Germ-line mosaicism has important implications for genetic counselling (p. 258).

UNIPARENTAL DISOMY

An individual normally inherits one of a pair of homologous chromosomes from each parent (p. 31). Over the last decade, with the advent of DNA technology, individuals have been identified who have been shown to have inherited both homologues of a chromosome pair from only one of their parents, so-called *uniparental disomy*. If an individual inherits two copies of the same homologue from one parent, through an error in meiosis II (p. 32), this is called *uniparental isodisomy*. If, however, the individual inherits the two different homologues from one parent through an error in meiosis I, this is termed *uniparental heterodisomy*. In either instance, it is presumed that the conceptus would originally be trisomic with loss of a chromosome leading to the 'normal' disomic state. One-third of such chromosome losses, if they occurred with equal frequency, would result in uniparental disomy. Alternatively, it is postulated that uniparental disomy could arise as a result of a gamete from one parent which is nullisomic being 'rescued' by fertilisation by a disomic gamete thereby restoring the disomic state in the zygote.

Using DNA techniques, uniparental disomy has been shown to be the cause of a father with haemophilia having an affected son and of a child with cystic fibrosis being born to a couple in which only the mother was a carrier (with proven paternity)! Uniparental paternal disomy has also been shown in some cases of the rare overgrowth syndrome known as the Beckwith–Wiedemann syndrome (p. 220).

GENOMIC IMPRINTING

Although it was originally believed that genes on homologous chromosomes were expressed equally, it is now recognised that different clinical features can result, depending on whether a gene is inherited from the father or from the mother. This 'parent of origin' effect is referred to as *genomic imprinting*. Although the mechanism by which differential expression of the maternally and paternally derived alleles in early development occurs was thought to involve differential methylation, at present there is no clear pattern of methylation observed when the active and inactive alleles of the imprinted genes are compared in all instances.

Genomic imprinting has been observed in two syndromes associated with mental handicap known as the Prader–Willi and Angelman syndromes.

The Prader–Willi and Angelman syndromes

The Prader–Willi syndrome, a disorder characterised by short stature, obesity and learning difficulty (Fig. 6.18), most frequently occurs as a result of an interstitial

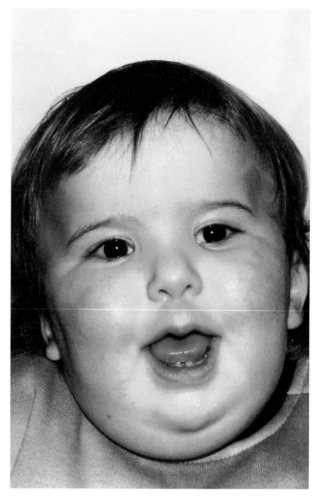

Fig. 6.18
Male child with the Prader–Willi syndrome.

deletion of the proximal portion of the short arm of chromosome 15 (p. 220). DNA analysis has revealed that the chromosome deleted is almost always the paternally derived homologue. A proportion of individuals with the Prader–Willi syndrome found not to have a chromosome deletion, have been shown to have *maternal uniparental disomy*. Of interest, is that individuals with another syndrome, the so-called Angelman syndrome (p. 220), characterised by epilepsy, severe learning difficulties, an unsteady or ataxic gait and a happy affect (Fig. 6.19), have also been shown in some instances to have an interstitial deletion of the same region of chromosome 15 or to have *paternal uniparental disomy*. Families have been reported in which a chromosomal translocation of the proximal portion of the long arm of chromosome 15 involved in these two syndromes is segregating. Depending on whether the translocation is transmitted by the father or mother, the affected offspring within the family have had either the Prader–Willi syndrome or the Angelman syndrome!.

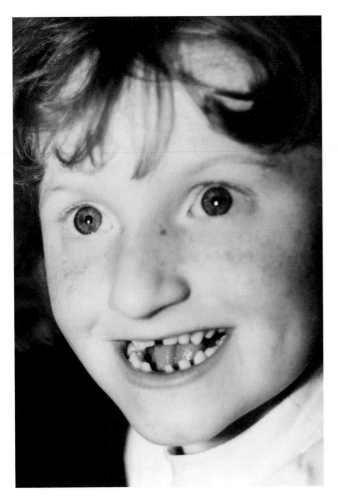

Fig. 6.19
Female child with the Angelman syndrome.

Recent findings have shown that only the paternally inherited allele of a critical region of the proximal portion of chromosome 15, including the gene for what is known as the small nuclear ribonucleoprotein polypeptide N (SNRPN), is expressed, i.e. the SNRPN gene is maternally imprinted. These findings are consistent with

the hypothesis that expression of a functional SNRPN gene product is lacking in the Prader–Willi syndrome and its deficiency could lead, in part, to the features of the Prader–Willi syndrome.

MITOCHONDRIAL INHERITANCE

The observation of disorders which affect both males and females but are transmitted only through females (Fig. 6.20) can be explained by the exclusive maternal contribution of mitochondrial DNA to offspring (p. 12). In humans, *cytoplasmic* or *mitochondrial* inheritance has been proposed as a possible explanation for the pattern of inheritance observed in some rare disorders an example of which is a particular type of hereditary blindness, Leber's optic atrophy. This has been shown to be due to a defect in the detoxification of cyanide due to mutations in the mitochondrial DNA of the gene for the electron transport protein NADH-coenzyme Q oxido-reductase. As mitochondria have an important role in cellular metabolism, it is not surprising that the organs most susceptible to mitochondrial mutation are the central nervous system, skeletal muscle and heart.

The pattern of inheritance of DNA sequence variants in mitochondrial DNA from the bones of nine persons found in a shallow grave 20 miles outside Ektarinburg has provided evidence supporting the reported fate of the Russian royal family and their party at the time of the Bolshevik uprising!

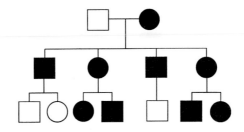

Fig. 6.20
Family tree consistent with mitochondrial inheritance.

ELEMENTS

1 Family studies are often necessary to determine the mode of inheritance of a trait or disorder and to give appropriate genetic counselling. A standard short-hand convention exists for pedigree documentation of the family history.

2 Mendelian disorders can be inherited in four ways: autosomal dominant, autosomal recessive, X-linked dominant and X-linked recessive.

3 Autosomal dominant alleles are manifest in the heterozygous state and are usually transmitted from one generation to the next but can occasionally arise as a new mutation. They usually affect both males and females equally. Each offspring of a parent with an autosomal dominant gene has a 1 in 2 chance of inheriting it from the affected parent. Autosomal dominant alleles can exhibit reduced penetrance, variable expressivity and sex limitation.

4 Autosomal recessive disorders are only manifest in the homozygous state and normally only affect individuals in one generation, usually in one sibship in a family. They affect both males and females equally. Offspring of parents who are heterozygous for the same autosomal recessive allele have a 1 in 4 chance of being homozygous for that allele. The less common an autosomal recessive allele, the greater the likelihood that the parents of a homozygote are consanguineous.

5 X-linked recessive alleles are normally only manifest in males. Offspring of females heterozygous for an X-linked recessive allele have a 1 in 2 chance of inheriting the allele from their mother. Daughters of males with an X-linked recessive allele are obligate heterozygotes whilst sons cannot inherit the allele. Rarely, females manifest an X-linked recessive trait because they are homozygous for the allele, have a single X chromosome, have a structural rearrangement of one of their X chromosomes, or are heterozygous but show skewed or non-random X-inactivation.

6 There are only a few disorders known to be inherited in an X-linked dominant manner. In X-linked dominant disorders hemizygous males are more severely affected than heterozygous females.

7 Unusual patterns of inheritance can be explained by phenomena such as genetic heterogeneity, mosaicism, anticipation, imprinting, uniparental disomy and mitochondrial mutations.

FURTHER READING

Bateson W, Saunders E R 1902 Experimental studies in the physiology of heredity. Royal Society Reports to the Evolution Committee, pp 132–134
Early observations on Mendelian inheritance.
Hall J G 1988 Somatic mosaicism: observations related to clinical genetics. Am J Hum Genet 43: 355–363
Good review of findings due to somatic mosaicism in clinical genetics.
Hall J G 1990 Genomic imprinting: review and relevance to human diseases. Am J Hum Genet 46: 857–873
Extensive review of examples of imprinting in inherited diseases in humans.
Kingston H M 1994 An ABC of clinical genetics, 2nd edn. British Medical Association, London
A simple outline primer of the basic principles of clinical genetics.
Vogel F, Motulsky A G 1986 Human genetics, 2nd edn. Springer-Verlag, Berlin
This text has detailed explanations of many of the concepts in human genetics outlined in this chapter.

Mathematical and population genetics

In the previous chapter we have considered the different ways in which genetic disorders can be inherited and begun to explore the concept of genetic risks, a subject which will be discussed in greater detail (Ch. 20). In this chapter we shall consider some of the more mathematical aspects of the ways in which genes are inherited and extend our horizons beyond the individual to look at how genes are distributed in populations. This branch of the subject is known as *population genetics*.

By its very nature genetics lends itself to a numerical approach with many of the most influential pioneering figures in human genetics having come from a mathematical background. They were particularly attracted by the challenges of trying to determine the frequencies of genes in populations and the rates at which they mutate. Much of this early work still has implications for medical practice and by the completion of this chapter it is hoped that the interested student will have a better understanding of the following issues:

1. Why does a dominant trait not increase in a population at the expense of a recessive one?
2. Knowing the incidence of a disorder, how can we estimate the carrier frequency and the *mutation rate* of the relevant gene?
3. How can a particular genetic disorder be more common in one population or community than in another?
4. How can we confirm that a genetic disorder shows a particular pattern of inheritance?
5. What is genetic linkage and how does this differ from linkage disequilibrium?
6. What will be the effects of medical intervention on the allele frequencies and the incidence of genetic disorders?

ALLELE FREQUENCIES IN POPULATIONS

At first sight it would seem reasonable to expect that dominant traits would increase in the population at the expense of recessive ones. After all, on average, three-quarters of the progeny of two heterozygotes will mani-fest the dominant trait, but only one quarter will have the recessive trait. It could be concluded therefore that eventually almost everyone in the population will have the dominant trait. However it can be shown that in a large randomly mating population, in which there is no disturbance by outside influences, dominant traits do not increase at the expense of recessive ones. In fact, in such a population, the relative proportions of the different genotypes remain constant from one generation to another. This is known as the *Hardy–Weinberg principle* as it was proposed, independently, by an English mathematician, G. H. Hardy, and a German physician, W. Weinberg in 1908. This is one of the most fundamental principles in human genetics.

THE HARDY—WEINBERG PRINCIPLE

Consider an 'ideal' population in which there is a gene locus with two alleles A and a, which have frequencies of p and q respectively. These are the only alleles found at this locus so that p + q = 100% or 1. The frequency of each genotype in the population can be determined by construction of a Punnett's square which shows how the different genes can combine (Fig. 7.1)

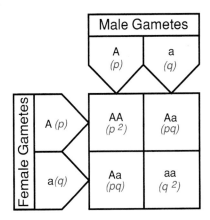

Fig. 7.1
Punnett's square showing the allele frequencies and resulting genotype frequencies for a two allele system in the first generation.

From Figure 7.1 it can be seen that the frequencies of the different genotypes are:

Genotype	Phenotype	Frequency
AA	A	p^2
Aa	A	$2pq$
aa	a	q^2

We have now established that if there is random mating of sperm and ova the frequencies of the different genotypes in the first generation will be as shown above. Next consider that these individuals mate with each other to produce a second generation. Once again a Punnett's square is used to show the different matings and their frequencies (Fig. 7.2).

From Figure 7.2 a table is drawn up to calculate the total frequency for each genotype in the second generation (Table 7.1).

This reveals that the relative frequency or proportion of each genotype is the same in the second generation as in the first. In fact it can be shown that no matter how many generations are studied the relative frequencies will remain constant and in a state of *equilibrium*.

FACTORS WHICH CAN DISTURB THE HARDY–WEINBERG EQUILIBRIUM

The discussion above relates to an 'ideal' population. By definition such a population is large and shows random mating with no new mutations and no selection for or against any particular genotype. For some human characteristics, such as *neutral genes* for blood groups or enzyme variants, these criteria can be fulfilled. However, in genetic disorders, several factors can disturb the *Hardy–Weinberg*

Table 7.1 Shows the frequency of the various types of offspring from the matings shown in Figure 7.2

Mating type	Frequency	Frequency of offspring		
		AA	Aa	aa
AA × AA	p^4	p^4	–	–
AA × Aa	$4p^3q$	$2p^3q$	$2p^3q$	–
Aa × Aa	$4p^2q^2$	p^2q^2	$2p^2q^2$	p^2q^2
AA × aa	$2p^2q^2$	–	$2p^2q^2$	–
Aa × aa	$4pq^3$	–	$2pq^3$	$2pq^3$
aa × aa	q^4	–	–	q^4
Total		$p^2(p^2+2pq+q^2)$	$2pq(p^2+2pq+q^2)$	$q^2(p^2+2pq+q^2)$
Relative frequency		p^2	$2pq$	q^2

equilibrium by influencing either the distribution of genes in the population or by altering the gene frequencies. These potentially disturbing factors include:

1. Non-random mating
2. Mutation
3. Selection
4. Small population size
5. Gene flow (migration).

Non-random mating

Random mating, or *panmixis*, refers to the selection of a partner regardless of that partner's genotype. *Non-random mating* can lead to an increase in the frequency of affected homozygotes by two mechanisms, either assortative mating or consanguinity.

Assortative mating

Assortative mating is the tendency for human beings to chose partners who share characteristics such as height, intelligence and racial origin. If assortative mating extends to conditions such as autosomal recessive deafness, which accounts for a large proportion of all congenital hearing loss, then this will lead to a small increase in the frequency of affected homozygotes.

Consanguinity

Consanguinity is the term used to describe marriage between blood relatives who have at least one common ancestor no more remote than a great-great grandparent. Widespread consanguinity in a community will lead to a relative increase in the frequency of affected homozygotes with a relative decrease in the frequency of heterozygotes.

Mutation

The validity of the Hardy–Weinberg principle is based on the assumption that no new mutations occur. If a particular locus shows a high mutation rate then there will be a

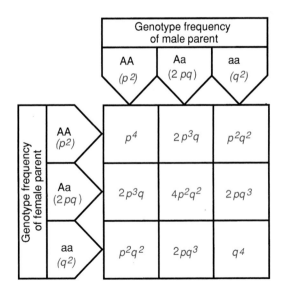

Fig. 7.2
Punnett's square showing the frequencies of the different matings in the second generation.

steady increase in the proportion of mutant alleles in a population. In practice mutations do occur at almost all loci, albeit at different rates, but the effect of their introduction is usually balanced by the loss of mutant alleles due to reduced fitness of affected individuals. If a population is found to be in Hardy–Weinberg equilibrium, it is generally assumed that these two opposing factors have roughly equal effects. This is discussed further in the section which follows on the estimation of mutation rates.

Selection

In the 'ideal' population there is no *selection* for or against any particular genotype. For deleterious characteristics there is likely to be negative selection with affected individuals having reduced reproductive (= biological = genetic) *fitness*. This infers that they do not have as many offspring as unaffected control members of the same population. In the absence of new mutations this reduction in fitness will lead to a reduction in the frequency of the mutant allele.

Selection can act in the opposite direction by increasing fitness. For some autosomal recessive disorders there is evidence that heterozygotes show a slight increase in biological fitness as compared with unaffected homozygotes. This is referred to as *heterozygote advantage*. The best understood example is sickle-cell disease in which affected homozygotes have severe anaemia and often show persistent ill-health. However, heterozygotes are relatively immune to *Plasmodium falciparum* malaria because if their red blood cells are invaded by the parasite they undergo sickling and are rapidly destroyed. In areas in which this form of malaria is endemic, carriers of sickle-cell anaemia, who are described as having *sickle-cell trait*, are at a biological advantage as compared with unaffected homozygotes. Therefore, in these communities, there will tend to be more heterozygotes and fewer affected homozygotes than would be predicted by the Hardy–Weinberg principle.

Small population size

In a large population the numbers of children produced by individuals with different genotypes, assuming no alteration in fitness for any particular genotype, will tend to balance out, so that gene frequencies will remain stable. However, in a small population it is possible that one allele could be transmitted to a high proportion of offspring by chance, resulting in marked changes in allele frequency from one generation to the next, so that Hardy–Weinberg equilibrium is disturbed. This phenomenon is referred to as *random genetic drift*. If one allele is lost altogether then it is said to be *extinguished* and the other allele is described as having become *fixed* (Fig. 7.3).

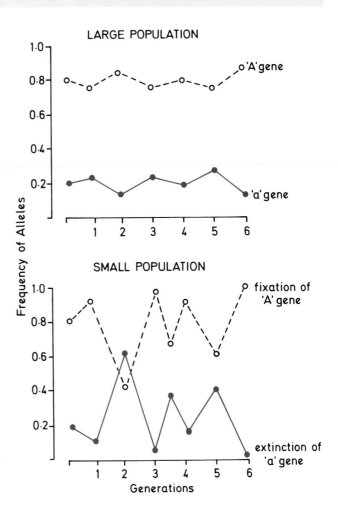

Fig. 7.3
The possible effects of random genetic drift in large and small populations.

Gene flow (migration)

If new alleles are introduced into a population as a consequence of migration with subsequent intermarriage, this will lead to a change in the relevant allele frequencies. This slow diffusion of alleles across a racial or geographical boundary is known as *gene flow*. The most widely quoted example is the gradient shown by the incidence of the B blood group allele throughout the world (Fig. 7.4). This allele is thought to have originated in Asia and spread slowly westward as a result of admixture through invasion.

Other examples of gene flow include the ΔF508 cystic fibrosis mutation (p. 236) and the Pi Z a_1-antitrypsin deficiency allele (p. 140), both of which show their highest incidence in Scandinavia with declining frequencies across Europe. Presumably this is a reflection of over-social Viking activity!

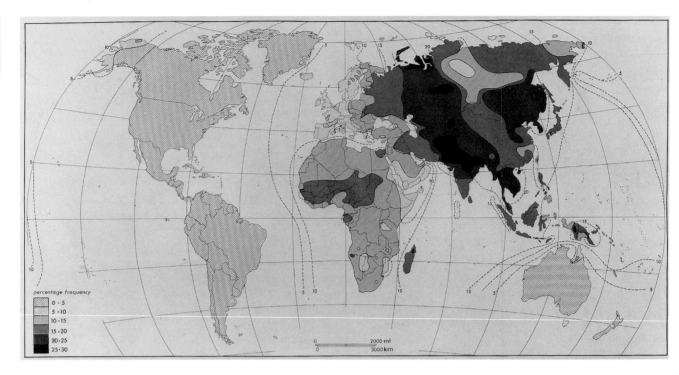

Fig. 7.4
Distribution of blood group B throughout the world (from Mourant, Kopéc & Domianiewska-Sobczaz 1976 The Distribution of the Human Blood Groups and Other Polymorphisms, 2nd edn. Oxford University Press, with permission).

VALIDITY OF THE HARDY–WEINBERG EQUILIBRIUM

It is relatively simple to establish whether a population is in Hardy–Weinberg equilibrium for a particular trait if all possible genotypes can be identified. Consider a system with two alleles A and a, with three resulting genotypes AA, Aa/aA and aa. Amongst 1000 individuals selected at random, the following genotype distributions are observed:

AA	800
Aa/aA	185
aa	15

From these figures the incidence of the A allele (p) equals $[(2 \times 800) + 185]/2000 = 0.8925$ and the incidence of the a allele (q) equals $[185 + (2 \times 15)]/2000 = 0.1075$.

Now consider what the expected genotype frequencies would be if the population is in Hardy–Weinberg equilibrium and compare these with the observed values.

Genotypes	Observed	Expected
AA	800	796.5 ($p^2 \times 1000$)
Aa/aA	185	192 ($2pq \times 1000$)
aa	15	11.5 ($q^2 \times 1000$).

These observed and expected values correspond closely and formal statistical analysis with a χ^2 test would confirm that the observed values do not differ significantly from those expected if the population is in equilibrium.

Next consider a different system with two alleles B and b. Amongst 1000 randomly selected individuals the observed genotype distributions are:

BB	430
Bb/bB	540
bb	30

From these figures the incidence of the B allele (p) equals $[(2 \times 430) + 540]/2000 = 0.7$ and the incidence of the b allele (q) equals $[540 + (2 \times 30)]/2000 = 0.3$.

Using these values for p and q the observed and expected genotype distributions can be compared.

Genotype	Observed	Expected
BB	430	490 ($p^2 \times 1000$)
Bb/bB	540	420 ($2pq \times 1000$)
bb	30	90 ($q^2 \times 1000$)

These values differ considerably with an increased number of heterozygotes at the expense of homozygotes. Deviation such as this from Hardy–Weinberg equilibrium should prompt a search for factors which could result in increased numbers of heterozygotes such as heterozygote advantage or negative assortative mating, i.e. the attraction of opposites!

Unless there is strong evidence to the contrary it is usually assumed that most populations are in equilibrium for most genetic traits, despite the number of factors which can disturb this equilibrium, as it is very unusual to find a population in which genotype frequencies show significant deviation from those which would be expected.

APPLICATIONS OF THE HARDY–WEINBERG EQUILIBRIUM

Estimation of carrier frequencies

If the incidence of an autosomal recessive disorder is known then it is possible to calculate the carrier frequency using some relatively simple algebra. If, for example, the disease incidence equals 1 in 10 000, then $q^2 = 1/10\,000$ and therefore $q = 1/100$. As $p + q = 1$, therefore $p = 99/100$. The carrier frequency can then be calculated as $2 \times 99/100 \times 1/100$, i.e. $2pq$, which approximates to 1 in 50. Thus a rough approximation of the carrier frequency can be obtained by doubling the square root of the disease incidence. Approximate values for gene frequency and carrier frequency derived from the disease incidence can be extremely useful when calculating risks for genetic counselling (p. 257) (Table 7.2).

Estimation of mutation rates

Direct method

If an autosomal dominant disorder shows full penetrance and is therefore always expressed in heterozygotes, an estimate of its *mutation rate* can be made relatively easily by counting the number of new cases in a defined number of births. Consider a sample of 100 000 children, 12 of whom have a particular autosomal dominant disorder. Only 2 of these children have an affected parent so that the remaining 10 must have their disorder as a result of new mutations. Therefore 10 new mutations have occurred amongst the 200 000 genes inherited by these children (each child inherits 2 genes) giving a mutation rate of 1 per 20 000 gametes per generation.

Indirect method

For an autosomal dominant disorder with reproductive fitness (f) equal to zero, all cases must result from new

mutations. If the incidence of the disorder is denoted as I and the mutation rate as μ, as each child inherits 2 genes and a mutation on either will cause the disorder, therefore $I = 2\mu$.

If fitness is greater than zero, and the disorder is in Hardy–Weinberg equilibrium, then genes lost through reduced fitness must be counterbalanced by new mutations. Therefore, $2\mu = I(1-f)$ or $\mu = [I(1-f)]/2$.

Thus if an estimate of genetic fitness can be made by comparing the average number of offspring born to affected patients as compared with controls such as their unaffected siblings, it will be possible to calculate the mutation rate.

A similar approach can be used to estimate mutation rates for autosomal recessive and sex-linked recessive disorders. With an autosomal recessive condition, 2 genes will be lost for each homozygote who fails to reproduce. These will be balanced by new mutations. Therefore, $2\mu = I(1-f) \times 2$ or $\mu = I(1-f)$.

For a sex-linked recessive condition with incidence in males equal to I^M, 3 X chromosomes are transmitted per couple per generation. Therefore, $3\mu = I^M (1-f)$ or $\mu = [I^M(1-f)]/3$.

Why is it helpful to know mutation rates?

At first sight it could seem that knowledge of these formulae linking mutation rates with disease incidence and fitness is of little practical value. However there are several ways in which this information can be useful.

Estimation of gene size

If a disorder has a high mutation rate this could yield information about the structure of the gene which would help expedite its isolation and characterisation. For example, the gene could contain a high proportion of GC residues which are thought to be particularly prone to copy error (p. 62), or it could contain a high proportion of repeat sequences (p. 55) which could predispose to misalignment in meiosis resulting in deletion and duplication, or it could simply be that the gene is very large.

Determination of mutagenic potential

If valuable information is to be gained about the potential mutagenic effects of nuclear accidents such as Chernobyl, it will be necessary to have accurate methods for determining mutation rates and how these are related to observed changes in disease incidence (p. 18).

Consequences of treatment of genetic disease

Understanding of the relationship between disease incidence, fitness and mutation rate will be necessary to

Table 7.2 Approximate values for gene frequency and carrier frequency calculated from the disease incidence assuming Hardy – Weinberg equilibrium

Disease incidence ($q2$)	Gene frequency (q)	Carrier frequency ($2pq$)
1/1000	1/32	1/16
1/2000	1/45	1/23
1/5000	1/71	1/36
1/10 000	1/100	1/50
1/50 000	1/224	1/112
1/100 000	1/316	1/158

determine the likely effects of improved treatment for serious genetic disorders. This is discussed further towards the end of this chapter.

WHY ARE SOME GENETIC DISORDERS MORE COMMON THAN OTHERS?

It is axiomatic that if a gene shows a high mutation rate, then this will usually result in a high incidence of the relevant disease. However factors other than the mutation rate and the fitness of affected individuals can also be involved. Mention has already been made of some of the mechanisms which can account for a high gene frequency of a particular disorder in a specific population. These will now be considered in the context of population size.

Small populations

Several rare autosomal recessive disorders show a relatively high incidence in certain populations and communities (Table 7.3). The most likely explanation for most of these observations is that the high allele frequency has resulted from a combination of a *founder effect* coupled with social, religious or geographical isolation of the relevant group. Such groups are referred to as *genetic isolates*. In some of the smaller populations genetic drift could also have played a role.

For example, several otherwise very rare autosomal recessive disorders have been found to occur at a relatively high frequency in the Old Order Amish, a religious isolate of European origin now living in Pennsylvania. Presumably, by chance, one or two original founders of the group carried these alleles which became established at relatively high frequency because of the restricted number of partners available to members of the religious sect.

A founder effect can also be observed for autosomal dominant disorders. Variegate porphyria, which is characterised by photosensitivity and drug induced neurovisceral disturbance, has a much higher incidence in the Afrikaner population of South Africa than in any other country or race. This is thought to be due to one of the early Dutch settlers having the condition and transmitting it to a large number of his or her descendants (p. 78).

One particularly unusual explanation for a high gene frequency in a small population is provided by the Hopi Indians of Arizona, who show a high incidence of albinism. Affected males were protected from outdoor farming activity because of their susceptibility to bright sunlight and it seems that this provided them with opportunity for reproductive activity in the absence of their unaffected peers. It is worth noting that several famous historical figures were affected with albinism: these include Noah and the Reverend William Spooner who was famous for transposing the initial letters of words – hence 'Spoonerism'.

Table 7.3 Rare recessive disorders which are relatively common in certain groups of people

Group	Disorder	Clinicial features
Finns	Congenital nephrotic syndrome	oedema, proteinuria, susceptibility to infection
	Aspartylglycosaminuria	progressive mental and motor deterioration, coarse features
	MULIBREY – nanism	MUscle, LIver, BRain and EYe involvement
	Congenital chloride diarrhoea	reduced Cl – absorption, diarrhoea
Amish	Cartilage–hair hypoplasia	dwarfism, fine, light-coloured and sparse hair
	Ellis–van Creveld syndrome	dwarfism, polydactyly, congenital heart disease
Hopi and San Blas Indians	Albinism	lack of pigmentation
Ashkenazi Jews	Tay–Sachs disease	progressive mental and motor deterioration, blindness
	Gaucher's disease	hepatosplenomegaly, bone lesions, skin pigmentation
	Dysautonomia	indifference to pain, emotional lability, lack of tears, hyperhidrosis
Karaite Jews	Werdnig–Hoffmann disease	infantile spinal muscular atrophy
Afrikaners	Sclerosteosis	increased stature, syndactyly, cranial nerve palsies
	Lipoid proteinosis	thickening of skin and mucous membranes
Ryukyan islands (off Japan)	'Ryukyan' spinal muscular atrophy	muscle weakness, club foot, scoliosis

Large populations

When a serious autosomal recessive disorder, which results in reduced fitness in affected homozygotes, has a high incidence in a large population, the explanation must lie in either a very high mutation rate or in heterozygote advantage. The latter explanation is the more probable for most autosomal recessive disorders (Table 7.4).

Heterozygote advantage

For sickle-cell anaemia and β thalassaemia there is good evidence that heterozygote advantage results from reduced susceptibility to *Plasmodium falciparum* malaria. The mechanism by which this is thought to occur is that the red cells of heterozygotes for sickle-cell can more effectively

Table 7.4 Presumed increased resistance in heterozygotes which could account for the maintenance of various genetic disorders in certain populations (AR = autosomal recessive; XR = X-linked recessive; AD = autosomal dominant)

Disorder	Genetics	Region	Resistance or advantage
Sickle–cell disease	AR	Tropical Africa	falciparum malaria
β–thalassaemia	AR	Mediterranean	falciparum malaria
G6PD deficiency	XR	Mediterranean	falciparum malaria
Cystic fibrosis	AR	Western Europe	tuberculosis the plague? cholera?
Tay–Sachs disease	AR	Eastern European Jews	tuberculosis
Congenital adrenal hyperplasia	AR	Yupik Eskimo	influenza B
Non-insulin dependent diabetes	AD	Pima Indians and others	periodic starvation
Phenylketonuria	AR	Western Europe	spontaneous abortion rate lower?

express malarial or altered self antigens which will result in more rapid removal of parasitised cells from the circulation. Americans of Afro-Caribbean origin are no longer exposed to malaria so it would be expected that the frequency of the sickle-cell allele amongst these individuals would gradually decline. It is hard to disentangle this effect on the allele frequency from admixture with other populations.

For several autosomal recessive disorders the mechanisms proposed for heterozygote advantage are largely speculative (Table 7.4). The recent discovery of the cystic fibrosis gene, with the subsequent elucidation of the role of its protein product in membrane permeability (p. 237), supports the hypothesis of selective advantage through increased resistance to the effects of gastro-intestinal infections such as cholera and dysentery in the heterozygote. This relative resistance could result from reduced loss of fluid and electrolytes. It could be that this selective advantage was most valuable several hundred years ago when these infections were endemic in Western Europe. If this is so then a gradual decline in the incidence of cystic fibrosis would be expected.

An alternative and entirely speculative mechanism for the high incidence of a condition such as cystic fibrosis is that of increased viability of sperm bearing the mutant gene. Molecular studies of families in which cystic fibrosis is segregating will soon reveal whether this is indeed a possibility.

A major practical problem when studying heterozygote advantage is that even a tiny increase in heterozygote fitness as compared with the fitness of unaffected homozygotes can be sufficient to sustain a high allele frequency. For example in cystic fibrosis, with an allele frequency of approximately 1 in 44, a heterozygote advantage of between 2% and 3% would be sufficient to account for the high allele frequency.

GENETIC POLYMORPHISM

A *polymorphism* is defined as the occurrence in a population of two or more genetically determined forms in such frequencies that the rarest of them could not be maintained by mutation alone. By convention, a polymorphic locus is one at which there are at least two alleles each with frequencies greater than 1%. Alleles with frequencies of less than 1% are referred to as rare *variants*.

Studies of enzyme and protein variability have shown that in humans at least 30% of structural gene loci are polymorphic, with each individual being heterozygous at between 10% and 20% of all structural loci. Known polymorphic protein systems include the ABO blood groups and many serum proteins. A large number of enzymes exhibit polymorphic electrophoretic differences or what are known as *isozymes*.

Polymorphism at the DNA level has proved particularly valuable in the positional cloning studies which have led to the isolation of many disease genes (p. 243). Polymorphic DNA markers are also of use in gene tracking (p. 54), which has facilitated preclinical diagnosis, prenatal diagnosis and carrier detection for over 200 single gene disorders. The value of a particular polymorphic system is assessed by determining its *polymorphic information content* (PIC). The higher the PIC value, the more likely it is that a polymorphic marker will be of value in linkage analysis and gene tracking.

Finally mention should be made of the distinction between *balanced* and *transient polymorphisms*. In a balanced polymorphism, two or more different forms are maintained by a balance between the selective advantage of the heterozygote and the reduced fitness of the affected homozygote. Thus the high incidence of the sickle-cell allele in areas where malaria is endemic is an example of a balanced polymorphism. However, as has already been discussed, the incidence of the sickle-cell allele is likely to decline in populations which are no longer exposed to malaria, so that in these situations the polymorphism can be considered as *transient*.

CHAPTER

7

SEGREGATION ANALYSIS

Segregation analysis refers to the study of the way in which a disorder is transmitted in families so as to establish the underlying mode of inheritance. The mathematical aspects of segregation analysis are extremely complex and fall far beyond the scope of this book and most doctors! However, it is important that those who encounter families with genetic disease have some understanding of the principles involved in segregation analysis as well as an awareness of some of the pitfalls and problems.

AUTOSOMAL DOMINANT INHERITANCE

For an autosomal dominant disorder the simplest approach is to compare the observed numbers of affected offspring born to affected parents with what would be expected based on the disease penetrance, i.e. 50% if penetrance is complete. A χ^2 test can be used to see if the observed and expected numbers differ significantly. As long as care is taken to ensure that families are not ascertained because of affected children, which would introduce a bias, this is usually a straightforward exercise.

AUTOSOMAL RECESSIVE INHERITANCE

For disorders believed to show autosomal recessive inheritance, formal segregation analysis is much more difficult. Consider 64 possible sibships of size 3 in which both parents are carriers, drawn from a large hypothetical population (Table 7.5). The sibship structure is what would be expected on average, assuming that the birth of an affected child does not deter the parents from having further children.

In this population, on average, 27 of these 64 sibships will not contain any affected individuals. This can be calculated simply by cubing 3/4, i.e. $3/4 \times 3/4 \times 3/4 =$

Table 7.5 Shows the expected sibship structure in a hypothetical population which contains 64 sibships each of size 3, in which both parents are carriers of an autosomal recessive disorder. If no allowance is made for truncate ascertainment, in that the 27 sibships with no affected cases will not be ascertained, then a falsely high segregation ratio of 48/111 (= 0.43) will be obtained.

No. of affected in sibship	Structure of sibship	No. of sibships	No. of affected	Total no. of sibs
3	■ ■ ■	1	3	3
2	■ ■ □	3	6	9
	□ ■ ■	3	6	9
	■ □ ■	3	6	9
1	■ □ □	9	9	27
	□ ■ □	9	9	27
	□ □ ■	9	9	27
0	□ □ □	27	0	81
	TOTAL	64	48	192

27/64. Therefore when the families are analysed these 27 sibships containing only healthy individuals will not be ascertained. This is referred to as *truncate* or *incomplete ascertainment*. If this is not taken into account, a falsely high *segregation ratio* of 0.43 will be obtained instead of the correct figure of 0.25.

Mathematical methods have been devised to accommodate for truncate ascertainment, but analysis is usually further complicated by the problems associated with achieving full or complete ascertainment. In practice it can actually be very difficult to 'prove' that a disorder shows autosomal recessive inheritance unless accurate molecular or biochemical methods are available for carrier detection. A high incidence of parental consanguinity provides strong supportive evidence for autosomal recessive inheritance, a point first noted by Bateson and Garrod as long ago as 1902 (p. 81).

GENETIC LINKAGE

Mendel's third law, the principle of independent assortment, states that members of different gene pairs assort to gametes independently of one another (p. 4). Stated more simply, genes at different loci segregate independently. Whilst this is true of genes on different chromosomes, it is not always true for genes which are located on the same chromosome.

If two loci are positioned so close together on the same chromosome, or what is termed *syntenic*, that alleles at these loci are inherited together more often than not, then these loci are said to be *linked*. In effect the two loci are sufficiently close together for it to be unlikely that they will be separated by a crossover or recombination in meiosis (Fig. 7.5).

Linked alleles on the same chromosome are said to be in *coupling*, whereas those on opposite homologous chromosomes are described as being in *repulsion*. This is known as the linkage *phase*.

RECOMBINATION FRACTION

The *recombination fraction*, which is usually designated as θ (Greek theta) is a measure of the distance separating two loci, or more precisely an indication of the likelihood that a crossover will occur between them. If two loci are not linked then θ equals 0.5, as on average genes at unlinked loci will segregate together during 50% of all meioses. If θ equals 0.05, this means that on average the syntenic alleles will segregate together 19 times out of 20: a crossover will occur between them during on average only 1 in 20 meioses.

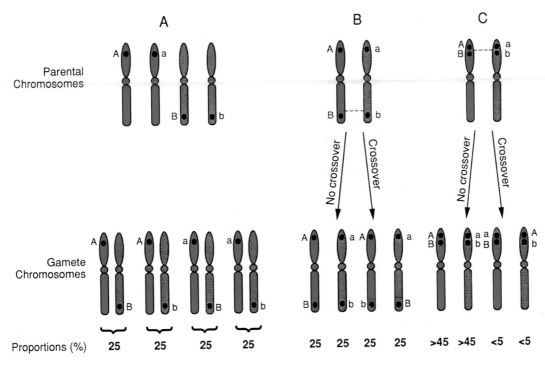

Fig. 7.5
Segregation at meiosis of alleles at two loci. In A the loci are on different chromosomes and in B they are on the same chromosome but widely separated. Hence these loci are not linked and there is independent assortment. In C the loci are closely adjacent so that separation by a crossover is unlikely i.e. the loci are linked.

CENTIMORGANS

The unit of measurement for genetic linkage is known as a *map unit* or *centiMorgan* (cM). If two loci are one cM apart, then a crossover occurs between them during on average only 1 in every 100 meioses, i.e. $\theta = 0.01$. CentiMorgans are a measure of the genetic or linkage distance between two loci. This is not the same as physical distance which is measured in base pairs.

The human genome has been estimated by recombination studies to be about 3000 cM in length. As the physical length of the haploid human genome is approximately 3×10^9 base pairs, 1cM corresponds to approximately 10^6 base pairs (or 1000 kilobases). However, the relationship between linkage map units and physical length is not linear. Some chromosome regions appear to be particularly prone to recombination, so-called 'hot spots', and for reasons which are not understood, recombination tends to occur more often during meiosis in the female than in the male. As a rough guide, during meiosis I large chromosomes would be expected to show an average of three crossovers, medium sized chromosomes two crossovers and small chromosomes one crossover.

LINKAGE ANALYSIS

Linkage analysis has proved to be an extremely valuable tool for mapping gene loci (p. 60). The basic methodology involves study of the segregation of the disease in large families with polymorphic markers from each chromosome. Eventually a marker will be identified which cosegregates with the disease more often than would be expected by chance, i.e. the loci are linked. The mathematical analysis tends to be very complex, particularly if lots of closely adjacent markers are being used as in *multipoint linkage analysis*. However the underlying principle is relatively straightforward and involves the use of likelihood ratios, the logarithms of which are known as *Lod scores*.

LOD SCORES

When studying the segregation of alleles at two loci which could be linked, a series of likelihood ratios is calculated for different values of the recombination fraction (θ), ranging from $\theta = 0$ to $\theta = 0.5$. The likelihood ratio at a given value of θ equals the likelihood of the observed data if the loci are linked at recombination value of θ divided by the likelihood of the observed data if the loci are not linked ($\theta = 0.5$). The logarithm to the base 10 of this ratio is known as the lod score (Z). Logarithms are used because they allow results from different families to be added together.

Therefore when a research paper reports that linkage of a disease with a DNA marker has been identified with a lod score (Z) of 4 at recombination fraction (θ) 0.05, this means that in the families which have been studied the results indicate that it is 10 000 (10^4) times more likely that the disease and marker loci are closely linked (i.e. 5cM apart) than that they are unlinked. It is generally agreed that a lod score of +3 or greater is confirmation of linkage. In fact this ratio of 1000 to 1 reduces to 20 to 1 because the prior probability of observing linkage is only 1 in 50. The importance of taking prior probabilities into account in probability theory is discussed in the section on Bayes' theorem (p. 253).

A 'simple' example

Consider a three generation family in which several members have an autosomal dominant disorder (Fig 7.6). A and B are alleles at a locus which could or could not be linked to the disease locus.

To establish whether it is likely that these two loci are linked, the lod score is calculated for various values of θ. The value of θ which gives the highest lod score is taken as the best estimate of the recombination fraction. This is known as a *maximum likelihood method*.

To demonstrate the underlying principle, the lod score will be calculated for a value of θ equal to 0.05. If θ equals 0.05 then the loci are linked, in which case the disease gene and the B marker must be on the same chromosome in II_2, as both of these characteristics have been inherited from the mother. Thus in II_2 the linkage phase is known – the disease allele and the B allele are in coupling. Therefore the probability that III_1 would be affected and would also inherit the B marker equals 0.95, i.e. $1-\theta$. A similar result is obtained for the remaining three members of the sibship in generation III, giving a value for the numerator of $(0.95)^4$. If the loci are not linked, then the likelihood of observing both the disease and marker B in III_1 equals 0.5. A similar result is obtained

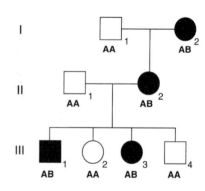

Fig. 7.6
A three generation pedigree showing segregation of an autosomal dominant disorder and alleles (A and B) at a locus which may or may not be linked to the disease locus.

for his three siblings, giving a value for the denominator of $(0.5)^4$.

Therefore the lod score for this family given a value of $\theta = 0.05$ equals $\log_{10} 0.95^4/0.5^4 = \log_{10} 13.032 = 1.15$.

To confirm linkage other families would have to be studied until by pooling all the results a lod score of +3 or greater is obtained. A lod score of –2 or less is taken as proof that the loci are not linked. This less stringent requirement for proof of non-linkage, i.e. a lod score of –2 as compared with +3 for proof of linkage, is due to the high prior probability of 49/50 that any two loci are not linked.

LINKAGE DISEQUILIBRIUM

This is defined formally as the association of two linked alleles more frequently than would be expected by chance. In the family which has just been analysed (Fig. 7.6) support was obtained for linkage of the disease gene with the B marker allele. Assume that further studies confirm linkage of these loci and that the A and B alleles have an equal frequency of 0.5. It would be reasonable to expect that the disease gene would be in coupling with allele A in approximately 50% of families and with allele B in the remaining 50%. If, however, the disease allele was found to be in coupling almost exclusively with one particular marker allele this would be an example of *linkage disequilibrium*.

The demonstration of linkage disequilibrium in a particular disease suggests that the mutation which has caused the disease has occurred relatively recently and that the marker locus being studied is very closely linked to the disease locus. For example, one of the very small number of the original mutations for sickle-cell disease occurred in a β globin gene which was closely adjacent to a very rare syntenic RFLP (p. 57) (Fig. 4.19). Selection for this sickle-cell mutation, with only very rare recombination having occurred between it and the adjacent tightly linked locus, has resulted in a very high proportion of present day sickle-cell alleles being in coupling with this otherwise rare RFLP.

Other disorders in which linkage disequilibrium has been identified include Huntington's disease (p. 86), myotonic dystrophy (p. 249), cystic fibrosis (p. 236), phenylketonuria (p. 130) and the Fragile X syndrome (p. 223).

MEDICAL AND SOCIETAL INTERVENTION

Recent developments in molecular biology, such as the human genome project (p. 284) and pilot studies using gene therapy (p. 278), have reawakened concern that future generations could have to cope with an ever increasing burden of genetic disease. The term *eugenics* was first used by Charles Darwin's cousin, Francis Galton, to refer to the improvement of a population by selective breeding. The notion that this should be applied to human populations became popular during the early years of this century, culminating in the profoundly distasteful and totally unacceptable practices of Nazi Germany. Ensuing revulsion led to the total abandonment of eugenic programmes in humans with universal condemnation and agreement that these have no place in modern medical practice.

Nevertheless, doctors who care for patients and families with hereditary disease are faced with a dilemma. On the one hand, by helping patients with serious genetic disease to survive and reproduce they are indeed increasing the numbers of 'bad genes' in society, thereby potentially adding to mankind's future genetic load. Such behaviour could be interpreted as dysgenic. On the other hand, most medical practitioners would argue that their responsibility to an individual patient far outweighs their obligation to either contemporary society or to future generations.

Before returning to this ethical debate it is worth considering the possible long term effects of artificial selection for or against genetic disorders.

AUTOSOMAL DOMINANT DISORDERS

If everyone with an autosomal dominant disorder was successfully encouraged not to reproduce, then the incidence of that disorder would decline rapidly with all future cases only being due to new mutations. This would have a particularly striking effect on the incidence of relatively mild conditions such as familial hypercholesterolaemia in which genetic fitness is close to 1.

Alternatively, if successful treatment became available for all patients with a serious autosomal dominant disorder which at present is associated with a marked reduction in genetic fitness, then there would be an immediate increase in the frequency of the disease gene followed by a more gradual levelling off at a new equilibrium level. If, at one time, all those with a serious autosomal dominant disorder died in childhood (f = 0) then the incidence of affected individuals would be 2μ. If treatment raised the fitness from 0 to 0.9, then the incidence of affected children in the next generation would rise to 2μ due to new mutations plus 1.8μ inherited which equals 3.8μ. Eventually a new equilibrium would be reached by which time the disease incidence would have risen ten-fold to 20μ. This can be calculated relatively easily using the formula $\mu = [I(1–f)]/2$ (p. 95). The net result would be that the proportion of affected children who die would be less (100% → 10%), but the total number affected would be much greater, although the actual number who die from the disease would remain unchanged at 2μ.

AUTOSOMAL RECESSIVE DISORDERS

In contrast to an autosomal dominant disorder, artificial selection against an autosomal recessive condition will have only a very slow effect.

The reason for this difference is that in autosomal recessive conditions most of the genes in a population are present in healthy heterozygotes who would not be affected by eugenic measures. It can be shown that if there is complete selection against an autosomal recessive disorder so that no homozygotes reproduce, then the number of generations (n) required to change the allele frequency from q_o to q_n equals $1/q_n - 1/q_o$. Therefore, for a condition with an incidence of approximately 1 in 2000 and an allele frequency of roughly 1 in 45, if all affected patients refrained from reproduction then it would take over 500 years (18 generations) to reduce the disease incidence by half. With rarer conditions it would take even longer!

Now consider the opposite situation where selection operating against a serious autosomal recessive disorder is relaxed because of improvement in medical treatment. More affected individuals will reach adult life and transmit the mutant allele to their offspring. The result will be that the frequency of the mutant allele will increase until a new equilibrium is reached. Using the formula $\mu = I(1-f)$ (p. 95), it can be shown that when the new equilibrium is eventually reached, an increase in fitness from 0 to 0.9 will have resulted in a tenfold increase in the disease incidence.

SEX-LINKED RECESSIVE DISORDERS

When considering the effects of selection against these disorders, it is necessary to take into account the fact that a large proportion of the relevant genes are present in entirely healthy female carriers, who are often unaware of their carrier status. For a very serious condition with fitness equal to 0 in affected males, selection will have no effect unless female carriers choose to limit their families. If all female carriers opted not to have any children, then the incidence would be reduced by two thirds, i.e. from 3μ to μ.

A much more plausible possibility is that effective treatment will be forthcoming for these disorders. This will result in a steady increase in the disease incidence. For example an increase in fitness from 0 to 0.5 will lead to a doubling of the disease incidence by the time a new equilibrium has been established. This can be calculated using the formula $\mu = [I^M(1-f)]/3$ (p. 95).

CONCLUSION

In reality it is extremely difficult to predict the long term impact of medical intervention on the incidence and burden of genetic disease. Non-directive genetic counselling could lead to a reduction in the number of affected children being born, but it is quite likely that many of these children will be 'replaced' by carrier siblings, either by such couples compensating by having large families, or, more recently, by the use of prenatal diagnosis, so that the overall effects on gene frequency are almost impossible to determine. Whilst it is true that improvements in medical treatment could result in an increase in genetic load in future generations, it is equally possible that successful gene therapy will have eased the overall burden of these disorders in terms of human suffering. Some of these arguments could have been made many years ago for other major medical developments such as the discovery of insulin and antibiotics which have had overwhelming financial implications in terms of burgeoning pharmaceutical costs and an increasingly geriatric population. Ultimately it can reasonably be argued that it is how a society copes with these challenges that gives a true measure of the validity of its claim to be civilised.

ELEMENTS

1 According to the Hardy–Weinberg principle the relative proportions of the possible genotypes at a particular locus remain constant from one generation to the next.

2 Factors which may disturb Hardy–Weinberg equilibrium are non-random mating, a change in the number of mutant alleles in the population, selection for or against a particular genotype, small population size, and migration.

3 If an autosomal recessive disorder is in Hardy–Weinberg equilibrium the carrier frequency can be estimated by doubling the square root of the disease incidence.

4 The mutation rate for an autosomal dominant disorder can be measured directly by estimating the proportion of new mutations among all members of one generation. Indirect estimates of mutation rates can be made using the formulae:

$\mu = [I(1-f)]/2$ for autosomal dominant inheritance

$\mu = I(1-f)$ for autosomal recessive inheritance

$\mu = [I^M(1-f)]/3$ for sex-linked recessive inheritance.

5 Otherwise rare single gene disorders can show a high incidence in a small population because of a founder effect coupled with genetic isolation.

6 When a serious autosomal recessive disorder has a relatively high incidence in a large population this is likely to be due to heterozygote advantage.

7 Closely adjacent loci on the same chromosome are said to be linked if genes at these loci segregate together during more than 50% of meioses. The recombination fraction (θ) indicates how often two such genes will be separated (recombine) at meiosis.

8 The lod score is a mathematical indication of the relative likelihood that two loci are linked. A lod score of +3 or greater is taken as confirmation of linkage.

FURTHER READING

Allison A C 1954 Protection afforded by sickle-cell trait against subtertian malarial infection. Br Med J i: 290–294
A landmark paper providing clear evidence that the sickle-cell trait provides protection against parasitaemia by falciparum malaria.

Emery A E H 1986 Methodology in medical genetics, 2nd edn. Churchill Livingstone, Edinburgh
A useful handbook of basic population genetics and mathematical methods for analysing the results of genetic studies.

Haldane J B S 1935 The rate of spontaneous mutation of a human gene. J Genet 31: 317–326
The first estimate of the mutation rate for haemophilia using an indirect method.

Hardy G H 1908 Mendelian proportions in a mixed population. Science 28: 49–50
A short letter in which Hardy pointed out that in a large randomly mating population dominant 'characters' would not increase at the expense of recessives.

Khoury M J, Beaty T H, Cohen B H 1993 Fundamentals of genetic epidemiology. Oxford University Press, New York.
A comprehensive text-book of population genetics and its areas of overlap with epidemiology.

Vogel F, Motulsky A G 1986 Human genetics, problems and approaches, 2nd edn. Springer-Verlag, Berlin
The definitive text-book of human genetics with extensive coverage of mathematical aspects.

Polygenic and multifactorial inheritance

INTRODUCTION

Many disorders demonstrate familial clustering which does not conform to any recognised pattern of Mendelian inheritance. Examples include several of the most common congenital malformations and many of the common diseases of adult life (Table 8.1). These conditions show a definite familial tendency but the incidence in close relatives of affected individuals is usually around 2–4%, instead of the much higher figures which would be seen if these conditions were caused by mutations in single genes.

This pattern of inheritance is referred to as *multifactorial*. As it is likely that both genes and environment are implicated in the cause of these disorders, it is now generally accepted that multifactorial inheritance involves the interaction of adverse environmental factors with an underlying innate susceptibility determined by the additive effect of many genes.

It should be emphasised that the concept of multifactorial inheritance has been developed to explain the familial patterns observed for these conditions. Unlike single gene inheritance, firm scientific support for multifactorial inheritance is lacking. Several statistical models have been proposed. The underlying mathematical prin-

ciples are complex and to understand these models it is necessary to have a detailed knowledge of the statistics of the normal (Gaussian) distribution. In this chapter we shall focus on the most plausible and easily understood of these models. This was originally proposed by Falconer and is known as the *liability/threshold model*.

POLYGENIC INHERITANCE AND THE NORMAL DISTRIBUTION

Before considering the liability/threshold model in detail, it is necessary to outline briefly the scientific basis of what is known as *polygenic* or *quantitative* inheritance. This involves the inheritance and expression of a phenotype being determined by many genes at different loci, with each gene exerting a small additive effect. Additive implies that the effects of the genes are cumulative, i.e. no one gene is dominant or recessive to another.

Several human characteristics (Table 8.2) show a continuous distribution in the general population, which closely resembles a normal distribution. This takes the form of a symmetrical bell-shaped curve distributed evenly about a mean (Fig. 8.1). The spread of the distribution about the mean is determined by the standard deviation. Approximately 68%, 95% and 99.7% of observations fall within the mean plus or minus one, two or three standard deviations respectively.

It is possible to show that a phenotype with a normal distribution in the general population can be generated by polygenic inheritance involving the action of many genes at different loci, each of which exerts an equal

Table 8.1 Disorders which show multifactorial inheritance

Congenital malformations
  Cleft lip/palate
  Congenital dislocation of the hip
  Congenital heart defects
  Neural tube defects
  Pyloric stenosis
  Talipes
Adult onset diseases
  Diabetes mellitus
  Epilepsy
  Glaucoma
  Hypertension
  Ischaemic heart disease
  Manic depression
  Schizophrenia

Table 8.2 Human characteristics which show a continuous normal distribution

Blood pressure
Dermatoglyphics (ridge count)
Head circumference
Height
Intelligence
Skin colour

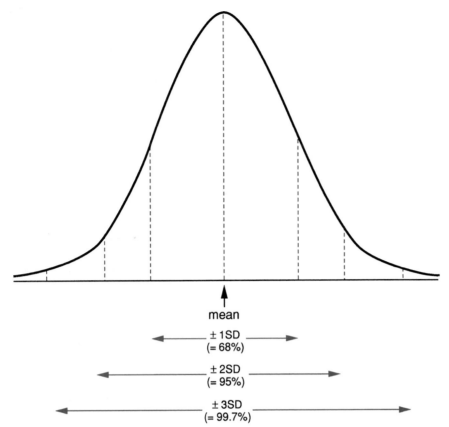

mean

±1SD
(= 68%)

±2SD
(= 95%)

±3SD
(= 99.7%)

Fig. 8.1
The normal (Gaussian) distribution.

additive effect. This can be illustrated by considering a trait such as height. If height were to be determined by two equally frequent alleles, a (tall) and b (short), at a single locus, then this would result in a discontinuous phenotype with three groups in a ratio of 1 (tall-aa) to 2 (average-ab/ba) to 1 (short-bb). If the same trait were to be determined by two alleles at each of two loci inter-acting in a simple additive way, then this would lead to a phenotypic distribution of five groups in a ratio of 1 (4 tall genes) to 4 (3 tall + 1 short) to 6 (2 tall + 2 short) to 4 (1 tall + 3 short) to 1 (4 short). For a system with three loci each with two alleles the phenotypic ratio would be 1–6–15–20–15–6–1 (Fig. 8.2).

It can be seen that as the number of loci increases, the distribution increasingly comes to resemble a normal curve, thereby lending support to the concept that characteristics such as height are determined by the ad-ditive effects of many genes at different loci. Further support for this concept comes from the study of familial correlations for characteristics such as height and, to a lesser extent, intelligence. *Correlation* is a statistical measure of the degree of association of variable pheno-mena, or in more simple terms a measure of the degree of resemblance or relationship between two parameters. As first degree relatives share on average 50% of their genes (Table 8.3), it would be reasonable to predict that, if a parameter such as height is polygenic, then the correlation between first degree relatives such as siblings

should be 0.5. Several studies have shown that the sib–sib correlation for height is indeed close to 0.5.

In reality, it is probable that human characteristics such as height and intelligence are also influenced by environment and possibly also by genes which are not additive in that they exert a dominant effect. These factors probably account for the observed tendency of offspring to show what is known as 'regression to the mean'. This is demonstrated by tall or intelligent parents (the two are not mutually exclusive!) having children whose average height or intelligence is slightly lower than the average parental value. Similarly, parents who are very short or of low intelligence tend to have children whose average height or intelligence is lower than the general popu-lation average, but higher than the average value of the parents. If a trait was to show true polygenic inheritance with no external influences then the measurements in offspring would be distributed evenly around the mean of the parents' values. Regression to the mean (i.e. the population mean) probably occurs mainly because of the modifying effects of the environment.

MULTIFACTORIAL INHERITANCE – THE LIABILITY/THRESHOLD MODEL

Efforts have been made to extend the polygenic theory for the inheritance of *continuous traits* to try to account

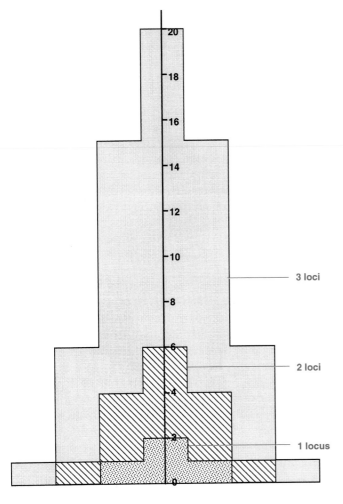

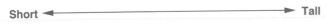

Short ⟵ ———————————— ⟶ Tall

Fig. 8.2
Shows the distribution of genotypes for a characteristic such as height with 1, 2 and 3 loci each with 2 alleles of equal frequency. The values for each genotype can be obtained from the binomial expansion $(p+q)^{2n}$ where $p = q = 1/2$ and n equals the number of loci.

Table 8.3 Degrees of relationship

Relationship	Proportion of genes shared
First degree	1/2
Parents	
Siblings	
Children	
Second degree	1/4
Uncles and aunts	
Nephews and nieces	
Grandparents	
Grandchildren	
Halfsiblings	
Third degree	1/8
First cousins	
Great grandparents	
Great grandchildren	

for *discontinuous* multifactorial disorders. According to the liability/threshold model, all of the factors which influence the development of a multifactorial disorder, whether genetic or environmental, can be considered as a single entity known as *liability*. The liabilities of all individuals in a population form a continuous variable, which has a normal distribution in both the general population and in relatives of affected individuals. However the curves for these relatives will be shifted to the right, with the extent to which they are shifted being directly related to the closeness of their relationship to the affected index case (Fig. 8.3).

To account for a discontinuous phenotype (i.e. affected or not affected) with an underlying continuous distribution, it is proposed that a threshold exists above which the abnormal phenotype is expressed. In the general population the proportion beyond the threshold is the population incidence and among relatives the proportion beyond the threshold is the familial incidence.

It is important to emphasise once again that liability includes all factors which contribute to the cause of the condition. Looked at very simply a deleterious liability can be viewed as consisting of a combination of several 'bad' genes and adverse environmental factors. Liability cannot be measured but the mean liability of a group can be determined from the incidence of the disease in that group using statistics of the normal distribution. The

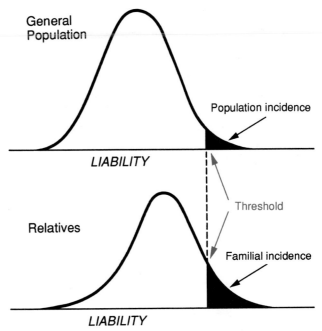

Fig. 8.3
Hypothetical liability curves in the general population and in relatives for a hereditary disorder in which the genetic predisposition is multifactorial.

units of measurement are standard deviations and these can be used to estimate the correlation between relatives.

CONSEQUENCES OF THE LIABILITY/THRESHOLD MODEL

Part of the attraction of this model is that it provides a simple explanation for the observed familial risks in conditions such as cleft lip/palate, pyloric stenosis and spina bifida:

1. The incidence of the condition is greatest amongst relatives of the most severely affected patients, presumably because they are the most extreme deviants along the liability curve. For example, in cleft lip/palate the proportion of affected first degree relatives (parents, siblings and offspring) is 6% if the index patient has bilateral cleft lip and palate, but only 2% if the index patient has a unilateral cleft lip (Fig. 8.4).

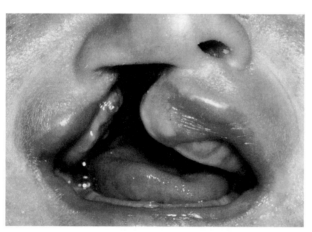

A

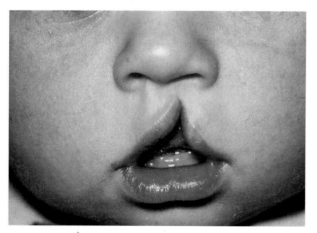

B

Fig. 8.4
(A) Severe and (B) mild forms of cleft lip/palate.

2. The risk is greatest amongst close relatives of the index case and decreases rapidly in more distant relatives. For example, in spina bifida the risks to first, second and third degree relatives of the index case are approximately 4%, 1% and less than 0.5% respectively.
3. If there is more than one affected close relative then the risks for other relatives are increased. In spina bifida, if two siblings are affected, the risk to a subsequent sibling is approximately 10%.
4. If the condition is more common in individuals of one particular sex, then relatives of an affected individual of the less frequently affected sex will be at higher risk than relatives of an affected individual of the more frequently affected sex. This is illustrated by the condition pyloric stenosis. Pyloric stenosis shows a male to female ratio of 5 to 1. The proportions of affected offspring of male index patients are 5.5% for sons and 2.4% for daughters, whereas the risks to the offspring of female index patients are 19.4% for sons and 7.3% for daughters. The probable explanation for these different risks is that in order for a female to be affected she has to lie at the extreme of the liability curve, so that her close relatives will also have a very high liability for developing the condition. As males are more susceptible to develop the disorder, risks in male offspring are higher than in female offspring regardless of the sex of the affected parent.

HERITABILITY

Though it is not possible to assess an individual's liability for a particular disorder, it is possible to estimate what proportion of the aetiology can be ascribed to genetic factors as opposed to environmental factors. This is referred to as *heritability*, which can be defined as the proportion of the total phenotypic variance of a condition which is caused by additive genetic variance. In statistical terms, variance equals the square of the standard deviation. Heritability is often depicted using the symbol h^2 and is expressed either as a proportion of 1 or as a percentage.

Estimates of the heritability of a condition or trait provide an indication of the relative importance of genetic factors in its causation, so that the greater the value for the heritability the greater the role of genetic factors.

Heritability is estimated from the degree of resemblance between relatives expressed in the form of a correlation coefficient which is calculated using statistics of the normal distribution. Alternatively, heritability can be calculated using data on the concordance rates in monozygotic and dizygotic twins. In practice it is desirable to try to derive heritability estimates using different types of relatives and to measure the disease incidence in relatives reared together and living apart so as to try to

Table 8.4 Estimates of heritability of various disorders

Disorder	Frequency (%)	Heritability
Schizophrenia	1	85
Asthma	4	80
Cleft lip +/− cleft palate	0.1	76
Pyloric stenosis	0.3	75
Ankylosing spondylitis	0.2	70
Club foot	0.1	68
Coronary artery disease	3	65
Hypertension (essential)	5	62
Congenital dislocation of the hip	0.1	60
Anencephaly and spina bifida	0.5	60
Peptic ulcer	4	37
Congenital heart disease	0.5	35

Table 8.5 Calculation of relative risk for a disease association

	Marker positive	Marker negative
Patients	a	b
Controls	c	d
Relative risk	= a/c ÷ b/d	
	= ad/bc	

disentangle the possible effects of common environmental factors.

Estimates of heritability for some common diseases are given in Table 8.4. These figures indicate that the genetic contribution to a condition such as pyloric stenosis is much greater than for peptic ulcer or congenital heart disease. These observations have important practical implications for both research and for patient management. If the heritability is high then a search for susceptibility genes is justified, whereas prevention of a multifactorial disorder with low heritability is more likely to be achieved by a search for, and subsequent avoidance of, adverse environmental factors.

IDENTIFYING GENES WHICH CAUSE MULTIFACTORIAL DISORDERS

Multifactorial disorders are common and make a major contribution to human morbidity and mortality (p. 7). It is therefore not surprising that vigorous efforts are being made to try to identify and isolate genes which contribute to their aetiology. Towards this end several strategies can be employed.

DISEASE ASSOCIATIONS

The study of disease associations is undertaken by comparing the incidence of a particular polymorphism in affected patients with the incidence in a carefully matched control group. If the incidences differ significantly, this provides evidence for a positive or negative association.

The polymorphic system which has been studied most often is the HLA histocompatibility complex on chromosome 6 (p. 160). One of the strongest known HLA associations is that between ankylosing spondylitis and the B27 allele. This is present in approximately 90% of all patients and in 5% of controls. The strength of an HLA

association is indicated by the ratio of the risk of developing the disease in those with the antigen to the risk of developing the disease in those without the antigen (Table 8.5). This is known as the *relative risk* and it gives an indication of how much more frequently the disease occurs in individuals with a specific marker than in those without that marker.

Progress in molecular biology has led to a huge increase in the number of polymorphic systems which can be studied in a search for disease associations. The many alleles at the *HLA complex* can now be studied at the molecular level using the polymerase chain reaction (p. 48). This has resulted in many more HLA associations being identified than was possible previously.

The potential value of molecular biology in the study of disease associations is illustrated by the most common form of senile dementia which is known as Alzheimer's disease. A very rare form of Alzheimer's disease shows early onset with autosomal dominant inheritance. In some of these families mutations have been identified in the amyloid precursor protein gene on chromosome 21 and it is believed that this observation is related in some way to the observed high incidence of Alzheimer's disease in adults with trisomy 21 or Down's syndrome (p. 216).

However, these early onset families account for less than 1% of all cases of Alzheimer's disease. Recent studies have shown that in the much more common late onset form of Alzheimer's disease, which shows only weak familial aggregation, there is a strong association with the ε4 allele of apolipoprotein E. This protein is encoded by a gene on chromosome 19 and acts as a ligand for the low density lipoprotein receptor (p. 135). The incidence of the ε4 allele is approximately 40% in patients with Alzheimer's disease, in contrast to 12% in age-related controls. The risk of developing Alzheimer's disease is particularly increased if an individual has two ε4 alleles.

The demonstration of a disease association can be of value in risk calculation for genetic counselling and, as in the case of Alzheimer's disease, can also help unravel genetic heterogeneity. The elucidation of a disease association can also reveal the identity of one of the 'polygenes' contributing to a multifactorial disorder. However, even for a condition such as Alzheimer's disease, many other factors, genetic and environmental, must be involved, as it has been estimated that the ε4 allele accounts for only 17% of the variance in the liability to develop the disease.

SIB-PAIR ANALYSIS

If affected siblings inherit a particular allele more often than would be expected by chance, this indicates that that allele or its locus is involved in some way in causing the disease.

Consider a set of parents with alleles AB (father) and CD (mother) at a particular locus. The probability that any two of their children will have both alleles in common is 1 in 4 (Fig. 8.5). The probability that they will have one allele in common is 1 in 2 and the probability that they will have no alleles in common equals 1 in 4. If siblings who are affected with a particular disease show deviation from this 1:2:1 ratio for a particular polymorphism, this implies that there is a causal relationship between the locus and the disease. In type 1 diabetes mellitus (p. 183) study of the HLA haplotypes in affected sib pairs showed significant deviation from this expected 1:2:1 ratio, indicating that alleles in the HLA complex are causally related in some way.

The nature of the causal relationship will not always be clear. It could reflect a disease association (p. 109), or linkage of a disease locus with the marker locus (p. 99), or even linkage disequilibrium (p. 101) between the marker locus and a closely adjacent locus which encodes a deleterious dominant or additive gene. In the case of type 1 diabetes mellitus, studies have indicated that the HLA association accounts for at least 50% of its heritability.

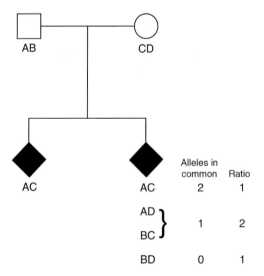

Fig. 8.5
The probability that siblings will have 2, 1 or 0 parental alleles in common. Significant deviation from the 1:2:1 ratio indicates that the locus is causally related to the disease.

LINKAGE ANALYSIS

Linkage analysis has proved extremely valuable in mapping single gene disorders by studying the cosegregation of polymorphisms with the disease until a linked marker has been identified (p. 100). However, this type of approach is much more difficult in multifactorial disorders for the following reasons:

1. If a multifactorial disorder has a polygenic underlying genetic susceptibility, then it is unlikely that alleles at a single locus will make a major contribution. It is extremely difficult mathematically to develop strategies for detecting linkage of additive 'polygenes' each of which makes only a small contribution to the phenotype.
2. Many multifactorial diseases show a variable age of onset so that the genetic status of unaffected family members cannot be known with certainty.
3. Most families in which a multifactorial disease is, or has been, present have only one or two living affected members so that the number of 'informative meioses' available for study is usually very small.
4. Some apparent multifactorial disorders such as coronary artery disease and schizophrenia are probably aetiologically heterogeneous, with different genetic and environmental mechanisms involved in different sub-types which cannot be easily distinguished at the phenotypic level.

Despite the initial enthusiasm that susceptibility loci had been identified for conditions such as bipolar depression and schizophrenia, this type of conventional linkage analysis has met with little success in identifying loci or alleles contributing to any of the common multifactorial disorders.

Linkage analysis has been successful, however, either directly or indirectly, in identifying genes or loci contributing to several multifactorial conditions using firstly candidate genes (p. 62) and secondly the *reductionist approach*. A candidate gene is one which a priori could be expected to be involved in causing a disease. For example, it would be reasonable to suppose that the insulin gene could be involved in causing diabetes mellitus, although in fact studies have shown that it is not. One success story for the candidate gene approach stems from the identification of chromosome 22 microdeletions in the DiGeorge syndrome (p. 221), in which affected infants usually have cardiac outflow tract malformations, which in isolation are thought to show multifactorial inheritance. Subsequent studies showed that DNA markers from the deleted region cosegregated with cardiac malformations in families showing aggregation of the relevant cardiac defects. This suggests that at least a proportion of these malformations are caused by a gene on chromosome 22 which exerts a major dominant effect on a polygenic/environmental background.

The reductionist approach involves identifying families in which an apparent multifactorial disorder is showing single gene inheritance and then isolating the gene by traditional positional cloning techniques (p. 61). Once isolated and characterised, a search for germ-line and somatic rearrangements can be made in patients who present as isolated cases of the same disorder. An example of how this technique has been successful is the discovery of deletions of the adenomatous polyposis coli (APC) gene in sporadically occurring carcinoma of the colon (p. 173). The APC gene is one of many involved in what could be regarded as a 'polygenic' multistage process of carcinogenesis (p. 174).

CONCLUSION

The term multifactorial has been coined to describe the large number of common disorders which show familial aggregation and are likely to result from the interaction of genetic factors and environment. The genetic mechanisms underlying these disorders are poorly understood and the liability/threshold model should be regarded as an attractive and plausible hypothesis rather than a proven scientific fact. In time molecular studies may reveal that some apparent multifactorial disorders are aetiologically heterogeneous, representing in some cases an admixture of single-gene disorders and environmental phenotypes. Alternatively, some conditions such as insulin dependent diabetes mellitus may be shown to be due to the action of one or two major genes interacting with a polygenic background and yet to be defined environmental insults.

When counselling families, empiric risks derived from family studies should be used (p. 259). These are preferable to theoretical risks obtained using complex mathematical models. It is important to remember that these models have been proposed to fit the observed facts, and while their use can be acceptable if no empiric risk data are available, it is always preferable to counsel on the basis of results obtained in original family studies.

ELEMENTS

1 The concept of multifactorial inheritance has been proposed to account for the common congenital malformations and adult-onset disorders which show non-Mendelian familial aggregation. These disorders are thought to result from the interaction of genetic and environmental factors.

2 Human characteristics such as height and intelligence, which show a normally distributed continuous distribution in the general population, are probably caused by the additive effects of many genes, i.e. polygenic inheritance.

3 According to the liability/threshold model for multifactorial inheritance the population's genetic and environmental susceptibility, which is known as liability, is normally distributed. Individuals are affected if their liability exceeds a threshold superimposed on the liability curve.

4 Recurrence risks to relatives for multifactorial disorders are influenced by the disease severity, the degree of relationship to the index case, the number of affected close relatives and, if there is a higher incidence in one particular sex, the sex of the index case.

5 Heritability is a measure of the proportion of the total variance of a character or disease which is due to the genetic variance.

6 Genes or loci which contribute to susceptibility for multifactorial disorders can sometimes be identified by a search for disease markers or sibpair or linkage analysis.

FURTHER READING

Falconer D S 1965 The inheritance of liability to certain diseases estimated from the incidence among relatives. Ann Hum Genet 29: 51–76
The original exposition of the liability/threshold model and how correlations between relatives can be used to calculate heritability.
Fraser F C 1980 Evolution of a palatable multifactorial threshold model. Am J Hum Genet, 32: 796–813
An amusing and 'reader-friendly' account of models proposed to explain multifactorial inheritance.
King R A, Rotter J I, Motulsky A G (eds) 1992 The genetic basis of common diseases. Oxford University Press, Oxford
A lengthy and detailed review of the genetic aspects of common adult onset disorders.

SECTION B | GENETICS IN MEDICINE

CHAPTER 9

Haemoglobin and the haemoglobinopathies

It has been estimated that more than a quarter of a million persons are born in the world each year with one of the disorders of the structure and synthesis of haemoglobin (Hb), the so-called *haemoglobinopathies*.

During the course of the last 40 years, the haemoglobinopathies have served as a model for our understanding of the pathology of inherited disease in humans at the clinical, protein and DNA level. It is necessary to consider the structure, function and synthesis of Hb in order to better understand the various types of haemoglobinopathies.

STRUCTURE OF HAEMOGLOBIN

Hb is the protein present in red blood cells responsible for oxygen transport. There are large quantities of Hb in blood making it amenable to analysis.

PROTEIN ANALYSIS

Ingram, in 1956, by fractionating the peptides from digestion of human Hb with the proteolytic enzyme, trypsin, found 30 discrete peptide fragments. Trypsin cuts polypeptide chains at the amino acids arginine and lysine. Analysis of the 580 amino acids of human Hb had previously shown there to be a total of 60 arginine and lysine residues. This suggested that Hb was made up of two identical peptide chains.

About the same time a family was reported in which two rare haemoglobin variants, Hb S and Hb Hopkins II, were both present in some family members. Several members of the family who possessed both variants had children with normal Hb, offspring who were heterozygous for only one Hb variant as well as offspring who, like their parents, were doubly heterozygous for the two Hb variants. This provided further support for the suggestion that there were at least two different genes involved in the production of human Hb.

Shortly thereafter, the amino-terminal amino-acid sequence of human Hb was determined and showed valine–leucine and valine–histidine sequences in

equimolar proportions with two moles of each of these sequences per mole of Hb. This suggested that human Hb was a tetramer consisting of two pairs of dissimilar polypeptides referred to as the α and β globin chains.

Analysis of the iron content of human Hb revealed it to constitute 0.35% of its weight, from which it was calculated that human Hb should have a minimum molecular weight of 16 000. In contrast, determination of the molecular weight of human Hb by physical methods gave values of the order of 64 000, consistent with the suggested tetrameric structure, $\alpha_2\beta_2$, with each of the globin chains having its own iron containing prosthetic group, haem.

Subsequent investigators demonstrated that Hb from normal adult individuals also contained a minor fraction, 2–3%, with an electrophoretic mobility different from Hb A. This was called Hb A_2. Subsequent studies revealed Hb A_2 to be a tetramer of two normal alpha globin chains and two other polypeptide chains whose amino acid sequence resembled most closely the beta globin chain. This was designated delta (δ).

DEVELOPMENTAL EXPRESSION OF HAEMOGLOBIN

Analysis of Hb from a human fetus revealed it to consist primarily of another type of Hb with a different electrophoretic mobility, which was called fetal Hb or Hb F. Subsequent analysis showed Hb F to be a tetramer of two alpha globin chains and two polypeptide chains whose sequence resembled the beta globin chain and which were designated gamma, γ. Trace amounts, 0.5%, of Hb F are found in the blood of normal adults.

Analysis of Hb from embryos earlier in gestation reveals there to be a succession of different embryonic Hbs, Hb Gower I and II, and Hb Portland, which are produced at different times of gestation. Subsequent analysis has revealed that these different Hbs, which are transiently expressed in development, are in fact tetramers of various combinations of alpha or alpha-like zeta (ζ) chains with beta or beta-like gamma and epsilon (ϵ)

Table 9.1 Human haemoglobins

Stage in development	Haemoglobin	Structure	Proportion (%) in normal adult
Embryonic	Gower I	$\zeta_2\varepsilon_2$	–
	Gower II	$\alpha_2\varepsilon_2$	–
	Portland I	$\zeta_2\gamma_2$	–
Fetal	F	$\alpha_2\gamma_2$	<1
Adult	A	$\alpha_2\beta_2$	97–98
	A$_2$	$\alpha_2\delta_2$	2–3

globin chains (Table 9.1). Apart from the transient expression of the zeta chain early in embryonic life, the alpha globin chain gene is expressed throughout development. Similarly, epsilon globin chain expression occurs early in embryonic life with gamma chain expression occurring throughout fetal life followed by increasing levels of expression of the beta globin chain towards the end of fetal life. The ordered expression of these chains results in the various Hb tetramers seen during development (Fig. 9.1).

GLOBIN CHAIN STRUCTURE

The analysis of the structure of the individual globin chains was initially at the protein level.

PROTEIN STUDIES

Amino acid sequencing of the various globin polypeptides, carried out in the 1960s by a number of different investigators, showed that the alpha globin chain was 141 amino acids in length whilst the beta chain contained 146 amino acids. The alpha and beta chains were found to have a similar sequence of amino acids but were by no means identical. Analysis of the amino acid

sequence of the delta chain showed it to differ by 10 amino acids from the beta globin chain. Similar analysis of the gamma globin chain showed that it also most closely resembled the beta globin chain, differing by 39 amino acids. In addition, it was found that there were two types of fetal Hb in which the gamma chain contained either the amino acid glycine or alanine at position 136, $^G\gamma$ and $^A\gamma$ respectively. More recently, partial sequence analyses of the zeta and epsilon chains of embryonic Hb suggest the former to be similar in amino acid sequence to the alpha chain, whilst the latter resembles the beta chain.

Thus, it appears that there are two groups of globin chains, the alpha-like and beta-like, all of which seem to be derived from an ancestral primordial Hb gene, which has undergone a number of gene duplications, and to have diverged during the course of evolution.

GLOBIN GENE MAPPING

The first evidence for the arrangement of the various globin structural genes on the human chromosomes was provided by analysis of the Hb electrophoretic variant, Hb Lepore. Comparison of trypsin digests of Hb Lepore with Hb from normal persons, revealed that the alpha chains were normal, whereas the non-alpha chains appeared to consist of an amino terminal delta-like sequence and a carboxy terminal beta-like sequence.

It was therefore proposed that Hb Lepore could represent a 'fusion' globin chain which had arisen as a result of a cross-over occurring coincidentally with mispairing of the delta and beta globin genes during meiosis due to the sequence similarity of the two genes and the close proximity of the delta and beta globin genes on the same chromosome (Fig. 9.2). If this hypothesis was correct, it was argued that there should also be an 'anti-Lepore' Hb, i.e. a beta–delta fusion product in which the non-alpha globin chains contained beta chain residues at the amino terminal end and delta chain residues at the

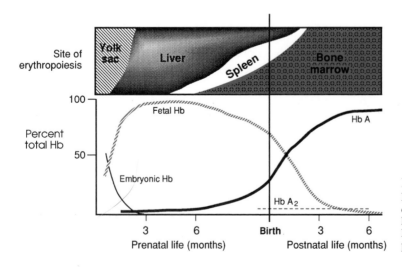

Fig. 9.1
Haemoglobin synthesis during prenatal and postnatal development. There are several embryonic haemoglobins (after Huehns E R, Shooter E M 1965 Human Haemoglobins. J Med Genet 2: 48–90, with permission).

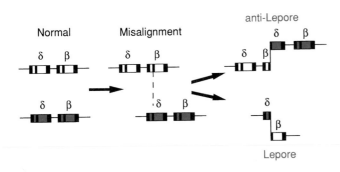

Fig. 9.2
Mechanism of unequal crossing over which generates Hb Lepore and anti-Lepore (adapted from Weatherall & Clegg).

carboxy terminal end. In the late 1960s, a new Hb electrophoretic variant, Hb Miyada, was indeed identified by investigators in Japan in which analysis of trypsin digests showed it to contain a beta chain sequence at the amino terminal end and a delta chain sequence at the carboxy terminal end, as predicted.

Further evidence at the protein level for mapping of the human globin genes was provided by the report of another Hb electrophoretic variant, Hb Kenya. Subsequent analysis of this variant suggested that it was a gamma–beta fusion product with a cross-over having occurred somewhere between amino acids 81 and 86 in the globin chain. It was suggested that, in order for this fusion polypeptide to have occurred, the gamma globin structural gene must also be in close physical proximity to the beta globin gene.

Little evidence was forthcoming from protein studies about the mapping of the alpha globin genes. The presence of normal Hb A in individuals who, by family studies, should have been homozygous for a particular alpha chain variant or obligate compound heterozygotes (p. 81), suggested that there could be more than one alpha globin gene. In addition, the proportion of the total Hb made up by the alpha globin chain variant, in persons heterozygous for those variants, was consistently lower (less than 20%) than that seen with the beta globin chain variants (usually more than 30%), suggesting that there could be more than one alpha globin structural gene.

DNA STUDIES

Detailed information on the structure of the globin genes has been made possible by DNA techniques (p. 53). Immature red blood cells, reticulocytes, provide a ready source of mRNA rich in globin message because they synthesise little else! Use of beta globin cDNA for restriction mapping studies of DNA from normal persons in conjunction with gene mapping studies has revealed that the non-alpha or beta-like globin genes are located in a 50 kilobase stretch on the short arm of chromosome 11 (Fig. 9.3). The whole of this 50 kilobase stretch has been cloned and the nucleotide sequence of each of these structural genes is known. Of particular interest are regions with sequences similar to the globin structural genes but which are non-functional and do not produce an identifiable message or protein product, i.e. pseudogenes (p. 11).

Similar studies of the alpha globin structural genes have revealed that there are, in fact, two alpha globin structural genes, α_1 and α_2 located on chromosome 16 (Fig. 9.3). DNA sequence analysis has revealed differences between these two structural genes even though the alpha globin chains produced have an identical amino acid sequence – further evidence of the 'degeneracy' of the genetic code. In addition, there are pseudo-alpha, pseudo-zeta and zeta genes to the 5' side of the alpha globin genes as well as a recently discovered theta (θ) globin gene to the 3' side of the α1 globin gene. This latter gene, whose function is unknown, is of interest because, unlike the pseudoglobin genes, its structure contains no apparent defects to prevent expression. It has been suggested that it could be expressed in early erythroid tissue such as the fetal liver and yolk sac.

SYNTHESIS AND CONTROL OF HAEMOGLOBIN EXPRESSION

From in vitro translation studies with reticulocyte mRNA from normal persons it is known that alpha and beta globin chains are synthesised in roughly equal proportions. In vitro studies of globin chain synthesis have shown, however, that beta globin mRNA is more

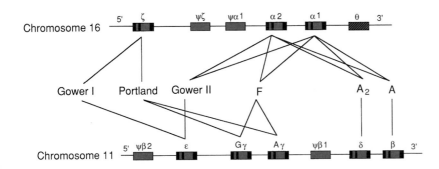

Fig. 9.3
The alpha and beta globin regions on chromosomes 16 and 11 showing the structural genes and pseudogenes (ψ) and the various haemoglobins produced (adapted from Carrell R W & Lehman H 1985 The haemoglobinopathies. In: Dawson A M, Besser G, Compston N (eds) Recent Advances in Medicine 19. Churchill Livingstone, Edinburgh, pp. 223–225).

efficient in protein synthesis than alpha globin mRNA and that this difference is compensated for in the red blood cell precursors by a relative excess of alpha globin mRNA. It seems that the most important level of regulation of expression of the globin genes and possibly other eukaryotic genes is likely to occur at the level of transcription (p. 13).

DISORDERS OF HAEMOGLOBIN STRUCTURE

The disorders of human Hb can be divided into two main groups, structural globin chain variants and disorders of synthesis of the globin chains, the *thalassaemias*.

STRUCTURAL VARIANTS

In 1975, Ingram demonstrated that the difference between Hb A and Hb S lay in the substitution of valine for glutamic acid in the beta globin chain. Since then more than 300 Hb electrophoretic variants have been described. The variety of types of mutations responsible for these

Hb variants is as diverse as those observed in microbial genetics (Table 9.2). Some 200 of these electrophoretic variants are single amino acid substitutions resulting from a point mutation. The majority of these are rare, but a few are polymorphic in certain populations, i.e. occurring in more than 1% of persons.

Types of mutation

Deletion

There are a number of Hb variants in which one or more amino acids of one of the globin chains is missing or deleted.

Insertion

Conversely, there are variants in which the globin chains are longer than normal due to *insertions*.

Frame-shift mutation

Frame-shift mutations involve disruption of the normal triplet reading frame, i.e. addition or removal of a

Table 9.2 Structural variants of haemoglobin [*residues are either added (+) or lost (–)]

Type of mutation	Examples	Chain/residue(s)/alteration
Point (over 200 variants)	Hb S Hb C Hb E	beta, 6 glu to val beta, 6 glu to lys beta, 26 glu to lys
Deletion (shortened chain)	Hb Freiburg Hb Lyon Hb Leiden Hb Gun Hill	beta, 23 to 0 beta, 17–18 to 0 beta, 6 or 7 to 0 beta, 92–96 or 93–97 to 0
Insertion (elongated chain)	Hb Grady	alpha, 116–118 (glu, phe, thr) duplicated
Frameshift (insertion/deletion of other than multiples of 3 base-pairs)	Hb Tak Hb Cranston Hb Wayne	*beta, + 11 residues, loss of termination codon, insertion of 2 base-pairs in codon 146/147 *alpha, + 5 residues, due to loss of termination codon by single base-pair deletion in codon 138/139
Chain termination	Hb Constant Spring Hb McKees Rock	*alpha, + 31 residues, point mutation in termination codon *beta, – 2 residues, point mutation in 145, generating premature termination codon
Fusion chain (unequal crossing-over)	Hb Lepore/anti-Lepore Hb Kenya/anti-Kenya	non-alpha, delta-like residues at N–terminal end and beta-like residues at C–terminal end, vice versa, respectively non-alpha, gamma-like residues at N–terminal end and beta-like residues at C–terminal end, vice versa, respectively

number of bases which are not a multiple of three (p. 17). In this instance, translation of the mRNA continues until a termination codon is read 'in frame'. These variants can result in either an elongated or shortened globin chain.

Point mutation

A point mutation which generates a chain terminating codon (p. 16), results in a shortened globin chain, whereas a mutation in the terminating codon results in an elongated chain.

Fusion polypeptides

The last type of structural variants are the *fusion poly-peptides*, Hbs Lepore and Kenya, which result from unequal cross-over events in meiosis (p. 116).

Clinical aspects

Some of the haemoglobin variants are associated with disease but many are harmless and do not interfere with normal function, having been identified only in the course of electrophoretic surveys of Hb in large populations. A number, however, do interfere in a variety of ways, with the normal function of Hb (Table 9.3). If the mutation is on the inside of the globin subunits, in close proximity to the haem pockets or at the interchain contact areas, this can produce an unstable Hb molecule which precipitates in the red blood cell, damaging the membrane and resulting in haemolysis. Alternatively, mutations can interfere with the normal oxygen transport function of Hb leading either to an enhanced or reduced oxygen affinity or to a Hb which is stable in its reduced form, so-called *methaemoglobin*.

Table 9.3 Functional abnormalities of structural variants of haemoglobin

Clinical features (types)	Example
Haemolytic anaemia	
Sickling disorders	Hb S
	Hb C
	Hb E
Unstable haemoglobin	Hb Köln
	Hb Gun Hill
	Hb Bristol
Cyanosis	
Haemoglobin M (methaemoglobinaemia)	Hb M (Boston)
	Hb M (Hyde Park)
Low O_2 affinity	Hb Kansas
Polycythaemia	
High O_2 affinity	Hb Chesapeake
	Hb Heathrow

The structural variants of Hb identified by electrophoretic techniques probably represent a minority of the total number of variants that exist since it is predicted that only one-third of the possible Hb mutations which could occur will produce an altered charge in the Hb molecule and thereby be detectable by electrophoresis (Fig. 9.4).

SICKLE-CELL DISEASE

Although the severe hereditary haemolytic anaemia, *sickle-cell disease*, was first recognised just after the turn of the century, it was only in 1940 that the red blood cells from persons with sickle-cell disease were noted to appear birefringent when viewed in polarised light under the microscope, as well as to be distorted in shape under

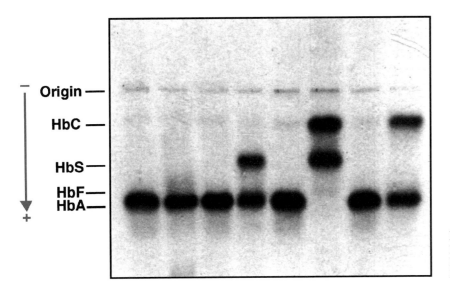

Origin —

HbC —

HbS —

HbF —
HbA —

+

Fig. 9.4
Haemoglobin electrophoresis showing haemoglobin A, C and S (courtesy of Dr D. Norfolk, The General Infirmary at Leeds).

deoxygenated conditions, so-called *sickling* (Fig. 9.5). Pauling, in 1949, analysing Hb from patients with sickle-cell disease by electrophoresis, demonstrated that it had a different mobility when compared to normal Hb, Hb A, and called it Hb S for sickle.

Clinical aspects

Sickle-cell disease is the most common haemo-globinopathy and the clinical manifestations are very numerous including cerebral symptoms, kidney failure, 'pneumonia', heart failure, weakness and lassitude. All of these manifestations can be traced back to the action of the mutant allele. Hb S is less soluble than normal haemoglobin and tends to crystallize out, causing the sickle-shaped deformation of the red cells. Sickle cells are less stable, having a shorter survival time in the circulation, leading to a more rapid red cell turnover with consequent anaemia. In addition the sickle-cells have a reduced deformability tending to obstruct small arteries, resulting in an inadequate oxygen supply to the tissues (Fig. 9.6).

Persons with sickle-cell disease can present acutely unwell with a sudden onset of chest, back, or limb pain, fever and dark urine due to the presence of free haemo-globin in the urine, a so-called *sickle-cell crisis*.

When compared to the general population, persons with sickle-cell disease have an increased risk of early death, although earlier recognition and treatment of the known complications of sickle-cell disease, as well as prophylactic measures, have resulted in improved life expectancy. Some simple measures, such as prophylactic penicillin to prevent the risk of overwhelming sepsis due to splenic infarction, have met with limited success in treating specific complications. It is fair to state that although there is an understanding of the molecular basis of sickle-cell disease, none of the various thera-peutic approaches to prevent the sickling process have had any clear benefit as yet.

SICKLE-CELL TRAIT

The heterozygous or carrier state for the sickle-cell allele is known as *sickle-cell trait* and is not thought, in general, to be associated with any significant risk to health. There are, however, reports suggesting a small risk of sudden death in military recruits after strenuous exercise. In addition, there is continuing controversy about whether there are risks from hypoxia in persons with sickle-cell trait in relation to airplane flights.

Mutational basis

In sickle-cell disease, knowledge of the genetic code (p. 14) suggested that the substitution of valine at the sixth position of the beta globin chain was due to an alteration in the second base of the triplet coding for glutamic acid, i.e. GAG to GTG. Using the restriction

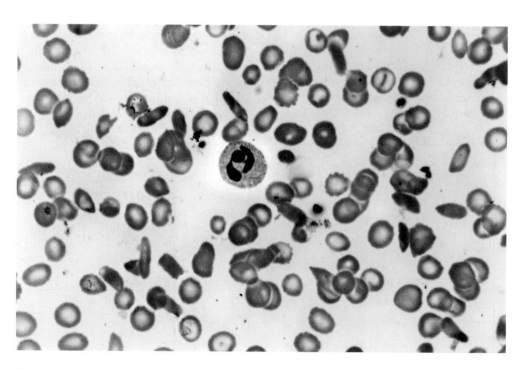

Fig. 9.5
Blood film showing sickling of red cells in sickle-cell disease (courtesy of Dr D. Norfolk, The General Infirmary at Leeds).

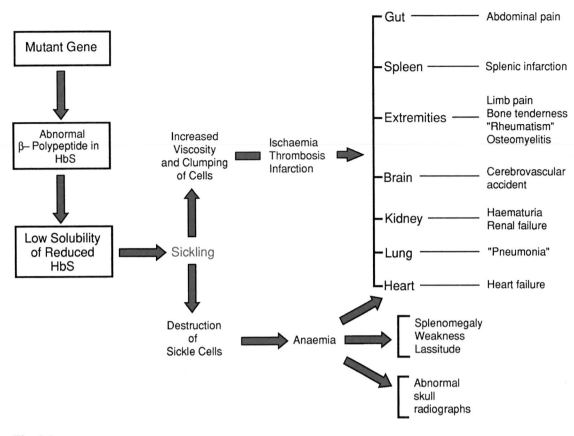

Fig. 9.6
The pleiotropic effects of the gene for sickle-cell disease.

enzyme, Mst II, whose nucleotide recognition sequence is abolished by the point mutation in Hb S, it is possible to demonstrate a difference between persons with sickle-cell disease and normal persons in the restriction fragments when hybridised with a radioactively labelled beta globin probe (Fig. 4.13, p. 54).

This means of identification of a particular mutation is possible with a few other Hb structural variants, e.g. Hb E using the restriction enzymes Hph I or Mn II. It is rare, however, for the mutation in a structural Hb variant to be within the nucleotide recognition sequence of a restriction enzyme (p. 46). Family studies of linked polymorphic DNA sequence variants can be used for carrier testing and prenatal diagnosis of the other haemoglobinopathies (p. 57).

DNA studies of the beta globin genes and flanking regions have revealed that, in addition to promoter sequences in the 5' flanking regions of the various globin genes, there are sequences 6 to 20 kb 5' to the epsilon globin gene necessary for the expression of the various beta-like globin genes. This region has been called the *locus control region, lcr,* and is involved in the timing and tissue specificity of expression or *switching* of the beta-like globin genes in development.

DISORDERS OF HAEMOGLOBIN SYNTHESIS

The *thalassaemias* are the commonest single group of inherited disorders in humans occurring in persons from the Mediterranean area, the Middle East, the Indian subcontinent and South-East Asia. They are a heterogeneous group of disorders and are classified according to the particular globin chain or chains synthesised in reduced amounts, i.e. alpha, beta, delta-beta or gamma-delta-beta thalassaemia.

The pathophysiology is similar in all forms of thalassaemia. An imbalance of globin chain production results in the accumulation of free globin chains in the red blood cell precursors. These are very insoluble and precipitate resulting in the haemolysis of the red blood cells, i.e. a haemolytic anaemia, with consequent compensatory hyperplasia of the bone marrow.

ALPHA THALASSAEMIA

Alpha thalassaemia is due to an underproduction of alpha chains. It occurs most commonly in persons from South-East Asia. There are two main types of alpha thalassaemia which differ in their severity. The severe form, in which no alpha globin chains are produced, is associated with death of the fetus in utero, due to massive oedema as a result of heart failure from the severe in utero anaemia, so-called hydrops fetalis (Fig. 9.7). Analysis of the Hb present reveals it to be a tetramer of gamma globin chains, so-called *Hb Barts*. In the milder form of alpha thalassaemia, although some alpha globin chains are produced, there is still a relative excess of beta globin chains which results in the production of the beta globin tetramer, *Hb H*. Both these tetramers have an oxygen affinity similar to that of myoglobin and do not release oxygen normally in the peripheral tissues. In addition, Hb H is unstable and precipitates, resulting in haemolysis of the red blood cells.

Mutational basis

In vitro translation studies using mRNA from reticulocytes from fetuses with hydrops fetalis show no synthesis of alpha globin. However, when mRNA from reticulocytes of persons with the milder form of alpha thalassaemia, Hb H disease, is used, alpha globin is produced but in reduced amounts when compared to the quantity produced by mRNA from reticulocytes from normal persons. Studies comparing the quantitative hybridisation of radioactively labelled alpha globin cDNA to DNA from fetuses with hydrops fetalis, persons with Hb H disease and normal persons are consistent with this type of thalassaemia being due to deletions of the alpha globin genes. Restriction mapping studies of the alpha globin region of chromosome 16 reveal that there are two alpha globin structural genes on each chromosome 16. The various forms of alpha thalassaemia have been shown to be due to deletions of one or more of these structural genes (Fig. 9.8).

The deletions of the alpha thalassaemia genes are believed to have arisen as a result of unequal cross-over events in meiosis which are thought to be more likely to occur where genes with homologous sequences are in close proximity. Support for this hypothesis comes from the finding of the other product of such an event, i.e. persons with three alpha globin structural genes located on one chromosome.

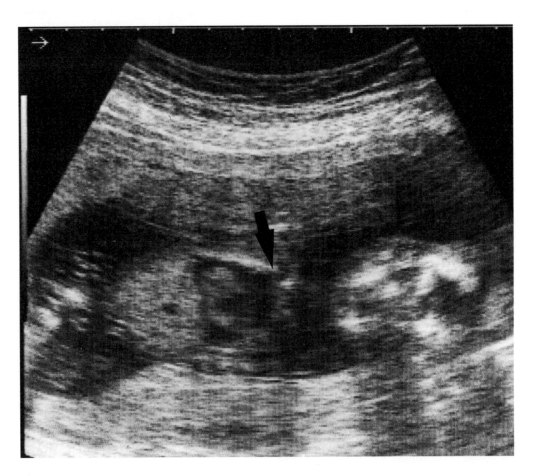

Fig. 9.7
Longitudinal ultrasound scan of a coronal section of the head (to the right) and thorax of a fetus with hydrops fetalis due to the severe form of alpha-thalassaemia, Hb Barts, showing a large pleural effusion (arrowed) (courtesy of Mr J. Campbell, St James's Hospital, Leeds).

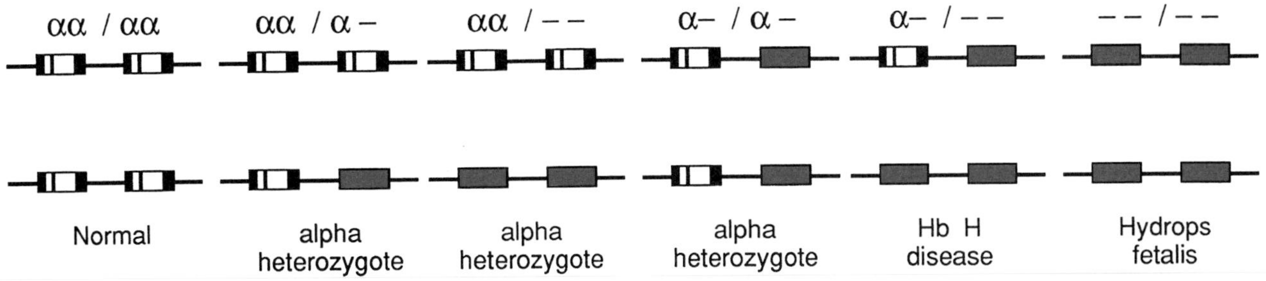

αα / αα   αα / α –   αα / – –   α– / α –   α– / – –   – – / – –

Normal   alpha   alpha   alpha   Hb H   Hydrops
           heterozygote heterozygote heterozygote disease   fetalis

Fig. 9.8
Representation of the structure of the normal ▬█▮█▬ and deleted ▬███▬ alpha-globin structural genes in the various forms of alpha thalassaemia (adapted from Emery, A E H 1984, revised & reprinted 1985. An introduction to recombinant DNA. John Wiley, Chichester).

These observations resulted in the recognition of two other milder forms of alpha thalassaemia not associated with anaemia, which can only be detected by the transient presence in the immediate newborn period of Hb Barts. The results of the DNA mapping studies of the alpha globin genes have shown that these milder forms of alpha thalassaemia are due to the deletion of one or two of the alpha globin genes. Non-deletion forms of alpha thalassaemia have also been found but these are fairly uncommon.

An exception to this classification of the alpha thalassaemias is the Hb variant Constant Spring, named after the town in the USA where the original patient came from. This was detected as an electrophoretic variant in a person with Hb H disease, i.e. alpha thalassaemia. Hb Constant Spring is due to an abnormally long alpha chain which is the result of a mutation in the normal termination codon at position 142 in the alpha globin gene. Translation of this alpha globin mRNA continues until the occurrence of another termination codon, resulting in the abnormally long alpha globin chain variant. In addition, this abnormal alpha globin mRNA molecule is unstable with a consequent relative deficiency of alpha globin chains, resulting in the presence of the beta globin tetramer, Hb H.

BETA THALASSAEMIA

Beta thalassaemia is due to underproduction of the beta globin chain of haemoglobin. In thalassaemia major, or Cooley's anaemia as it was known, the child usually presents in the first year of life with a severe transfusion dependent anaemia. Unless the child is adequately transfused compensatory expansion of the bone marrow results in an unusually-shaped face and skull (Fig. 9.9). Although persons with thalassaemia major used to die in their late teens or early twenties as a result of complications due to iron overload from repeated transfusions, the regular daily use of iron-chelating drugs, such as desferrioxamine has improved their long-term survival.

Mutational basis

Restriction mapping studies have shown that beta thalassaemia is rarely due to a deletion. DNA sequencing has often been necessary to reveal the molecular

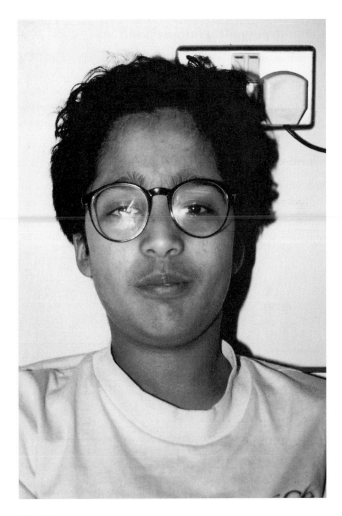

Fig. 9.9
Facies of a child with β thalassaemia showing prominence of the forehead due to changes in skull shape as a result of bone marrow hypertrophy (courtesy of Dr D. Norfolk, The General Infirmary at Leeds).

pathology in beta thalassaemia. A wide variety of different mutations, which include point mutations, insertions and deletions of one or more bases, have been shown to be responsible. These occur at a number of places, both within the coding and non-coding portions of the beta globin genes as well as in the 5′ flanking promoter region, the 5′ capping sequences (p. 15) and the 3′ polyadenylation sequences (p. 15) (Fig. 9.10).

The various types of mutations causing beta thalassaemia are often unique to certain population groups and can be considered to fall into 4 main functional types.

Promoter mutations

Mutations in the 5′ flanking promoter region of the beta globin gene result in reduced transcription levels of the beta globin mRNA, this being proof that they are involved in the control of transcription.

Capping/polyadenylation mutations

Mutations in the 5′ and 3′ DNA sequences, involved respectively in the capping (p. 15) and polyadenylation (p. 15) of the mRNA, can result in abnormal processing and transportation of the beta globin mRNA to the cytoplasm with consequent reduced levels of translation.

Chain termination mutations

Insertions, deletions and point mutations can all generate a nonsense or chain termination codon, resulting in the premature termination of translation of the beta globin

mRNA. This will result in the majority of instances in a shortened beta globin mRNA which is often unstable and rapidly degraded with reduced levels of translation of an abnormal beta globin.

mRNA splicing mutations

Mutations involving the invariant 5′ GT or 3′ AG dinucleotides of the introns in the beta globin gene or the consensus donor or acceptor sequences (p. 15) result in abnormal splicing with consequent reduced levels of beta globin mRNA. In the most common beta thalassaemia mutation in persons from the Mediterranean region, the mutation leads to the creation of a new acceptor AG dinucleotide splice site sequence in the first intron of the beta globin gene creating a so-called *cryptic splice site*. The cryptic splice site competes with the normal splice site leading to reduced levels of the normal beta globin mRNA. Mutations in the coding regions of the beta globin region can also lead to cryptic splice sites.

Clinical aspects

In vitro translation studies using mRNA from persons with beta thalassaemia due to these different types of mutations show either reduced or absent production of beta globin chains, beta$^+$ and beta^0 respectively.

Persons homozygous for beta^0 thalassaemia mutations have a severe transfusion dependent anaemia. Individuals heterozygous for beta thalassaemia have *thalassaemia trait* or *thalassaemia minor* and usually experience no symptoms. They do have, however, a mild hypochromic, microcytic anaemia. Because of the marked mutational

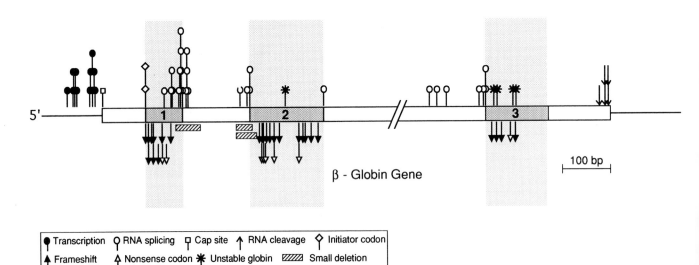

Fig. 9.10
Location and some of the types of mutation in the beta globin gene and flanking region which result in beta thalassaemia (IVS-intervening sequence or intron)(adapted from Orkin S H, Kazazian H H, 1984 The mutation and polymorphism of the human beta-globin gene and its surrounding DNA. In: Roman H L, Campbell A, Sandler L M (eds) Annu Rev Genet 18: 131–171).

heterogeneity seen in beta thalassaemia, affected individuals are often compound heterozygotes (p. 81), i.e. have different mutations in their beta globin genes, leading to a wide range of severity of the disorder. One form of beta thalassaemia of intermediate severity requires less frequent transfusions, and is known as *thalassaemia intermedia*. In addition, due to the prevalence of some of the structural variants of haemoglobins in certain populations, individuals presenting with severe anaemia are found who are heterozygous for both Hb S and beta thalassaemia. In addition, it is also not unusual for individuals from populations in which the haemoglobinopathies are prevalent, to have mutations in both the alpha and beta globin genes, i.e. they represent double heterozygotes (p. 81).

DELTA-BETA THALASSAEMIA

In *delta-beta thalassaemia* there is underproduction of both the delta and beta globin chains. Persons homozygous for delta-beta thalassaemia produce no delta or beta globin chains. Although one would expect such persons to have a fairly profound illness, they are only mildly anaemic, due to increased production of gamma globin chains, with Hb F levels being much higher than the mild compensatory increase seen in homozygotes for beta thalassaemia.

Mutational basis

Delta-beta thalassaemia has been shown to be due to extensive deletions in the beta globin region involving the delta and beta globin structural genes (Fig. 9.11). Some deletions extend to include the $^{A}\gamma$ globin gene so that only the $^{G}\gamma$ globin chain is synthesised.

HEREDITARY PERSISTENCE OF FETAL HAEMOGLOBIN

Hereditary persistence of fetal Hb, HPFH, in which there is persistence of the production of fetal Hb into childhood and adult life is included in the thalassaemias. Most forms of HPFH are, in fact, a form of delta-beta thalassaemia in which continued gamma chain synthesis compensates for the lack of production of delta and beta globin chains. Persons with hereditary persistence of fetal Hb continue to produce significant amounts of fetal Hb after birth accounting for 20–30% of total Hb in heterozygotes and 100% in homozygotes. This is not associated with any medical problems and was originally considered more of a scientific curiosity than anything else.

Mutational basis

Some forms of HPFH have been shown to be due to deletions of the delta and beta globin genes. Analysis of the non-deletion forms of HPFH has shown point mutations in the 5' flanking promoter region of either the Gγ or Aγ globin genes near the CAT box sequences involved in the control of expression of the haemoglobin genes.

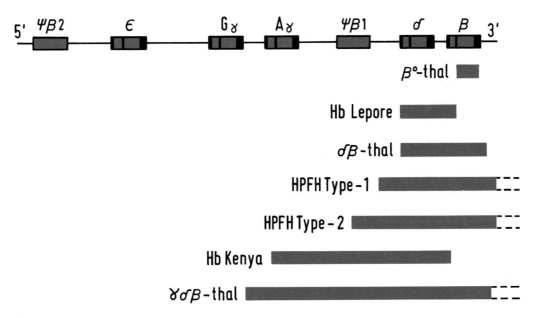

Fig. 9.11
Some of the deletions in the beta globin region which result in some forms of thalassaemia and hereditary persistence of fetal haemoglobin.

CLINICAL VARIATION

Finally, in certain populations many of the haemoglobinopathies are relatively 'common' and, not unexpectedly, persons are reported who have two different disorders of Hb. Understandably, in the past, recognition of such individuals was often quite difficult. Certain combinations of haemoglobinopathies can result in a previously unexplained mild form of what is normally thought to be an invariably severe disease. For example, deletion of one or two of the alpha globin genes in a person homozygous for beta$^+$ thalassaemia results in a milder illness because there is less of an imbalance in globin chain production. Similarly, the presence of one of the forms of HPFH in a person homozygous for beta thalassaemia can contribute to amelioration of the disease as the increased production of gamma globin chains compensates for the deficient beta globin chain production.

ELEMENTS

1 Hb, the protein present in red blood cells responsible for oxygen transport, is a tetramer made up of two dissimilar pairs of polypeptide chains and the iron-containing prosthetic molecule, haem.

2 Human Hb is heterogeneous. During development it comprises a succession of different globin chains which are differentially expressed during embryonic, fetal and adult life, i.e. $\alpha_2\epsilon_2$, $\alpha_2\gamma_2$, $\alpha_2\delta_2$, $\alpha_2\beta_2$, etc.

3 The disorders of Hb, the haemoglobinopathies, can be divided into two main groups, the structural variants, e.g. sickle-cell Hb or Hb S, and disorders of synthesis, the thalassaemias. The former can be subdivided by the way in which they interfere with the normal function of Hb and/or the red blood cell, e.g. abnormal oxygen affinity or haemolytic anaemia. The latter can be subdivided according to which globin chain is synthesised abnormally, i.e. alpha, beta or delta-beta thalassaemia.

4 Family studies of the various disorders of human Hb and analysis of the mutations responsible for these at the protein and DNA level have led to an understanding of the normal structure, function and synthesis of Hb. This has allowed demonstration of the molecular pathology of these disorders and prenatal diagnosis of a number of the inherited disorders of human Hb is possible.

FURTHER READING

Cooley T B, Lee P 1925 A series of cases of splenomegaly in children with anemia and peculiar bone changes. Trans Am Pediat Soc 37: 29–40
The original decription of beta thalassaemia.
Kazazian H H 1990 The thalassaemia syndromes. Molecular basis and prenatal diagnosis in 1990. In: Miescher L A, Jaffe E R (eds) Seminars in Haematology 27:3, Saunders, London, pp. 209–228
A good review of the molecular basis of the thalassemia syndromes.
Pauling L, Itano H A, Singer S J, Wells I C 1949 Sickle-cell anaemia, a molecular disease. Science 110: 543–548
The first genetic disease in which a molecular basis was described, leading to a Nobel prize.
Serjeant G R 1992 Sickle cell disease, 2nd edn. Oxford University Press, Oxford
Excellent comprehensive text covering all aspects of this important disorder.
Stamatoyannopoulos G, Nienhuis A W, Leder P, Majerus F W (eds) 1987 The molecular basis of blood diseases. Saunders, Philadelphia
A textbook which covers the molecular basis of haematology in general.
Weatherall D J, Clegg J B 1981 The thalassaemia syndromes. Blackwell Scientific Publications, Oxford
Detailed clinical information along with good historical information about the discovery of the genetics of the disorders of haemoglobin. A new edition would be welcome.

CHAPTER 10

Biochemical genetics

In previous chapters the biochemistry and mode of action of genes have been considered at the DNA level. In this chapter we shall consider the more 'peripheral' biochemical effects of gene action.

Garrod at the beginning of the century introduced the concept of 'chemical individuality', leading to the concept of the *inborn error of metabolism*. Beadle and Tatum later developed the idea that metabolic processes, whether in humans or any other organism, proceed by steps. They proposed that each step was controlled by a particular enzyme and that this, in turn, was the product of a particular gene. This was referred to as the *one gene–one enzyme* concept.

THE INBORN ERRORS OF METABOLISM

In excess of 200 inborn errors of metabolism are known and the characteristics of a number of these are summarised in Table 10.1. They can be grouped either by the metabolite, metabolic pathway, function of the enzyme or cellular organelle involved.

Most inborn errors of metabolism are inherited in an autosomal recessive or X-linked manner with only a few being inherited in an autosomal dominant manner. This is because the defective protein in most inborn errors is an enzyme which is diffusible and there is sufficient residual activity in the heterozygous state for it to function as normal in most situations. If, however, the reaction catalysed by an enzyme is rate-limiting or the gene product acts as an inhibitor of other reactions, the disorder can manifest in the heterozygous state, i.e. be dominantly inherited.

DISORDERS OF AMINO ACID METABOLISM

PHENYLKETONURIA

Children with phenylketonuria (PKU), if untreated, are severely mentally retarded, frequently have convulsions, and in the past were often placed in institutional care. In these children, the particular enzyme necessary for the conversion of phenylalanine to tyrosine, phenylalanine hydroxylase (PAH) is deficient; that is, there is a 'genetic block' in the metabolic pathway (Fig. 10.1). This was, in fact, the first genetic disorder in humans shown to be due to a specific enzyme defect by Jervis in 1953. As a result of the enzyme defect, phenylalanine accumulates and some is converted into phenylpyruvic acid and other metabolites which are excreted in the urine. The enzyme block leads to a deficiency of tyrosine with a consequent reduction in melanin formation. Affected children therefore often have blond hair and blue eyes (Fig. 10.2) and areas of the brain which are usually pigmented, e.g. the substantia nigra, can also lack pigment.

Treatment

An obvious method for treating children with PKU would be to give the missing enzyme but this cannot be done simply by any conventional means of treatment (p. 277). Bickel, only a year after the enzyme deficiency had been identified, suggested that phenylalanine could be removed from the diet, which has proved to be an effective treatment. If PKU is detected early enough in childhood, mental retardation can be prevented by giving a diet containing a restricted amount of phenylalanine. Phenylalanine is, however, an essential amino acid and therefore cannot be entirely removed from the diet. By monitoring the level of phenylalanine in the blood, it is possible to supply sufficient amounts to meet normal requirements and avoid levels which result in mental retardation.

It is felt that the mental retardation seen in children with phenylketonuria is most likely due to an elevation of phenylalanine and/or its metabolites rather than a deficiency of tyrosine, since an adequate amount of the latter amino acid is available in a normal diet. It has been suggested that the reduced ability of the mother of a child with PKU, who will be an obligate heterozygote, to deliver an appropriate amount of tyrosine to her fetus in utero could result in reduced fetal brain growth. It could well be that there are both prenatal as well as postnatal factors responsible for the mental retardation in persons

Table 10.1 Characteristics of some inborn errors of metabolism (AR and AD = autosomal recessive or dominant. XR and XD = X-linked recessive or dominant)

Type of defect	Genetics	Deficient enzyme	Main clinical features
Amino acid metabolism			
Oculocutaneous albinism	AR	tyrosinase	lack of skin and pigment, eye defects
Alkaptonuria	AR	homogentisic acid oxidase	arthritis
Homocystinuria	AR	Cystathione β-synthetase	mental retardation, dislocation of lens, thrombosis, skeletal abnormalities
Maple syrup urine disease	AR	branched chain alpha-ketoacid decarboxylase	mental retardation
Phenylketonuria	AR	phenylalanine hydroxylase	mental retardation, fair skin, eczema, epilepsy
Amino acid transport			
Cystinuria	AR	renal transport defect of cystine	kidney stones
Urea cycle disorders			
Ornithine transcarbamylase deficiency	XD	ornithine carbamyl transferase	hyperammonaemia, death in early infancy
Carbohydrate metabolism			
Galactosaemia	AR	Galactose-1-phosphate uridyl transferase	cataracts, mental retardation, cirrhosis
Glycogen storage diseases			
McArdle's disease	AR	muscle phosphorylase	muscle cramps
Pompe's disease	AR	lysosomal α-1,4 glucosidase	heart failure, muscle weakness
Steroid metabolism			
Congenital adrenal hyperplasia	AR	21-hydroxylase, 11 β-hydroxylase, 3 β-dehydrogenase	virilisation, salt-loss
Testicular feminisation	XR	androgen binding protein	female external genitalia, male internal genitalia, male chromosomes
Lipoprotein metabolism			
Familial hypercholesterolaemia	AD	low-density lipoprotein receptor	early coronary artery disease
Lysosomal storage diseases			
Mucopolysaccharidoses			
Hunter's syndrome	XR	sulphoiduronate sulphatase	mental retardation, skeletal abnormalities, hepatosplenomegaly
Hurler's syndrome	AR	iduronidase	as Hunter's syndrome, plus corneal clouding
Sphingolipidoses			
Tay–Sachs disease	AR	Hexosaminidase-A	mental retardation, blindness, deafness
Gaucher's disease	AR	β-glucosidase	joint and limb pains, splenomegaly
Purine/pyrimidine metabolism			
Lesch–Nyhan disease	XR	hypoxanthine guanine phosphoribosyl transferase	mental retardation, uncontrolled movements, self-mutilation

Type of defect	Genetics	Deficient enzyme	Main clinical features
Porphyrin metabolism			
Hepatic porphyrias			
Acute intermittent porphyria (AIP)	AD	uroporphyrinogen I synthetase	abdominal pain, CNS effects
Hereditary coproporphyria	AD	coproporphyrinogen oxidase	as for AIP, photosensitivity
Porphyria variegata	AD	?	photosensitivity, as for AIP
Eythropoietic porphyrias			
Congenital erythropoietic porphyria	AR	?	haemolytic anaemia, photosensitivity
Organic acid disorders			
Methylmalonic acidaemia	AR	methylmalonyl-CoA mutase	hypotonia, poor feeding, developmental delay
Propionic acidaemia	AR	propionyl-CoA carboxylase	poor feeding, failure to thrive, vomiting, acidosis, hypoglycaemia
Copper metabolism			
Wilson's disease	AR	?	spasticity, rigidity, dysphagia, cirrhosis
Menkes' disease	XR	?	failure to thrive, neurological deterioration
Thyroid hormone biosynthesis			
Congenital hypothyroidism (dyshormonogenesis)	AR	dehalogenase, peroxidase	mental retardation
Peroxisomal disorders			
Zellweger's syndrome	AR	all peroxisomal enzymes	dysmorphic features, hypotonia, large liver, renal cysts
Adrenoleukodystrophy	XR	very long chain fatty acid-CoA synthetase	mental deterioration, fits, behavioural changes, adrenal failure
Miscellaneous			
α_1-antitrypsin deficiency	AR	α_1-antitrypsin	pulmonary emphysema, liver cirrhosis
Hereditary angioneurotic oedema	AD	C1 inhibitor	recurrent swelling of skin, throat, gut
Vitamin D-resistant rickets	XD	renal defect of phosphate reabsorption	rickets

with untreated PKU. The reports of children born to phenylketonuric mothers having an increased risk of mental retardation even when their mothers are on closely controlled dietary restriction provides further support for this concept (p. 203).

Diagnosis

PKU can be screened for by tests which detect the presence of the metabolite of phenylalanine, phenylpyruvic acid, in the urine by its reaction with ferric chloride or through elevated levels of phenylalanine in the blood in the Guthrie test. The latter test involves taking blood samples from children in the first week of life and comparing the amount of growth induced by the sample with standards in a strain of the bacteria *Bacillus*

subtilis which requires phenylalanine for growth. This technique has been replaced in most centres by use of direct fluorescent or immunological assays of phenylalanine levels.

Heterogeneity of phenylketonuria

Not all infants with elevated phenylalanine levels in the newborn period have PKU. A small percentage of newborn infants have a benign condition called hyperphenylalaninaemia and do not require treatment as they are not at risk of developing mental retardation. In some infants this is due to a transient inability of liver cells to metabolise phenylalanine; in others the levels remain elevated. It appears that the latter group have lower than normal levels of phenylalanine hydroxylase activity but

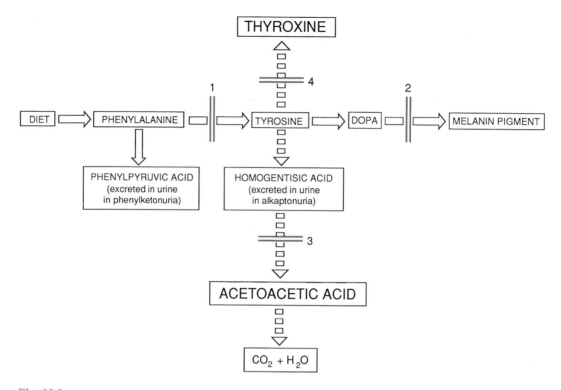

Fig. 10.1
Diagram indicating the sites of 'biochemical block' in (1) phenylketonuria, (2) albinism, (3) alkaptonuria and (4) congenital thyroxine deficiency (dyshormonogenesis).

have a low risk of developing mental retardation for reasons that are not clear.

The situation is made more complicated by the fact that there are also two rare variants of PKU in which the deficient enzyme is not phenylalanine hydroxylase but dihydropteridine reductase or dihydrobiopterin synthetase, two enzymes involved in the synthesis of tetra-hydrobiopterin, a cofactor of phenylalanine hydroxylase. Both disorders are more serious than classical PKU because there is a high likelihood of developing mental handicap despite satisfactory management of phenylalanine levels.

Mutational basis

Although all cases of classical PKU are due to a deficiency of phenylalanine hydroxylase, many different mutations of the PAH gene have now been identified (p. 59), most of which involve base substitutions in exons. Furthermore, at least 46 distinct RFLP haplotypes (p. 58) have been identified in association with these mutations, although four of these account for over 80% of PKU mutations in persons of Western European origin. Direct mutation identification or RFLP haplotype analysis provides a means of diagnosing PKU prenatally (p. 261).

ALKAPTONURIA

Alkaptonuria was the original inborn error of metabolism described by Garrod. In alkaptonuria there is a block in the breakdown of homogentisic acid, a metabolite of tyrosine (Fig. 10.1). As a consequence, homogentisic acid accumulates and is excreted in the urine, to which it imparts a dark colour on exposure to air (Plate 10). Dark pigment is also deposited in certain tissues such as the cartilage of ears (Plate 11) and joints, or what is known as ochronosis, which in the latter location can lead to arthritis later in life.

OCULOCUTANEOUS ALBINISM

Oculocutaneous albinism (OCA) involves the failure to synthesise the enzyme tyrosinase, which is necessary for the formation of melanin pigment from tyrosine (Fig. 10.1). In persons with OCA there is a lack of pigment in the skin, hair, iris and ocular fundus (Fig. 10.3). The lack of pigment in the eye, for reasons not totally clear, results in serious visual problems with very poor visual acuity and typical uncontrolled pendular eye movement (nystagmus).

Oculocutaneous albinism is biochemically heterogeneous. Cells from persons with classical albinism have no

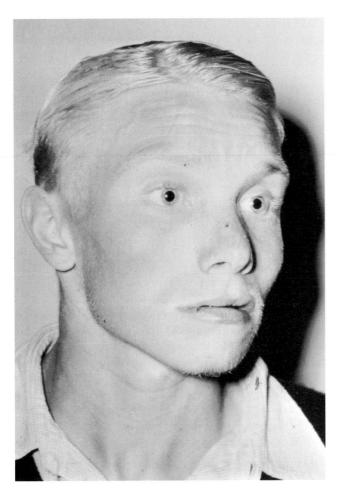

Fig. 10.2
Facies of a male with phenylketonuria; note the fair complexion.

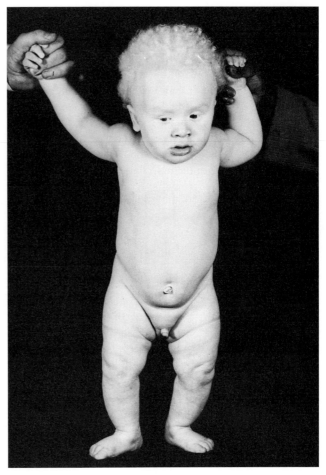

Fig. 10.3
Albinism in a child of Afro-Caribbean origin (by courtesy of Dr V.A. McKusick).

measurable tyrosinase activity, this being the so-called tyrosinase-negative form. However, cells from some persons with albinism show residual tyrosinase activity and are termed tyrosinase-positive. This is usually reflected clinically by variable development of pigmentation of hair and skin with age.

DNA studies have revealed the situation to be even more complex. The defect in classical tyrosinase-negative and some tyrosinase-positive families with oculocutaneous albinism has been shown to be due to mutations in the tyrosinase gene on the long arm of chromosome 11. Some of the families with tyrosinase-positive oculocutaneous albinism, however, have been shown *not* to be linked to that locus. A number of these families, interestingly, have a mutation in the P gene, the human homologue of a gene in the mouse called *pink-eyed dilution*, or pink-eye for short, located on the long arm of chromosome 15. In addition, a proportion of families with oculocutaneous albinism have been shown not to be linked to either of these two loci.

HOMOCYSTINURIA

Homocystinuria is an inborn error of sulphur amino acid metabolism characterised by mental retardation, fits, thrombotic episodes, osteoporosis and a tendency to dislocation of the lenses. It is due to a deficiency of the enzyme cystathionine β-synthetase. The disorder can be screened for by means of a positive cyanide nitro-prusside test which detects the presence of increased levels of homocystine in the urine. The diagnosis is confirmed by plasma amino acid analysis showing elevated homo-cystine levels and fibroblast cultures exhibiting reduced enzyme activity. Treatment involves a low methionine diet with cystine supplementation. A proportion of affected persons are responsive to the cofactor, vitamin B6, pyridoxine.

MAPLE SYRUP URINE DISEASE

Newborn infants with this disorder present in the first week of life with vomiting, then alternating decreased and increased tone proceeding on to death within a few weeks if left untreated. There is a characteristic odour of the urine likened to the smell of maple syrup. The disorder is due to a deficiency of the branched chain ketoacid decarboxylase producing increased excretion of the branched chain amino acids valine, leucine and isoleucine in the urine. The diagnosis is suggested by the presence of these amino acids in the urine and blood and is confirmed by demonstration of the enzyme deficiency in white blood cells. Treatment involves a diet limiting the intake of the 3 branched chain amino acids to the amount necessary for growth.

DISORDERS OF AMINO ACID TRANSPORT

CYSTINURIA

Persons with cystinuria present with symptoms due to kidney stones which can occur at different ages and which often, although not invariably, consist of cystine. The disorder is due to an excessive loss in the urine of the four dibasic amino acids, cystine, lysine, ornithine and arginine due to their reduced reabsorption in the renal tubules. Treatment is with D-penicillamine which reacts with cystine, the product being more soluble than free cystine. Although D-penicillamine has revolutionised treatment, it is not without the risk of side-effects as many persons are hypersensitive to it and it can also cause kidney damage.

UREA CYCLE DISORDERS

The urea cycle is a five-step metabolic pathway which takes place in liver cells for the removal of waste nitrogen from the amino groups of amino acids arising from the turnover of protein and DNA. It converts two molecules of ammonia and one of bicarbonate into urea. Deficiencies of enzymes in the urea cycle result in intolerance to protein due to the accumulation of ammonia in the body, or what is known as hyperammonaemia. This is deleterious to the central nervous system resulting in coma and, with some of the urea cycle disorders, death.

ORNITHINE TRANSCARBAMYLASE DEFICIENCY

Ornithine transcarbamylase deficiency is an X-linked dominant disorder in which affected hemizygous male infants present in the newborn period with poor feeding and lethargy which rapidly progresses to coma and death usually within the first month. Normal protein turnover results in marked hyperammonaemia which cannot be controlled except in the occasional affected male with a partial deficiency of the enzyme. Heterozygous females have a variable course depending on X-inactivation (p. 72) but often have protein intolerance.

DISORDERS OF CARBOHYDRATE METABOLISM

GALACTOSAEMIA

Newborn infants with galactosaemia present with vomiting, lethargy, failure to thrive and jaundice in the second week of life. If untreated, they go on to develop complications which include severe mental retardation, cataracts and cirrhosis of the liver. Galactosaemia can be screened for by the presence of reducing substances in the urine which can be confirmed on further testing to be galactose. A definitive diagnosis of galactosaemia is achieved by demonstration of a deficiency of the enzyme galactose-l-phosphate uridyl transferase, necessary for the metabolism of the sugar, galactose. The complications of galactosaemia can be prevented by feeding affected infants commercially available milk substitutes which do not contain galactose or lactose, the sugar found in milk which is broken down into galactose. Early diagnosis and treatment are essential if the severe complications are to be prevented.

GLYCOGEN STORAGE DISEASES

In this group of disorders glycogen accumulates in excessive amounts in skeletal muscle, cardiac muscle and liver. In addition, because of the metabolic block, glycogen is unavailable as a normal glucose source. This can result in hypoglycaemia, impairment of liver function and neurological abnormalities. In each of the eleven recognised different types of glycogen storage disease there is a specific enzyme defect involving one of the steps in the complex metabolic pathways of glycogen synthesis or degradation. The various types differ in which systems of the body glycogen accumulates and whether the structure of the glycogen produced is normal or not.

McArdle's disease

Persons with this disorder can present with muscle cramps on exercise or weakness in the teenage years. It is due to a deficiency of the glycogen phosphorylase specific to muscle. There is no effective form of treatment although the muscle cramps tend to decline if the exercise is continued, probably due to other energy sources becoming available from alternative metabolic pathways.

Pompe's disease

Infants with this disorder usually present in the first few months of life with hypotonia and delay of gross motor milestones due to muscle weakness. They develop an enlarged heart and will often die of cardiac failure by the age of 1 year. Voluntary and cardiac muscle is full of glycogen which accumulates due to the deficiency of the lysozomal enzyme α-glucosidase needed to break down glycogen. The diagnosis can be confirmed by enzyme assay on white blood cells or fibroblasts. The disorder is untreatable.

DISORDERS OF STEROID METABOLISM

There are a number of disorders of steroid metabolism which can lead to virilization of a female fetus due to a block in the biosynthetic pathways of cortisol as well as a disorder of salt loss due to deficiency of aldosterone (Fig 10.4).

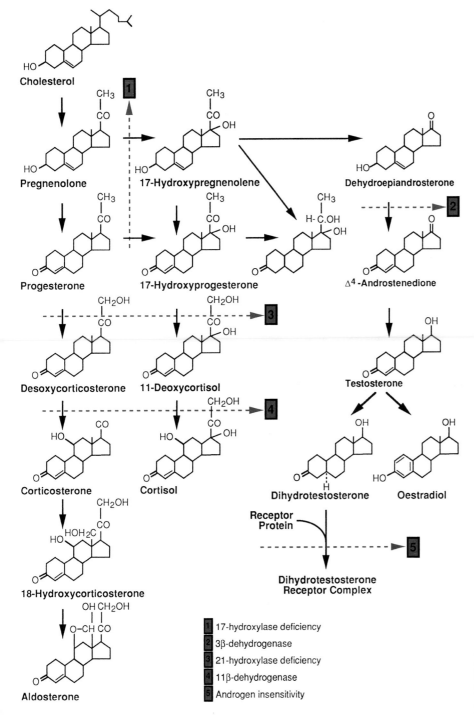

1 17-hydroxylase deficiency
2 3β-dehydrogenase
3 21-hydroxylase deficiency
4 11β-dehydrogenase
5 Androgen insensitivity

Fig. 10.4
Steroid biosynthesis indicating the sites of the common inborn errors of steroid biosynthesis (adapted from Benson and Fensom).

CONGENITAL ADRENAL HYPERPLASIA

The diagnosis of congenital adrenal hyperplasia should be considered in any newborn female infant presenting with virilization of the external genitalia (p. 226) (Fig. 10.5). It should not be forgotten, however, that males can also be affected. This is particularly important since approximately two-thirds of infants with the most common form of the adrenogenital syndrome due to 21-hydroxylase deficiency will also be salt losing. These infants can present in the second week of life with circulatory collapse.

The virilization in affected females is due to an accumulation of the adrenocortical steroids proximal to the enzyme block in the steroid biosynthetic pathway, many of which have testosterone-like activity (Fig. 10.4). Affected infants are treated with replacement cortisol along with fludrocortisone if they are also salt losing. Steroid replacement is lifelong and needs to be increased during intercurrent illness or times of stress, e.g. for surgery.

The commonest cause of the adrenogenital syndrome is deficiency of the enzyme 21-hydroxylase which accounts for 90% of cases in Western Europe. Congenital adrenal hyperplasia is less commonly due to deficiency of the enzymes 11 β-hydroxylase or 3 β-dehydrogenase and very rarely occurs as a result of an enzyme deficiency in another part of the steroid metabolic pathway.

TESTICULAR FEMINISATION

Individuals with testicular feminisation have normal female external genitalia, and undergo breast development in puberty (p. 226). They classically present either with primary amenorrhoea, which is lack of onset of menstrual periods, or with an inguinal hernia containing a gonad which turns out to be a testis. There is often scanty secondary sexual hair and examination of the internal genitalia reveals the uterus and fallopian tubes to be absent. Androgen production by the testes is normal but skin fibroblasts from affected individuals do not bind androgen normally due to abnormal androgen receptors (Fig. 10.4). Affected individuals usually have a female sexual orientation but obviously will be sterile. They require removal of their testes because of an increased risk of developing a testicular malignancy and should be placed on oestrogen for secondary sexual development and to prevent osteoporosis in the longer term.

LIPOPROTEIN METABOLISM

FAMILIAL HYPERCHOLESTEROLAEMIA

Familial hypercholesterolaemia (FH), the commonest single gene disorder in Western society, is one of the few

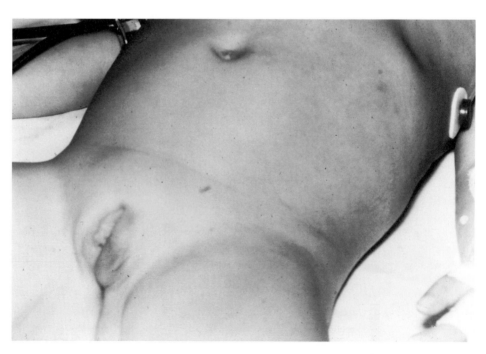

Fig. 10.5
Virilized external genitalia in a female with congenital adrenal hyperplasia.

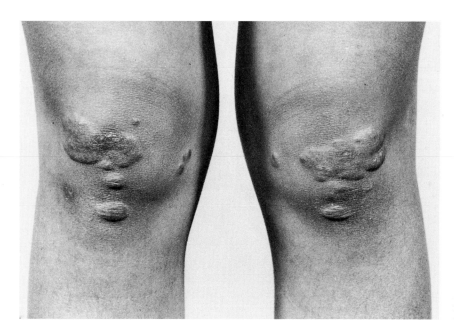

Fig. 10.6
Legs of a person homozygous for familial hypercholesterolaemia, showing multiple xanthomata (courtesy of Dr E. Wraith, Royal Manchester Children's Hospital, Manchester).

inborn errors inherited as an autosomal dominant trait. Persons with this disorder have elevated cholesterol levels and have a significant risk of developing early coronary artery disease (p. 188). In addition, persons with familial hypercholesterolaemia can present with subcutaneous deposition of lipid, known as *xanthomata* (Fig. 10.6). Starting with families who presented with early coronary artery disease, Brown and Goldstein unravelled the biology of the low density lipoprotein receptor (p. 7).

Cells normally derive their cholesterol from either endogenous cholesterol synthesis or by uptake of dietary cholesterol from the plasma via low density lipoprotein receptors on the cell surface. Intracellular cholesterol levels are maintained by free cholesterol inhibiting LDL receptor synthesis as well as reducing the level of de novo endogenous cholesterol synthesis.

The high cholesterol levels in persons with FH are due to high levels of low density lipoprotein as a consequence of deficient or defective function of the low-density lipoprotein receptors. Four main functional types or classes of mutation in the low density lipoprotein receptor have been identified; reduced or defective biosynthesis of the receptor, reduced or defective transport of the receptor from the endoplasmic reticulum to the Golgi apparatus, abnormal binding of the low density lipoprotein by the receptor and abnormal internalization of the low density lipoprotein by the receptor (Fig. 10.7).

Dietary restriction and drug treatment with agents such as cholestyramine, which sequesters cholesterol from the enterohepatic circulation, can lower cholesterol levels and, it is hoped, in the longer term reduce the risk of coronary artery disease. The recent detailed elucidation of the metabolic and biosynthetic pathways of cholesterol

has provided further therapeutic measures which involve blocking the secondary endogenous synthesis of cholesterol. It is hoped that these will be more effective than existing measures.

LYSOSOMAL STORAGE DISORDERS

In addition to the inborn errors of metabolism, in which an enzyme defect leads to deficiency of an essential metabolite and accumulation of intermediate metabolic precursors, there are a number of disorders in which a deficiency in one of the lysosomal enzymes involved in the degradation of complex macromolecules, such as the proteoglycans, leads to their accumulation. This accumulation occurs because macromolecules are normally in a constant state of flux with a delicate balance between their rates of synthesis and breakdown. Children born with this type of disorder are usually normal at birth but with the passage of time commence a downhill course of differing duration.

MUCOPOLYSACCHARIDOSES

Individuals with one of this group of disorders present with problems in their skeletal, vascular and often central nervous systems along with coarsening of the facial features. This is due to progressive accumulation of sulphated polysaccharides (also known as glycosaminoglycans) caused by defective degradation of the carbohydrate side chain of acid mucopolysaccharide. Twelve different mucopolysaccharidoses have now been recognised, based on clinical and genetic differences. Each type of mucopolysaccharidosis has a characteristic

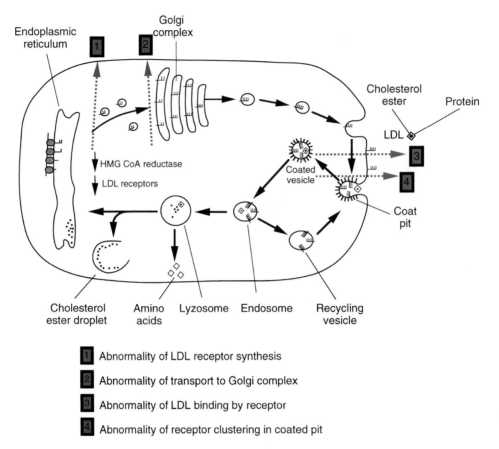

1 Abnormality of LDL receptor synthesis

2 Abnormality of transport to Golgi complex

3 Abnormality of LDL binding by receptor

4 Abnormality of receptor clustering in coated pit

Fig. 10.7
A diagram of the stages in cholesterol biosynthesis and in the metabolism of low density lipoprotein receptors indicating the type of mutations in familial hypercholesterolaemia (adapted from Brown M S, Goldstein J L 1986 A receptor-mediated pathway for cholesterol homeostasis. Science 232: 34–47).

pattern of excretion in the urine of the glycosamino-glycans, dermatan, heparan, keratan and chondroitin sulphate. Subsequent biochemical investigation has revealed the various types to be due to different enzyme deficiencies.

Hunter's syndrome

Males with this X-linked recessive disorder usually present between the ages of 2 to 5 years with hearing loss, a history of recurrent infection, diarrhoea and poor growth. Examination reveals a characteristic coarsening of their facial features (Fig. 10.8), along with enlargement of their liver and spleen and stiffness of their joints. X-rays of the spine reveal abnormalities in the shape of the vertebrae. There is progressive physical and mental deterioration with death usually in the teenage years.

The diagnosis can be confirmed by the presence of excess amounts of dermatan and heparan sulphate in the urine and deficient or decreased activity of the enzyme sulphoiduronate sulphatase in serum, white blood cells or fibroblasts.

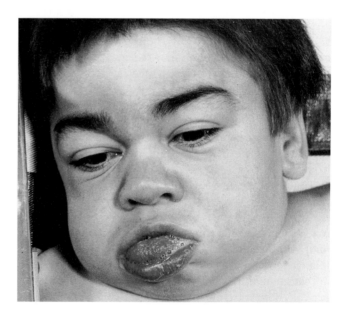

Fig. 10.8
Facies of a male with the mucopolysaccharidosis, Hunter's syndrome (courtesy of Dr E. Wraith, Royal Manchester Children's Hospital, Manchester).

Hurler's syndrome

This is the most severe of the mucopolysaccharidoses. Affected infants present in the first year with progressive corneal clouding, a characteristic curvature of the lower spine and subsequent poor growth. They develop hearing loss, coarse facial features, an enlarged liver and spleen, joint stiffness and vertebral changes in the second year. There is progression of these features along with mental handicap and death from a combination of cardiac failure and respiratory infections by the age of 10 years.

The diagnosis of the Hurler syndrome was initially made by demonstration of the presence of metachromatic granules in the cells, i.e. lysosomes distended by the storage material which is primarily dermatan sulphate. Increased urinary excretion of dermatan and heparan sulphate is commonly used as a screening test but confirmation of the diagnosis involves demonstration of the reduced activity of the lysosomal hydrolase α-L-iduronidase.

Treatment of the mucopolysaccharidoses has been attempted by enzyme replacement but there are a number of practical difficulties which have been responsible for its lack of success (p. 277). More recently, however, bone marrow transplantation has been attempted with varying reports of success biochemically and clinically as far as the skeletal and cerebral features are concerned (p. 278).

SPHINGOLIPIDOSES

In this group of disorders there is an inability to degrade sphingolipid, resulting in the progressive deposition of this material primarily in the brain, liver and spleen. Central nervous system involvement results in progressive mental deterioration, often with fits, resulting in death in childhood. There are at least ten different types with specific enzyme deficiencies.

Tay–Sachs disease

This is the best known sphingolipidosis and occurs most commonly in persons of Ashkenazi-Jewish extraction (p. 97). Affected infants usually present by 6 months of age with poor feeding, lethargy and floppiness. Loss of developmental milestones or developmental regression will usually become apparent in the second half of the first year. Feeding becomes increasingly difficult and the infant progressively deteriorates with deafness, visual impairment and spasticity proceeding to rigidity. Death usually occurs by the age of 3 years due to respiratory infection.

The diagnosis can be confirmed clinically by the presence of a 'cherry-red' spot in the centre of the macula of the fundus with biochemical confirmation of reduced hexosaminidase-A levels in serum, white blood cells or cultured fibroblasts.

Gaucher's disease

This is the commonest sphingolipidosis, and like Tay–Sachs disease, it occurs with an increased frequency amongst persons of Ashkenazi-Jewish ancestry. There are two main types based on the age of onset. In Type I, or the adult type of Gaucher's disease, affected persons present with febrile episodes with limb, joint or trunk pain. Clinical examination usually reveals an enlarged spleen and liver. Affected persons often show mild anaemia, a tendency to pathologic fractures, an arthropathy of the hip joint and X-ray changes in the vertebral bodies and proximal femora.

In type II, or infantile, Gaucher's disease infants usually present at 3 to 6 months of age with failure to thrive and hepatosplenomegaly. By 6 months of age they begin to show developmental regression and neurological deterioration with fits leading on to recurrent pulmonary infection and death in the second year.

The diagnosis of Gaucher's disease can be confirmed by reduced activity of the enzyme β-glucosidase in white blood cells and cultured fibroblasts. Treatment of individuals with the adult type of Gaucher's disease involves symptomatic relief of pain. In addition, it is often necessary to remove the enlarged spleen because it will often cause a secondary anaemia due to premature sequestering of red blood cells, a condition known as hypersplenism.

Attempts to treat persons with Gaucher's disease by enzyme replacement therapy (p. 278) have met with little success. However, modification of β-glucosidase by the addition of mannose-6-phosphate targets the enzyme to the lysosome where it can be functional. Treatment with this form of glucocerebrosidase has led to dramatic alleviation of symptoms and regression of the organomegaly in persons with the adult form of Gaucher's disease. The treatment is, however, expensive and other forms of therapy are being pursued.

PURINE/PYRIMIDINE METABOLISM

Gout is the disorder in humans which is classically associated with abnormalities of purine or pyrimidine metabolism. Joint pain, swelling and tenderness are a result of the inflammatory response of the body to deposits of crystals of a salt of uric acid. In fact, only in a minority of persons who present with gout is an inborn error of metabolism responsible. The most common cause is a combination of genetic and environmental factors. However, it is always important to consider disorders which can result in an increased turnover of purines (e.g.

a malignancy such as leukaemia) or reduced secretion of the metabolites (e.g. renal impairment) as a possible underlying precipitating cause.

LESCH–NYHAN SYNDROME

A particularly disabling disorder of purine metabolism is Lesch–Nyhan syndrome. This X-linked disorder is due to the deficiency of the enzyme hypoxanthine guanine phosphoribosyl transferase which results in increased levels of phosphoribosylpyrophosphate. The latter is normally a rate-limiting chemical in the synthesis of purines. Its excess leads to an increased rate of purine synthesis which results in an accumulation of excessive amounts of uric acid and some of its metabolic precursors. The main effect of this in the severe deficiency state is on the central nervous system, resulting in uncontrolled movements, spasticity, mental retardation and compulsive self-mutilation. Although drugs such as allopurinol, which inhibit uric acid formation, can lower uric acid levels, none yet offers any satisfactory treatment for the debilitating central nervous system effects.

PORPHYRIN METABOLISM

There are several different types of porphyria. These are due to abnormalities in the metabolism of porphyrins involved in the biosynthesis of haem. They are divided into two types depending on whether the excess production of porphyrins occurs predominantly in the liver or in the erythropoietic system.

HEPATIC PORPHYRIAS

Acute intermittent porphyria

Acute intermittent porphyria is characterised by attacks of abdominal pain, vomiting and mental disturbance in the form of confusion, emotional upset or hallucinations. Attacks can be precipitated by the administration of certain drugs. It is caused by a partial deficiency of the enzyme uroporphyrinogen I synthetase leading to increased excretion of the porphyrin precursors porphobilinogen and δ-aminolevulinic acid in urine. The step in the metabolic pathway of porphyrin involving this enzyme is rate-limiting so that even a partial deficiency results in clinical disease, particularly when stressed, or when certain drugs such as barbiturates are taken.

Hereditary coproporphyria

In hereditary coproporphyria, a related condition, also inherited as a dominant trait, there is a partial deficiency

of the enzyme coproporphyrinogen oxidase. The disorder is clinically indistinguishable from acute intermittent porphyria although approximately one-third of affected persons also have photo-sensitivity of their skin.

Porphyria variegata

Persons with this form of porphyria, prevalent in those of Afrikaner origin in South Africa (p. 78), have variable skin, neurological and visceral findings which can be triggered by drugs, as in acute intermittent porphyria. Although increased faecal excretion of the porphyrin precursors protoporphyrin and coproporphyrin can be demonstrated, a specific enzyme defect has not been identified as yet.

ERYTHROPOIETIC PORPHYRIAS
Congenital erythropoietic porphyria

The main feature of this type of porphyria is an extreme photosensitivity with blistering of the skin leading to extensive scarring, to the extent that most affected persons are unable to go out in normal daylight. In addition, many affected persons have a haemolytic anaemia requiring transfusion and frequently splenectomy. Further affected individuals have red-brown discolouration of their teeth, which show red fluorescence under ultraviolet light.

ORGANIC ACID DISORDERS

The inborn errors of the organic acids are a relatively recently recognised group of disorders. Affected individuals present with periodic episodes of poor feeding, vomiting and lethargy in association with a severe metabolic acidosis, low white cell (neutropaenia) and platelet (thrombocytopaenia) counts and often low blood sugar (hypoglycaemia) and high blood ammonia levels (hyperammonaemia). These episodes are often precipitated by intercurrent illness or increased protein intake and, after such an episode, affected children can show developmental regression. Analysis of blood from children at the time of these episodes reveals high levels of glycine, i.e. hyperglycinaemia. It was subsequently found that the acidosis in these episodes was often due to increased levels of the organic acids propionic or methylmalonic acid.

Deficiency of the enzyme methylmalonyl-CoA mutase, in methylmalonic acidaemia, and proprionyl-CoA carboxylase, in propionic acidaemia, results in accumulation of the toxic organic acid metabolites derived from deamination of certain amino acids, specific long-chain fatty acids and cholesterol side chains. Therapy of the acute episode involves treatment of any infection, fluid replacement, correction of the metabolic acidosis and stopping protein intake. Long-term prophylactic treatment involves protein restriction and rapid recognition and management of any intercurrent illness. A proportion of individuals with propionic acidaemia are responsive to biotin while some persons with methylmalonic acidaemia are responsive to vitamin B_{12}.

COPPER METABOLISM

There are two inborn errors of copper metabolism, Menkes' disease and Wilson's disease.

MENKES' DISEASE

Males with Menkes' disease usually present in the first few months of life with feeding difficulties, vomiting and poor weight gain. Subsequently floppinesss (hypotonia), fits and progressive neurological deterioration ensue with death due to recurrent respiratory infection usually occurring by the age of 3 years. A characteristic feature is the hair, which lacks pigment and is kinky and brittle and breaks easily. This was noted to resemble the wool of sheep suffering from copper deficiency. Abnormalities in serum copper and caeruloplasmin levels have been variably reported. Not surprisingly, the cloning of the gene for Menkes' disease has revealed it to code for a copper transport protein.

WILSON'S DISEASE

Persons affected with Wilson's disease commonly present in childhood or the early teenage years with fits, abnormal neurological findings, which can include spasticity, rigidity, dysarthria (difficulty in speaking) and dysphagia (difficulty with swallowing), and changes in behaviour or frank pyschiatric disturbance. Clinical examination can reveal the presence of what is called a Kayser-Fleischer ring, which is a golden brown or greenish collarette at the corneal margin (Plate 12). Investigation can reveal the presence of the third characteristic feature, abnormal liver function, which can lead on to cirrhosis.

High copper levels in the liver, decreased serum concentrations of the copper transport protein, caeruloplasmin, and abnormal copper loading tests have been used to confirm the diagnosis. The gene for Wilson's disease has recently been cloned and appears to be a copper transporting ATPase with sequence homology to the gene for Menkes' disease.

There are dramatic reports of striking improvement of the neurological features in persons with Wilson's disease using the chelating agents D-penicillamine and trientine, although these can cause side-effects (p. 132).

THYROID HORMONE BIOSYNTHESIS

CONGENITAL THYROXINE DEFICIENCY

Congenital hypothyroidism can be due to a deficiency of one of several enzymes involved in the production of the hormone thyroxine (Fig. 10.1). Simple hormone replacement can prevent the development of mental retardation, so-called 'cretinism', which occurs if children with this disorder are left untreated. In many areas of the United Kingdom congenital hypothyroidism is included as one of the inborn errors screened for in the newborn period (p. 272).

PEROXISOMAL DISORDERS

The peroxisomes are sub-cellular organelles bound by a single membrane present in all cells but especially abundant in liver and renal parenchymal cells. The organelle matrix has more than 40 enzymes which carry out a number of reactions involved in fatty acid oxidation and cholesterol biosynthesis interacting with metabolic pathways outside the peroxisomes. The enzymes of the peroxisomal matrix are synthesized on the polyribosomes, enter the cytosol and are transferred into the peroxisomes.

There are two main categories of peroxisomal disorders, disorders of peroxisome biogenesis, such as the Zellweger syndrome, and single peroxisomal enzyme defects, such as adrenoleukodystrophy.

ZELLWEGER'S SYNDROME

Newborn infants with Zellweger's syndrome present with hypotonia and weakness and have mildly dysmorphic facial features (Fig. 10.9) consisting of a prominent forehead and a large anterior fontanelle ('soft spot'). They can also have cataracts, and an enlarged liver. They usually go on to have fits with developmental regression and usually die by 1 year of age. Investigations usually reveal renal cysts and abnormal calcification in the cartilaginous growing ends of the long bones (Fig. 10.10). There is a range of severity of this disorder with different clinical diagnoses being given to the less severe types. The disorder appears to be due to a generalised failure to import the enzymes into the peroxisomes. The diagnosis can be confirmed by elevated levels of plasma long chain fatty acids. The gene for the Zellweger syndrome involves a protein involved in the peroxisome assembly.

It is unusual for inborn errors of metabolism to be associated with a dysmorphic syndrome (p. 198). In

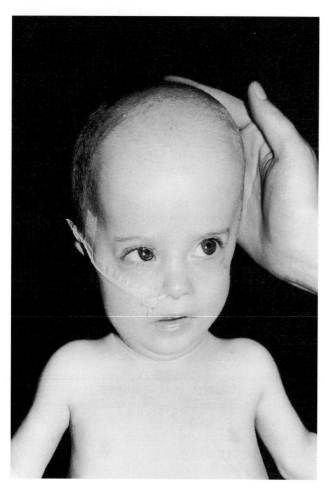

Fig. 10.9
Facies of an infant with Zellweger's syndrome showing a prominent forehead.

addition to the Zellweger syndrome, the Smith–Lemli–Opitz syndrome has recently been found to be due to an abnormality of cholesterol biosynthesis. There are a few other dysmorphic syndromes (p. 198) which have recently been recognised as being due to an inborn error.

ADRENOLEUKODYSTROPHY

Males with the X-linked disorder adrenoleukodystrophy (ALD) classically present in late childhood with deteriorating school performance, although affected males can present at any age and even, on occasion, be asymptomatic. A proportion of affected males can also present in adult life with less severe neurological features and adrenal insufficiency; this is known as adrenomyeloneuropathy. The disorder has been shown to be associated with a deficiency of the enzyme very long chain fatty acid (VLCFA) Co-A synthetase. The gene for ALD does not involve the gene for the enzyme VLCFA Co-A synthetase but has homology with a peroxisomal membrane protein.

Trials are being undertaken with a diet which uses as a source of fats an oil which has low levels of the very long chain fatty acids. This has been popularly called 'Lorenzo's oil' after a film of that title made about a child with adrenoleukodystrophy. The efficacy of this diet is, as yet, unclear.

MISCELLANEOUS INBORN ERRORS

α_1-ANTITRYPSIN DEFICIENCY

α_1-antitrypsin is one of the main serum proteins. It has an inhibitory activity for a number of proteolytic enzymes, including trypsin. Persons who are homozygous for the most common mutant allele of this protease inhibitor, Pi ZZ, have a greatly increased risk of developing pulmonary emphysema and cirrhosis of the liver (p. 182). There is conflicting evidence that persons heterozygous for α_1-antitrypsin deficiency have an increased risk of developing emphysema with exposure to environmental factors such as smoking or occupational chemicals (p. 148).

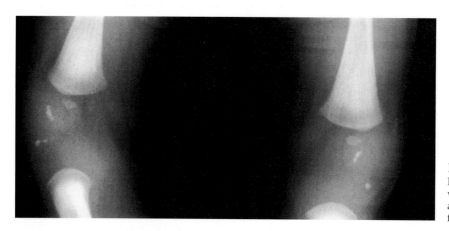

Fig. 10.10
Radiograph of the knee of a newborn infant with Zellweger's syndrome showing abnormal punctate calcification of the distal femoral epiphyses.

HEREDITARY ANGIONEUROTIC OEDEMA

This is a severe, sometimes fatal, disorder characterised by recurrent attacks of swelling (oedema) of the skin, throat and gut. Hereditary angioneurotic oedema is due to a specific deficiency of an inhibitor of the first component of complement, known as C1-INH (p. 157). There are two types of deficiency: in one, there is a reduction in the total amount of inhibitor; in the other, normal amounts of inhibitor are synthesised but it has little functional activity. Both types have been shown to be due to a variety of mutations of the C1-INH gene. Acute attacks can be treated with infusions of normal fresh-frozen plasma which contain the inhibitor. Attacks can also be prevented by treatment with epsilon aminocaproic acid and the androgenic drug danazol.

VITAMIN D-RESISTANT RICKETS

Individuals affected with vitamin D-resistant rickets usually present with short stature or deformities of growth of the lower limbs (p. 84). Persons with this disorder do not respond to the normal doses of vitamin D due to end organ insensitivity of the receptor to 1, 25-dihydroxycholecalciferol. As a consequence they have low serum phosphate levels due to reduced renal tubular reabsorption of phosphate. Treatment is with high levels of vitamin D although this can cause renal damage due to vitamin D toxicity.

PRENATAL DIAGNOSIS

In the majority of the inborn errors of metabolism in which an abnormal or deficient gene product can be identified, prenatal diagnosis is possible. Until recently this has been by biochemical analysis of cultured amniocytes obtained at mid-trimester amniocentesis. Techniques are now available for detection of many of the inborn errors of metabolism using direct or cultured chorionic villi, allowing first trimester diagnosis (p. 261). In addition, in many instances, this traditional biochemical approach is being replaced by the use of linked DNA sequence variants or specific mutational identification (p. 57). This latter approach is of particular value for the inborn errors of metabolism in which the biochemical basis has not yet been identified or the enzyme is not expressed in amniocytes or chorionic villi, e.g. phenylketonuria.

ELEMENTS

1 Metabolic processes in all species occur in steps, each being controlled by a particular enzyme which is the product of a specific gene, leading to the one gene–one enzyme concept.

2 A block in a metabolic pathway results in the accumulation of metabolic intermediates and/or a deficiency of the end product of the particular metabolic pathway concerned, a so-called inborn error of metabolism.

3 The majority of the inborn errors of metabolism are inherited as autosomal recessive or X-linked recessive traits. A few are inherited as autosomal dominant disorders involving rate-limiting enzymes or cell surface receptors.

4 A number of the inborn errors of metabolism can be screened for in the newborn period and successfully treated by dietary restriction or supplementation.

5 Prenatal diagnosis of many of the inborn errors of metabolism is possible by either conventional biochemical methods or the use of DNA markers.

FURTHER READING

Benson P F, Fensom A H 1985 Genetic biochemical disorders. Oxford University Press, Oxford
A good reference source for further information.
Cohn R M, Roth K S 1983 Metabolic disease: a guide to early recognition. Saunders, Philadelphia
Useful text as it considers the inborn errors from their mode of presentation rather than starting from the diagnosis.
Garrod A E 1908 Inborn errors of metabolism. Lancet ii: 1–7, 73–79, 142–148, 214–220
Reports of the first inborn errors of metabolism.
Moser H W 1992 Peroxisomal diseases. In: Harris H, Hirschhorn K (eds) Advances in human genetics. Plenum Press, London, pp 1–106.
A recent review of the expanding spectrum of this new group of inborn errors of metabolism.
Scriver C R, Beaudet A L, Sly W S, Valle D (eds) 1989 The metabolic basis of inherited disease, 6th edn. McGraw Hill, New York
A multi-author comprehensive detailed text with an exhaustive reference list.

CHAPTER 11 | Pharmacogenetics

DEFINITION

Some individuals can be especially sensitive to the effects of a particular drug, whereas others can be quite resistant. Such individual variation can be the result of factors which are not genetic. For example, both the young and the elderly are very sensitive to morphine and its derivatives, as are persons with liver disease. However, individual differences in response to drugs in humans can also be genetically determined.

The term *pharmacogenetics* was introduced by Vogel in 1959 for the study of genetically determined variations that are revealed solely by the effects of drugs. Such a definition would strictly exclude those hereditary disorders in which symptoms are usually only precipitated or aggravated by drugs. Many investigators, however, also include these latter disorders within the sphere of pharmacogenetics. Pharmacogenetics can be considered a separate branch of genetics and is likely to be of increasing importance in the future, particularly in relation to inherited differences in the biotransformation of environmental and occupational chemicals and carcinogens in relation to disease susceptibility.

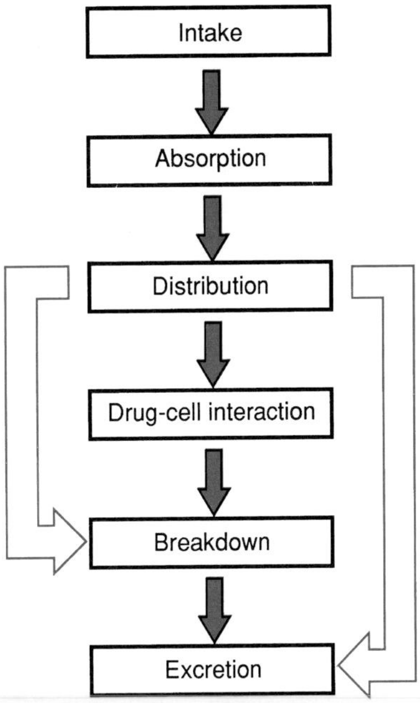

Fig. 11.1
Diagram of stages of metabolism of a drug.

GENETICS IN DRUG METABOLISM

DRUG METABOLISM

The metabolism of a drug usually follows a common sequence of events (Fig. 11.1). A drug is first absorbed from the gut, passes into the bloodstream, and so becomes distributed in the various tissues and tissue fluids. Only a small proportion of the total dose of a drug will be responsible for producing a specific pharmacological effect, most being broken down or excreted unchanged.

BIOCHEMICAL MODIFICATION

The actual breakdown process, which usually takes place in the liver, varies with different drugs. Some are completely oxidised to carbon dioxide which is exhaled. Others are excreted in modified forms either via the kidneys into the urine, or by the liver into the bile and thence the faeces. Many drugs undergo biochemical modifications increasing their solubility with the result that they are more readily excreted.

One important biochemical modification of many drugs is *conjugation*, which involves union with the carbohydrate glucuronic acid. Glucuronide conjugation occurs primarily in the liver. The elimination of morphine and its derivatives, such as codeine, is almost entirely dependent on this process. Isoniazid, used in the treatment of tuberculosis, and a number of other drugs, including the sulphonamides, are modified by the introduction of an acetyl group into the molecule, a process known as *acetylation* (Fig. 11.2).

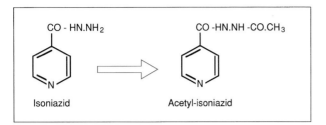

Fig. 11.2
Diagram of acetylation of the antituberculosis drug isoniazid.

KINETICS OF DRUG METABOLISM

The study of the metabolism and effects of a particular drug usually involves giving a standard dose of the drug and then after a suitable time interval determining the response. This can involve measuring the amount of the drug circulating in the blood or determining the rate at which it is metabolised. Such studies show that there is considerable variation in the way different individuals respond to certain drugs. This variability in response can be continuous or discontinuous.

If a test is carried out on a large number of subjects, their responses can be plotted (Fig. 11.3). In continuous variation the results form a bell-shaped or unimodal distribution. With discontinuous variation the curve is bimodal or sometimes trimodal. A discontinuous response suggests that the metabolism of the drug is under monogenic control. For example, if the normal metabolism of a drug is controlled by a dominant gene, R, and if some people are unable to metabolise the drug because they are homozygous for a recessive gene, r, there will be three classes of individuals: RR, Rr, and rr. If the responses of RR and Rr are indistinguishable, then a bimodal distribution will result. If RR and Rr are distinguishable, then a trimodal distribution will result, each peak or mode representing a different phenotype (Fig. 11.3). A unimodal distribution implies that the metabolism of the drug in question is under the control of many genes (p. 105) and the analysis of genetic factors in such cases is extremely complicated.

GENETIC VARIATIONS REVEALED SOLELY BY THE EFFECTS OF DRUGS

Among the best known examples of drugs which have been responsible for revealing genetic variability are hydrogen peroxide, isoniazid, succinylcholine, primaquine, certain anticoagulants and anaesthetic agents, the thiopurines, phenylbutazone, debrisoquine, and alcohol.

ACATALASIA

In 1946, Takahara, a Japanese otorhinolaryngologist, treated an 11-year-old girl for a gangrenous lesion of her

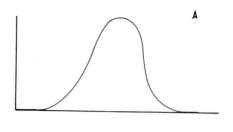

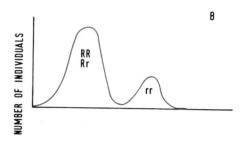

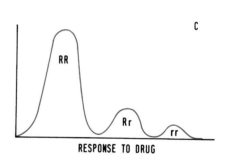

Fig. 11.3
Various types of response to different drugs; A. continuous variation, polygenic control of drug metabolism; B. and C. discontinuous variation, monogenic control of drug metabolism.

mouth. The infected tissue was excised and hydrogen peroxide was poured on the wound for sterilisation. Treatment of such a wound with hydrogen peroxide usually results in frothing of the blood which remains bright red. Takahara observed that treatment of the wound in this instance with hydrogen peroxide did not result in frothing and the blood turned brownish-black. He suggested that the patient could be deficient in the red cell enzyme catalase which breaks down hydrogen peroxide into water and oxygen. He argued that if this enzyme was absent then hydrogen peroxide would not be broken down, there would therefore be no frothing and the haemoglobin would be oxidised into methaemoglobin, which is brownish-black in colour.

Subsequent studies showed that this condition is indeed due to lack of the enzyme catalase and it has therefore been called acatalasia. Investigations of this girl's family and other families have shown that acatalasia is an autosomal recessive trait. Population studies of blood catalase activity have distinguished three classes of persons: those homozygous for the normal gene with normal levels of enzyme, those homozygous for the acatalasia allele with no enzyme in their blood, and heterozygous individuals with intermediate levels of the enzyme. Acatalasia is not limited to Japan but has since been described in other parts of the world. Only about half of those with acatalasia develop oral sepsis, the majority have no symptoms at all and are perfectly healthy.

ISONIAZID INACTIVATION

Isoniazid is one of the drugs which is used in the treatment of tuberculosis. It has been shown that isoniazid is rapidly absorbed from the gut, resulting in an initial high blood level which is slowly reduced as the drug is inactivated and excreted. The metabolism of isoniazid allows two groups to be distinguished, rapid and slow inactivators. In the former, blood levels of the drug fall rapidly after an oral dose; in the latter, blood levels remain high for some time. Family studies have shown that slow inactivators of isoniazid are homozygous for an autosomal recessive allele of the liver enzyme N-acetyl-transferase with lower activity levels. In the United States and Western Europe about 50% of the population are slow inactivators.

In some individuals, isoniazid can cause side-effects such as polyneuritis, a systemic lupus erythematosus-like disorder, or liver damage. Blood levels of isoniazid remain higher for longer periods in slow inactivators than in rapid inactivators on equivalent doses. One could expect side-effects to be more common in such individuals. Slow inactivators have a significantly greater risk of developing side-effects on doses which rapid inactivators require to ensure adequate blood levels for successful treatment of tuberculosis. Conversely, rapid inactivators have an increased risk of liver damage due to isoniazid.

Slow inactivators of isoniazid are also more likely to exhibit side-effects with hydralazine, an antihypertensive, and sulphasalazine, a sulphonamide derivative used to treat Crohn's disease, as these drugs are metabolised by the same enzyme.

DNA studies

Studies in other animal species have led to the cloning of the genes responsible for n-acetyl transferase activity in humans. This has revealed that there are three genes, one of which is not expressed and represents a pseudogene (NATP), one which does not exhibit differences in activity between individuals and has been termed monomorphic (NAT1), and a third which is polymorphic (NAT2).

SUCCINYLCHOLINE SENSITIVITY

Curare is a plant extract used by certain tribes of South American Indians. It produces profound muscular paralysis but with no loss of sensation. Medically, curare is used in surgical operations because of the muscular

relaxation which it produces. Succinylcholine, also known as suxamethonium, is another drug which produces muscular relaxation, though by a different mechanism from curare. Suxamethonium has the advantage over curare that its relaxation of skeletal and respiratory muscles and consequent apnoea (cessation of breathing) is only short-lived. The anaesthetist, therefore, needs to maintain respiration by artificial means for only 2 to 3 minutes before it returns spontaneously. However, about 1 patient in every 2000 has a period of apnoea which can last an hour or more. It was found that the apnoea in such instances can be corrected by transfusion of blood from a normal person. The anaesthetist, in these instances, has to maintain respiration until the effects of the drug have worn off. Succinylcholine is normally destroyed in the body by the plasma enzyme pseudocholinesterase. In patients who are highly sensitive to succinylcholine, the plasma pseudocholinesterase in their blood destroys the drug at a markedly slower rate than normal. In some very rare cases there is no enzyme. Family studies have shown that succinylcholine sensitivity is inherited as an autosomal recessive trait.

A refined method of studying plasma pseudocholinesterase in the blood involves determining the percentage inhibition of the enzyme by the local anaesthetic dibucaine (syn: cinchocaine). The result is termed the dibucaine number. The frequency distribution of dibucaine number values in families with succinylcholine sensitive individuals, gives a trimodal curve. The three modes represent the normal homozygotes, the heterozygotes and the affected homozygotes. Experimental evidence clearly indicates that there are at least two different forms of plasma pseudocholinesterase: the one in the normal homozygote and the one in the affected homozygote. The two enzymes differ not only in the way in which they are inhibited by dibucaine, the enzyme in the affected homozygote being less inhibited, but also in their enzyme kinetics, with the normal enzyme being more efficient than the abnormal enzyme in destroying acetylcholine and other choline esters.

GLUCOSE-6-PHOSPHATE DEHYDROGENASE VARIANTS

For many years, quinine was the drug of choice in the treatment of malaria. Although it has been very effective in acute attacks it is not very effective in preventing relapses. In 1926 primaquine was introduced and proved to be much better than quinine in preventing relapses. However, it was not long after primaquine was introduced that some people were found to be sensitive to the drug. The drug could be taken for a few days with no apparent ill effects, and then suddenly the patient would begin to pass very dark, often black, urine. Jaundice developed and the red cell count and haemoglobin concentration gradually fell as red blood cells were destroyed.

The patient usually recovered from such a haemolytic episode but occasionally the destruction of the red cells was extensive enough to be fatal. The cause of such cases of primaquine sensitivity was subsequently shown to be a deficiency in the red cells of the enzyme glucose-6-phosphate dehydrogenase (G6PD).

Family studies have shown that G6PD deficiency is inherited as an X-linked recessive trait (p. 82). G6PD deficiency is rare in most Caucasians but affects about 10% of Afro-Caribbean males and is also relatively common in males of Mediterranean origin. G6PD deficiency is thought to be relatively common as a result of conferring increased resistance to the malarial parasite. The red cell G6PD levels in persons of Mediterranean extraction with G6PD deficiency are very much lower than in persons of Afro-Caribbean origin with G6PD deficiency.

Persons with G6PD deficiency are sensitive not only to primaquine but also to many other compounds as well, such as phenacetin, nitrofurantoin and certain sulphonamides. These drugs should be used with caution in males of Afro-Caribbean and Mediterranean origin if their G6PD status is unknown, and in a person known to be G6PD deficient such drugs are absolutely contraindicated. Drug-induced haemolysis is uncommon in G6PD deficiency and, in fact, the main medical risk of G6PD deficiency is *favism*, in which a haemolytic crisis occurs after eating fava beans.

COUMARIN METABOLISM

The coumarin anticoagulant drugs are used in the treatment of a number of different disorders to prevent the blood from clotting. There is a discontinuous variation in the response of patients taking these drugs which involves an increased resistance to the effects of the drugs in some patients. This resistance appears to be transmitted as an autosomal dominant trait.

MALIGNANT HYPERTHERMIA

Malignant hyperthermia (MH) is a rare complication of anaesthesia. Susceptible individuals develop muscle rigidity as well as an increased temperature (hyperthermia), often as high as 42.3°C (108°F) during anaesthesia. This usually occurs when halothane is used as the anaesthetic agent, particularly when succinylcholine is used as the muscle relaxant for intubation. If it is not recognised rapidly and the affected person treated with vigorous cooling, the patient will die.

MH susceptibility appears to be inherited as an autosomal dominant trait affecting approximately 1 in 10 000 persons. Susceptible individuals can occasionally have a raised serum creatine kinase but this cannot be used as a reliable screening test of at risk family members. A more reliable prediction of an individual's susceptibility status can be carried out in vitro on a muscle biopsy by testing the response to halothane and caffeine. A person known or suspected of being susceptible to MH can undergo surgery provided that known precipitating anaesthetic agents are avoided. Should hyperthermia develop during surgery, it can be treated by intravenous procaine or procainamide but most effectively with dantrolene.

Polymorphic DNA markers linked to the malignant hyperthermia locus on chromosome 19 can be used to identify potentially susceptible individuals but MH is genetically heterogeneous (p. 81) with approximately only 50% of families linked to this locus.

THIOPURINE METABOLISM

A group of substances known as the thiopurines, which include 6-mercaptopurine, 6-thioguanine and azathioprine, are used extensively in the treatment of patients with various neoplasms as well as to prevent rejection in recipients of organ transplants. They are very effective drugs but have serious side effects such as leucopenia and severe liver damage. It has not been possible to predict either those who are likely to develop such side effects, or the possible therapeutic response in the individual patient, because the response to these drugs varies widely. An important step in the metabolism of these compounds is the process of methylation catalysed by the enzyme thiopurine methyltransferase (TPMT). It appears that erythrocyte TPMT activity is polymorphic, with roughly 0.3% of the population having undetectable activity. Individuals with these low levels could respond less well to these drugs but also be in danger of developing serious side effects. Those with high TPMT activity could be treated more aggressively with these drugs, resulting in a better therapeutic response which has been suggested to be the case in childhood leukaemia.

PHENYLBUTAZONE METABOLISM

Phenylbutazone is used in the treatment of the more severe forms of arthritis. The metabolism of this drug differs from the examples discussed so far in that it appears to be under polygenic control. Individuals who are relatively slow in metabolising phenylbutazone are more likely to develop drug-associated side effects such as hypoplastic anaemia.

DEBRISOQUINE METABOLISM

Debrisoquine is a drug which was frequently used in the treatment of hypertension. There is essentially a bimodal distribution in the response to the drug in the general population. Roughly 5–10% of British subjects are poor metabolisers, being homozygotes for an autosomal recessive gene with defective hydroxylation. Such individuals are more prone to overreact to the drug and develop hypotension during therapy. They are also more susceptible to adverse reactions to several other drugs such as the beta blockers, propranolol and metoprolol.

DNA studies

Molecular studies have now revealed that the gene involved in debrisoquine metabolism is one of the P450 family of genes on chromosome 22, known as CYP2D6. Surprisingly, the mutations responsible for the poor metaboliser phenotype occur in the introns, producing a series of incorrectly spliced messenger-RNAs (p. 15). It is postulated that these enzymes could be involved in the metabolism of plant toxins.

ALCOHOL METABOLISM

Under the heading of pharmacogentics we can also include a subject which in terms of its frequency and social implications dwarfs all others, namely, alcoholism and alcoholic cirrhosis, although some persons would debate whether alcohol should really be considered a drug. Alcoholism is clearly related to the amount consumed as well as to dietary and various social and economic factors. Nevertheless, evidence is gradually emerging which clearly indicates that genetic factors can also be involved. Some of this evidence is based on twin studies, which have shown high concordance rates (p. 182), and family studies, which have shown a high prevalence rate among relatives of alcoholics. Clearly, however, behaviour patterns within families could artificially inflate what would appear to be genetic factors. Similarly, apparent racial or ethnic differences in the incidence of alcoholism, such as the high incidence among certain American Indians and Eskimos, could well be affected by social factors.

Perhaps the most convincing evidence for the possible role of genetic factors in alcoholism comes from the study of the enzymes involved in alcohol metabolism. Alcohol is metabolised in the liver by alcohol dehydrogenase (ADH) to acetaldehyde, and then further degraded by acetaldehyde dehydrogenase (ALDH). Human ADH consists of dimers of various combinations of subunits of three different polypeptide units coded for by three loci, ADH1 coding for the alpha subunit, ADH2 for the beta subunit and ADH3 for the gamma subunit. ADH1 is primarily expressed in early fetal life, while ADH2 is expressed in adult life.

Persons of Far East Asian origin tolerate alcohol less well than persons of Caucasian origin and often exhibit an acute flushing reaction to alcohol (p. 185). It has been suggested that this sensitivity to alcohol could be due to differences in the rate of metabolism of acetaldehyde. There are two major acetaldehyde dehydrogenase variants

or *isozymes*, ALDH1 which is present in the cytosol and ALDH2 which is present in the mitochondria. The acute flushing reaction to alcohol in Far East Asians has been shown, in fact, to be due to absent ALDH2 activity. It has been suggested that this unpleasant reaction to alcohol could account for the reported lower incidence of alcoholism and alcohol related liver disease in that population.

HEREDITARY DISORDERS WITH ALTERED DRUG RESPONSE

It was pointed out at the beginning of this chapter that not all investigators include hereditary disorders with altered drug response within the sphere of pharmacogenetics. However, since it is a subject of immense importance in medical practice and touches on both genetics and pharmacology it is perhaps best discussed at this point. Similar precautions have to be borne in mind in several hereditary disorders in which severe exacerbations can be provoked by a particular drug.

PORPHYRIA VARIEGATA

Porphyria variegata, one of the several types of porphyria (p. 138), is inherited as an autosomal dominant trait. Some affected individuals have skin lesions particularly on exposed surfaces. Others have attacks of severe abdominal pain, muscular paralysis and even mental disturbance. During an acute attack the patient can die. It is recognised that in persons with porphyria an acute attack can be precipitated by barbiturates.

HAEMOGLOBINOPATHIES

Sulphonamides can cause severe haemolysis in individuals with certain haemoglobinopathies. This applies to persons with haemoglobin H, a haemoglobin which consists entirely of beta globin chains (p. 122), and with haemoglobin Zurich which was first described in members of a Swiss family in 1962. These haemoglobinopathies are, however, very rare conditions and are much less of a problem than porphyria and G6PD deficiency.

GOUT AND CHLOROTHIAZIDE

The treatment of congestive heart failure often involves the use of diuretics. These drugs increase the excretion of water and consequently reduce the amount of oedema. One of the most widely used is chlorothiazide. Not long after its initial use, it was realised that it could cause problems in persons who suffer from gout (p. 137). In genetically predisposed individuals attacks often follow dietary excesses which lead to an elevation in serum uric acid. Chlorothiazide has a similar effect by raising the serum level of uric acid in genetically predisposed individuals.

CRIGLER–NAJJAR SYNDROME

The Crigler–Najjar syndrome is characterised by a severe non-haemolytic jaundice often associated with deposition of unconjugated bilirubin in the central nervous system leading to neurological sequelae. The jaundice appears on the first or second day after birth and persists throughout life. Affected children often die in infancy. The condition is inherited as an autosomal recessive trait, the heterozygote being perfectly healthy. The basic defect appears to be the inability of the liver to conjugate bilirubin with glucuronides due to a deficiency of the enzyme glucuronyl transferase. When drugs, such as salicylates, are given to affected patients it is possible to show that they are unable to conjugate these substances.

NON-INSULIN DEPENDENT DIABETES

In non-insulin dependent diabetes inherited as an autosomal dominant trait (p. 185), it has been suggested that those at risk of developing the disease develop facial flushing after alcohol if they are first given the oral hypoglycaemic drug chlorpropamide. Although it was hoped that this could prove a useful test for familial susceptibility to diabetes, this has not been the case.

EVOLUTIONARY ORIGIN OF VARIATION IN DRUG RESPONSES

What is the evolutionary significance of genetic variations in response to certain drugs in particular ethnic groups (Table 11.1)? Man has been exposed to these drugs for no more than a few decades yet there is no doubt that mutations in genes conferring abnormal responses to these drugs arose, in many instances, many thousands of years ago. There is evidence in the case of G6PD deficiency that it can confer some protection against one form of malaria. With most hereditary variation in response to drugs we have very little idea of how or why it arose. A mutation which conferred selective advantage under certain dietary or environmental conditions in the past could be a possible explanation. Another possibility is that some mutations could have conferred resistance to particular infections.

ECOGENETICS

An extension of pharmacogenetics is the study of genetically determined differences in susceptibility to

Table 11.1 Ethnic variations in some pharmacogenetic disorders

Disorder	Ethnic group	Frequency (%)
Slow acetylation	Europeans	50
	Orientals	10
Pseudocholinesterase variants	Europeans	<1
	Eskimos	1–2
G6PD deficiency	N. Europeans	0
	S. Europeans	≤25
Hypolactasia	Europeans	<20
	Asians	100
Atypical ADH	Europeans	5
	Orientals	85

Table 11.2 Ecogenetics: genetic variation in susceptibility to environmental agents

Environmental agent	Genetic susceptibility	Disease
UV light	fair complexion	skin cancer
Drugs	(see text)	
Foods		
fats	hypercholesterolaemia	atherosclerosis
fava beans	G6PD deficiency	favism
gluten	gluten sensitivity	coeliac disease
salt	Na-K pump defective	hypertension
milk	lactase deficiency	lactose intolerance
alcohol	atypical ADH	alcoholism
oxalates	hyperoxaluria	renal stones
fortified flour	haemochromatosis	iron overload
Inhalants		
dust	α_1-antitrypsin deficiency	emphysema
smoking	AHH inducibility	lung cancer
allergens	atopy	asthma
Infections		
	defective immunity	diabetes mellitus? spondylitis?

the action of physical, chemical and infectious agents in the environment. This has been referred to as *ecogenetics*, a term first coined by Brewer in 1971. Such differences in susceptibility can be either unifactorial or multifactorial in causation (Table 11.2).

ORGANOPHOSPHATE METABOLISM

Paraoxonase is an enzyme which catalyses the breakdown of organophosphates. Some individuals have high serum enzyme activity and others low activity which results from a two allele polymorphic system. It could be that those who are homozygous for the low activity allele are predisposed to particular sensitivity to organophosphates, which are widely employed in agriculture and industry.

DISEASE SUSCEPTIBILITY

The field of ecogenetics could be particularly important in the possible identification of individuals at high risk from the effects of environmental mutagens and carcinogens (p. 163).

There are reports of an increased risk of bladder cancer in persons who are slow acetylators and who have had occupational exposure to aromatic amines. There is also the possibility of an increased risk of bladder cancer for slow acetylators in the general population in which no specific hazardous exposure has been recognised. Conversely, there are recent reports suggesting the possibility of an increased risk of colorectal cancer in rapid acetylators.

Recent studies have suggested that poor debrisoquine metaboliser status is less common than would be expected in persons with cancer of the lung. This is in contrast to another recently discovered activity level polymorphism for the enzyme glutathione S-transferase, GSTM1, which shows an increase in the incidence of the null phenotype, i.e. no activity, in persons with adenocarcinoma of the lung when compared to the general population. This enzyme is involved in the conjugation of glutathione with electrophilic compounds, including carcinogens such as benzpyrene, and could have a protective role against the development of cancer.

This susceptibility to disease is not just limited to cancer. Many of the common diseases in humans could be due to genetically determined differences in response to environmental agents or susceptibilities (p. 181). There are reports of a possible increased risk of developing Parkinson's disease due to differences in the detoxification of potential neurotoxins in association with a poor metaboliser phenotype in the hepatic cytochrome P450 CYP2D6 gene.

This area of medical genetics is very likely to become more important in the next few years as our attention turns more to the cause and prevention of common diseases. It raises, however, many social and ethical problems when our knowledge of genetic variation and susceptibility is translated into public policy (p. 269).

ELEMENTS

1 Pharmacogenetics is defined as the study of genetically determined variations revealed solely by the effects of drugs. Hereditary disorders in which symptoms can occur spontaneously but can be exacerbated or precipitated by drugs are often also included.

2 The metabolism of many drugs involves biochemical modification, often by conjugation with another molecule, which usually takes place in the liver. This biochemical transformation facilitates the excretion of the drug.

3 The ways in which many drugs are metabolised vary from person to person and can be genetically determined. In some instances, the biochemical basis is understood. For example, persons differ in the rate at which they inactivate the antituberculosis drug isoniazid by acetylation in the liver, being either rapid or slow inactivators. Slow inactivators have an increased risk of toxic side-effects associated with isoniazid therapy. Other examples include sensitivity to the muscle relaxant succinylcholine because of abnormal plasma pseudocholinesterase activity, and the development of a severe haemolytic anaemia when given the antimalarial drug primaquine (or a number of other drugs) due to deficiency of the enzyme glucose-6-phosphate dehydrogenase in red blood cells.

4 In other instances, genetic variation can be revealed by drugs but the precise biochemical basis is not yet known. One such example is malignant hyperthermia. This rare disorder is associated with the use of certain anaesthetic agents and muscle relaxants in general anaesthesia. The metabolism of a number of other drugs shows marked variation between persons, and family studies suggest a genetic causation, but the biochemical basis for this variation is yet to be fully elucidated.

5 The hereditary disorder porphyria variegata and some of the haemoglobinopathies are associated with altered drug response. With disorders such as diabetes and gout, where the aetiology is not clear, biochemical evidence of variation in response to drugs suggests a genetic contribution.

6 The term ecogenetics is used for the study of genetically determined differences between persons in their susceptibility to the action of physical, chemical and infectious agents in the environment.

FURTHER READING

Beutler E 1991 Glucose-6-phosphate dehydrogenase deficiency. N Eng J Med 324: 169–174
Recent review of an important ethnic pharmacogenetic polymorphism.

Ellis F R, Heffron J J A 1985 Clinical and biochemical aspects of malignant hyperpyrexia. In: Atkinson R S, Adams A P (eds) Recent advances in anaesthesia and analgesia. Churchill Livingstone, Edinburgh, pp 173–207
A rare but important disorder due to a pharmacogenetic susceptibility.

Kalow W, Spielberg S 1989 Human pharmacogenetics. In: Kalant H, Roschlau W H E (eds) Principles of medical pharmacology, 5th edn. Decker, Philadelphia, pp 119–127
An outline of the principles of pharmacogenetics.

Price Evans D A 1993 Genetic factors in drug therapy. Cambridge University Press, Cambridge
Up to date comprehensive textbook covering the field of pharmacogenetics.

Vogel F, Buselmaier W, Reichert W, Kellerman G, Berg P (eds) 1978 Human genetic variation in response to medical and environmental agents: Pharmacogenetics and ecogenetics. Springer-Verlag, Berlin
One of the early definitive outlines of the field of pharmacogenetics.

CHAPTER 12

Immunogenetics

THE IMMUNE SYSTEM

The immune system in humans can be divided into two parts: *cellular* and *humoral immunity*. During development, a lymphoid stem cell takes one of two pathways. The first involves the thymus gland as the primary lymphoid organ with differentiation into T lymphocytes in the secondary lymphoid organs which include the spleen and cortical regions of the lymph nodes. T lymphocytes are responsible for cellular immunity, i.e. transplantation immunity or *homograft* rejection and delayed hypersensitivity. T lymphocytes can be subdivided according to their function: *cytotoxic* or *killer lymphocytes* sensitised to destroy cells bearing antigens induced by virus infections; *helper lymphocytes* necessary for the induction of the

antibody response by B lymphocytes; and *suppressor lymphocytes* which inhibit or suppress the immune response.

Humoral immunity involves differentiation of lymphocyte stem cells into B lymphocytes. This occurs in the primary lymphoid organ sites of general haematopoesis, the fetal liver, spleen and later the bone marrow. The mature antibody producing cells, the plasma cells, are found in the secondary lymphoid organs which consist of the red pulp of the spleen and the medulla of the lymph nodes (Fig. 12.1).

When a T lymphocyte binds with antigen through its *T cell receptor* (p. 154) on the cell surface, in conjunction with the *major histocompatibility complex* (p. 160), it is activated to release a number of *lymphokines*. These include interleukin-2 (IL-2) which stimulates other T lymphocytes to divide and release further lymphokines, as well as

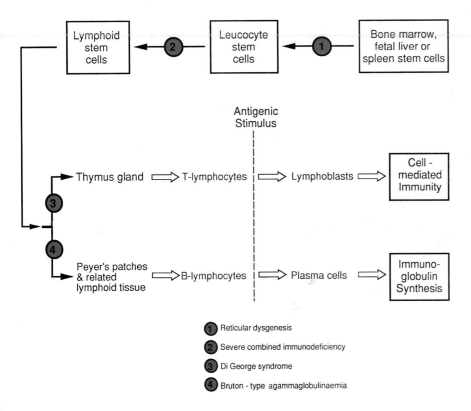

Fig. 12.1
Sites of hypothetical blocks in certain immunological deficiency diseases.

causing other white blood cells such as polymorpho-nuclear lymphocytes and macrophages to divide, and activating B lymphocytes to proliferate and divide.

IMMUNOGLOBULINS

The *immunoglobulins* (Ig), or antibodies, are one of the major classes of serum proteins and are part of the body's defence mechanism against infection. Their function, both in the recognition of antigenic variability and effector activities, has been revealed by protein and DNA studies of their structure.

IMMUNOGLOBULIN STRUCTURE

Papaine, a proteolytic enzyme, splits the immunoglobulin molecule into three fragments which can be separated by chromatography. Two of the fragments are similar, each containing an antibody site capable of combining with a specific antigen and therefore referred to as the *antigen-binding fragment* or *Fab*. The third fragment could be crystallised and was therefore called *Fc*. It binds complement and receptors on a number of different cell types involved in the immune response.

The immunoglobulin molecule is made up of four polypeptide chains: two 'light' (L) and two 'heavy' (H) chains of approximately 220 and 440 amino acids in length. They are held together in a Y-shape by disulphide bonds and non-covalent interactions. Each Fab fragment is composed of L-chains and parts of the H-chains, whereas each Fc fragment is composed only of parts of the H-chains (Fig. 12.2). Further analysis has revealed that the L-chains can be of two types, either kappa (κ) or lambda (λ). In addition there are five different classes of heavy chain designated respectively as γ, μ, α, δ and ε, one each respectively for the five major classes of the immunoglobulins IgG, IgM, IgA, IgD and IgE. The two types of light chain are common to all five classes of immunoglobulin. Thus the molecular formula for IgG is $\lambda_2\gamma_2$ or $\kappa_2\gamma_2$. The characteristics of the various classes of immunoglobulin are outlined in brief in Table 12.1.

IMMUNOGLOBULIN ALLOTYPES

The five classes of immunoglobulin occur in all normal individuals but genetically determined variants or *immunoglobulin allotypes* of these classes have also been identified. These are the *Gm* system associated with the heavy chain of IgG, the *Am* system associated with the IgA heavy chain, the *Km* and *Inv* systems associated with the kappa light chain, the *Oz* system for the lambda light

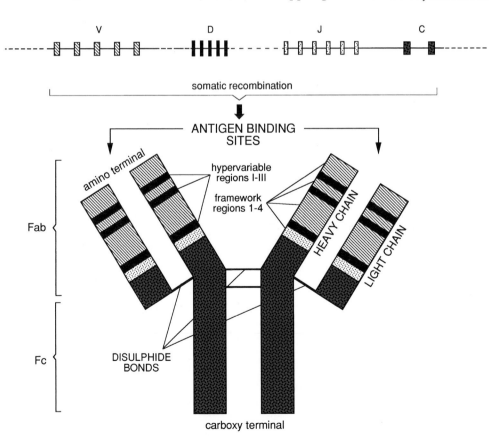

Fig. 12.2
Model of antibody molecule structure.

Table 12.1 Classes of human immunoglobulins

Class	Mol. wt	Serum concentration (mg/ml)	Antibody activity	Placental transfer
IgG	160 000	12.0	to bacteria and viruses (most antibodies)	+
IgM	900 000	1.0	to protein antigens (some blood groups and bacteria)	–
IgA	170 000+	2.5	in external secretions (local immunity)	+?
IgD	180 000	0.03	?	–
IgE	200 000	trace	in allergic reactions	–

chain and the *Em* allotype for the IgE heavy chain. The Gm and Km systems are independent of each other and are polymorphic (p. 97), the frequencies of the various alleles being different in various ethnic groups.

THE GENERATION OF ANTIBODY DIVERSITY

It could seem paradoxical for a single protein molecule to exhibit sufficient structural heterogeneity to be specific for a wide variety of antigens. Different combinations of heavy and light chains could, to some extent, account for this diversity. It would require, however, thousands of structural genes of each chain type to account for the large number of antibodies produced in response to the equally large number of antigens to which individuals can be exposed.

Persons with *multiple myeloma*, a cancer of antibody-producing plasma cells, make a single antibody species in large abundance. Persons with multiple myeloma excrete large quantities of this single or monoclonal protein in their urine. This protein, known as *Bence-Jones protein*, consists of an immunoglobulin light chain. Comparisons of this protein from different myeloma patients revealed the amino terminal ends of the molecule to be quite variable in their amino acid sequence whilst the carboxy terminal ends were relatively constant. These are called the *variable*, or V, and *constant*, or C, regions respectively. Further detailed analysis of the amino acid sequence of the V regions of different myeloma proteins showed four regions which vary little from one antibody to another, known as *framework regions* (1 to 4), and three markedly variable regions interspersed between these, known as *hypervariable regions* (I–III) (Fig. 12.2).

Dreyer and Bennett, as long ago as 1965, proposed that an antibody could be encoded for by separate 'genes' in germ line cells which undergo rearrangement, or, as they termed it, 'scrambling', in lymphocyte development.

DNA studies

Comparison of the restriction maps of the DNA segments coding for the C and V regions of the immunoglobulin λ light chains in embryonic and antibody producing cells revealed that they were far apart in the former whilst they were close together in the latter. More detailed analysis revealed that the DNA segments coding for the V and C regions of the light chain are separated by some 1500 base pairs in antibody producing cells. The intervening DNA segment was found to code for a *joining*, or J, region immediately adjacent to the V region of the light chain. The κ light chain was shown to have the same structure. Cloning and DNA sequencing of heavy-chain genes in germ line cells have revealed that they have a fourth region, called *diversity*, or D, between the V and J regions.

There are estimated to be 100 to 200 different DNA segments coding for the V region of the heavy chain, about 80 DNA segments coding for the V region of the κ light chain and 10 or so DNA segments coding for the λ light chain V region. Six functional DNA segments code for the J region of the heavy chain and five for the J region of the κ light chain, while each DNA segment coding for the C region of the λ light chain has its own DNA segment for the J region. A single DNA segment codes for the C region of the κ light chain, four DNA segments code for the C region of the λ light chain and nine functional DNA segments code for the C region of the different classes of heavy chain. There are also 2 functional DNA segments coding for the D region of the heavy chain (Fig. 12.3).

Estimation of the number of DNA segments coding for these various portions of the immunoglobulin molecule is confounded by the presence of a large number of unexpressed DNA sequences or pseudogenes (p. 11). Whilst the coding DNA segments for the various regions of the antibody molecule can be referred to as genes, use of this term in regard to antibodies themselves has deliberately been avoided because antibodies could be considered to be an exception to the general rule of 'one gene–one enzyme or protein' (p. 127).

IMMUNOGLOBULIN GENE REARRANGEMENT

The genes for the κ and λ light chains and the heavy chains in man have been assigned to chromosomes 2, 22 and 14 respectively. Only one of each of the relevant types of DNA segments is expressed in any single antibody molecule. The DNA coding segments for the various portions of the immunoglobulin chains on these chromosomes are separated by DNA which is non-coding. Somatic recombinational events involved in

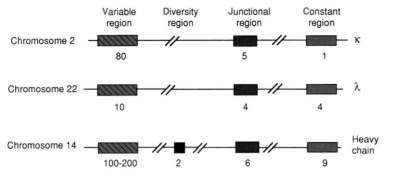

Fig. 12.3

Diagram of the estimated number of the various DNA segments coding for the κ, λ and various heavy chains.

antibody production involve short conserved joining nucleotide sequences and recombination recognition sequences that flank each germ line DNA segment (Fig. 12.4). Further diversity occurs by variable mRNA splicing at the V–J junction in RNA processing and by somatic mutation of the antibody genes. These mechanisms can easily account for the antibody diversity seen in nature. Although it probably involves some form of clonal selection, it is still not entirely clear, however, how particular DNA segments are selected to produce an antibody to a specific antigen.

'Gene shuffling' of this form is known to account for the marked variability seen in the surface antigens of the Trypanosome parasite and the different mating types in yeast.

CLASS SWITCHING

There is a normal switch of antibody class produced by B cells on continued or further exposure to antigen, usually from IgM the initial class of antibody produced in response to exposure to an antigen, to IgA or IgG.

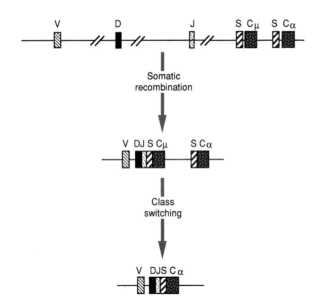

Fig. 12.4

Diagram of immunoglobulin heavy chain gene rearrangement and class switching.

This process, known as *class switching*, involves retention of the specificity of the antibody to the same antigen. Analysis of class switching in a population of cells derived from a single B cell has shown that both classes of antibody have the same antigen binding sites, having the same V region, and differ only in their C region. Class switching occurs by a somatic recombination event which involves DNA segments designated S (for switching) which lead to looping out and deletion of the intervening DNA. The result is to eliminate the DNA segment coding for the C region of the heavy chain of the IgM molecule and to bring the gene segment encoding the C region of the new class of heavy chain adjacent to the segment encoding the V region (Fig.12.4).

IMMUNOGLOBULIN SUPERFAMILY

Studies of the structure of other molecules involved in the immune response have shown a number to have structural and DNA sequence homology to the immunoglobulins. This involves a 110 amino acid sequence characterised by a centrally placed disulphide bridge which stabilises a series of antiparallel beta strands into what is called an antibody fold. This group of molecules with similar structure has been called the *immunoglobulin superfamily*. It consists of eight multigene families which, in addition to the κ and λ light chains and different classes of heavy chain, include the alpha, beta, gamma and delta chains of the T cell receptor, the class I and II major histocompatibility complex human leucocyte (HLA) antigens (p. 160) and β_2-microglobulin. The latter is a receptor for transporting certain classes of immunoglobulin across mucosal membranes. A series of other molecules show homology to the Ig superfamily. These include the T lymphocyte antigens CD4 and CD8, the epithelial cell polyimmunoglobulin receptor and proteins with quite different function such as the intercellular adhesion molecule, ICAM-1.

ANTIBODY ENGINEERING

The techniques of genetic engineering have led to the prospect of reshaping or designing human antibodies for specific therapeutic or diagnostic purposes. Recombinant antibodies can be constructed using the human variable region framework, the human constant regions of the heavy and light chains and the antigen-binding site of a mouse antibody. Persons treated with these 'engineered' antibodies do not mount an immune response to them, a problem met with in the use of rodent hybridoma-derived monoclonal antibodies. It is hoped that the use of human-derived myeloma cells for expression of these recombinant antibodies could overcome this difficulty.

IMMUNODEFICIENCY

Immunodeficiency can occur as a primary isolated abnormality or as a secondary or associated finding.

PRIMARY IMMUNODEFICIENCY DISORDERS

The manifestations of at least some of the primary immunological deficiency diseases in humans (Table 12.2) can be understood at a simple level by assuming that defects have occurred at specific points in the biology of the immune system (Fig. 12.1). It should be emphasised, however, that several rare immunological deficiency diseases do not fit into this simplified scheme.

Whenever cellular immunity (p. 151) is depressed this is associated with increased susceptibility to virus infections and can be shown experimentally in animals by prolonged survival of skin homografts. Whenever Ig synthesis is depressed this is associated with reduced resistance to bacterial infections which can lead to death in infancy as in severe combined immunodeficiency (SCID).

Severe combined immunodeficiency

Severe combined immunodeficiency (SCID), as the name indicates, is associated with an increased susceptibility to both viral and bacterial infections because of abnormal B- and T-cell function. Death usually occurs in infancy because of overwhelming infection, unless bone marrow transplantation is performed. SCID is known to be genetically heterogeneous and can be inherited either as an X-linked or autosomal recessive disorder. In approximately one-third to one-half of children with the autosomal recessive form, a deficiency of the enzymes adenosine deaminase or purine nucleoside phosphorylase can be demonstrated. These latter two types of SCID are, for all intents and purposes, inborn errors of metabolism which, for reasons that are not clear at present, specifically affect the immune system.

Reticular dysgenesis

Children with this very rare autosomal recessive form of immunodeficiency have abnormal cellular and humoral immunity and also have a deficiency of granulocytes. They usually die very early in the first year unless offered a bone marrow transplant.

DiGeorge syndrome

Children with the DiGeorge syndrome present with recurrent viral illnesses and are found to have markedly abnormal cellular immunity as characterised by severely reduced or absent T lymphocytes. This has been found to be due to their thymus gland being absent. They also usually have a number of characteristic congenital abnormalities which can include congenital heart disease and absent parathyroid glands. Because of the latter finding they can present in the newborn period with tetany due to low serum calcium levels secondary to low parathormone levels. This syndrome has been recognised to be part of the spectrum of phenotypes which can occur

Table 12.2 Some immunological deficiency diseases (Site of defect refers to Figure 12.1, AR = autosomal recessive; XR = X-linked recessive, BMT = bone marrow transplant)

Disorder	Site of defect	Thymus gland	Lymphocytes	Cell–mediated	Plasma cells	Ig synthesis	Genetics	Treatment
Reticular dysgenesis (absence of leucocytes)	1	absent	↓	↓	↓	↓	AR	BMT
Severe combined immunodeficiency	2	Vestigial	↓	↓	↓	↓	AR/XR	BMT, enzyme replacement for ADA deficiency
DiGeorge syndrome	3	absent (parathyroids absent as well)	+	↓	+	N	–	transplantation of fetal thymus
Bruton-type agamma-globulinaemia	4	+	+	N	↓	↓	XR	Ig injections and antibiotics

in relation to deletions of a region of the long arm of chromosome 22 (p. 221).

Bruton type agammaglobulinaemia

Male children with this X-linked immunodeficiency usually develop multiple recurrent bacterial infections of the respiratory tract and skin after the first few months of life, being protected initially by transplacental maternal IgG. Treatment of life-threatening infections with anti-biotics has improved survival prospects but these children can still die from respiratory failure due to complications of repeated lung infections. The diagnosis of this type of immunodeficiency is confirmed by demonstration of deficient immunoglobulins and absence of B lymphocytes.

SECONDARY OR ASSOCIATED IMMUNODEFICIENCY

There are also a number of hereditary disorders in which Ig abnormalities occur as one of a number of associated features as part of a syndrome (p. 198).

Ataxia telangiectasia

This is an autosomal recessive disorder in which children present in early childhood with difficulty in control of movement and balance (cerebellar ataxia), dilated blood vessels of the whites of the eyes (conjunctiva), ears and face (oculocutaneous telangiectasia), and a susceptibility to sinus and pulmonary infections. Persons with this disorder have low serum IgA levels and a hypoplastic thymus. The diagnosis of ataxia telangiectasia can be confirmed by demonstration of low or absent serum IgA and IgG and characteristic chromosome abnormalities on culture of peripheral blood lymphocytes, so-called chromosome instability (p. 226). In addition, individuals affected with ataxia telangiectasia have an increased risk of developing leukaemia or lymphoid malignancies.

Wiskott–Aldrich syndrome

In this X-linked recessive disorder affected boys have eczema, diarrhoea, recurrent infections, a low platelet count (thrombocytopaenia) and, usually, low serum IgM levels. Until the advent of bone marrow transplantation, these boys died in childhood from haemorrhage or B cell malignancies.

DNA STUDIES

The availability of closely linked DNA markers on the X chromosome for the Wiskott–Aldrich syndrome, Bruton type hypogammaglobulinaemia and X-linked SCID allows carrier testing for females at risk of being carriers by conventional DNA restriction mapping studies in families with more than one affected male.

If, however, there is a single affected male or if, as in the case of SCID, the disorder can show X-linked or autosomal recessive inheritance, then DNA studies of the pattern of X-inactivation (p. 72) in the lymphocytes of females at risk of being carriers can provide information on carrier status. In the case of severe combined immunodeficiency, DNA markers linked to the X-linked gene can be used to look for a pattern of X-inactivation in the T-lymphocyte population which is non-random. The finding in the mother of a sporadically affected male that all her peripheral blood T lymphocytes have the same chromosome inactivated, would confirm her to be a carrier for the X-linked form of SCID. This is represented in Figure 12.5.

The carrier (C) and non-carrier (NC) are both heterozygous for an Hpa II/Msp I restriction site polymorphism. Hpa II and Msp I recognise the same nucleotide recognition sequence but Msp I cuts double-stranded DNA whether it is methylated or not, while Hpa II will only cut unmethylated DNA, i.e. only the active X chromosome. In the carrier female the mutation in the SCID gene is on the X chromosome on which the Hpa II/Msp I restriction site is present. Eco RI/Msp I double digests of T lymphocytes result in 6, 4 and 2 kb DNA fragments on gel analysis of the restriction fragments for both the carrier and non-carrier females. Eco RI/Hpa II double digests of T lymphocyte DNA result, however, in a single 6 kb fragment in the carrier female. This is because in a carrier the only T cells to survive will be those in which the normal gene is on the active unmethylated X

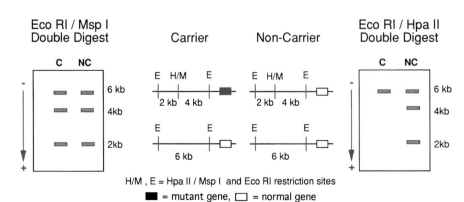

Fig. 12.5
Diagram showing non-random inactivation in T lymphocytes for carrier testing in X-linked SCID.

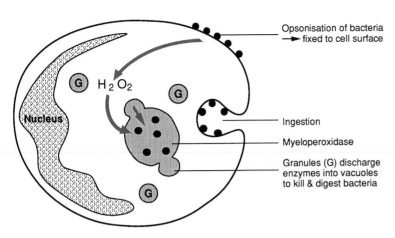

Opsonisation of bacteria
→ fixed to cell surface

Ingestion

Myeloperoxidase

Granules (G) discharge
enzymes into vacuoles
to kill & digest bacteria

Fig. 12.6
Diagrammatic representation of phagocytosis and the
pathways involved in intracellular killing of
microorganisms.

chromosome. Thus in a carrier, inactivation appears non-random although strictly speaking it is cell population survival which is non-random.

A mixed pattern of X-inactivation is consistent with either the disorder having arisen as a new X-linked mutation or being due to the autosomal recessive form. Similar X-inactivation studies of the peripheral blood B-lymphocyte population can be used to determine the carrier status of women at risk for Bruton type agammaglobulinaemia and the Wiskott–Aldrich syndrome.

DISORDERS OF PHAGOCYTIC FUNCTION

Humoral antibodies and lymphocyte cellular immunity are not the only defence against infection. A very important mechanism involves chemotaxis, phagocytosis and subsequent cell mediated killing of microorganisms (Fig. 12.6).

Chronic granulomatous disease

The best known example of a disorder of phagocytic function is chronic granulomatous disease, which can be inherited in an X-linked or autosomal recessive manner. This is associated with recurrent bacterial or fungal infections, often by commensal microorganisms which, until the advent of supportive treatment in the form of infection related and prophylactic antibiotics, conveyed a high childhood mortality.

Leucocyte adhesion deficiency

More recently, a second rare autosomal recessive disorder of phagocytic function known as leucocyte adhesion deficiency has been recognised. Affected individuals present with life threatening bacterial infections of the skin and mucous membranes with impaired pus formation. The increased susceptibility to infections occurs because of a lack of migration of phagocytic cells due to abnormal adhesion-related functions such as chemotaxis

and phagocytosis. This is due to absence of the β_2 integrin receptor subfamily of leucocyte cell surface glycoproteins. The disorder is fatal unless antibiotics are given both for infection and prophylactically until bone marrow transplant can be offered.

THE COMPLEMENT SYSTEM

Complement is a group of serum proteins which are activated either through the *classical pathway*, by antibody binding with antigen, or by the *alternative pathway* with the third component, C3, being activated by the cell membranes of invading microorganisms. The various components of complement interact in sequence, resulting in increased inflammation and vascular permeability. They also attract phagocytes and enhance phagocytosis, ultimately bringing about the destruction of cellular antigens (Fig. 12.7).

Relatively common genetic polymorphisms based on electrophoretic differences have been identified in the C3 and C4 components of complement. The C2 and C7 components of complement are also polymorphic but the frequency of the second allele is much lower.

A number of genetic defects of complement have been described, the most common and best known being deficiency of the Cl inhibitor of the complement system which causes hereditary angioneurotic oedema (p. 141). Persons with angioneurotic oedema periodically develop swelling of subcutaneous tissues which lasts for 48 to 72 hours. If this involves the upper respiratory tract it can lead to upper airways obstruction which can be potentially life-threatening and is difficult to treat.

Defects of the other components of complement are associated with an increased susceptibility to bacterial infections or a predisposition to a systemic lupus erythematosus-like disorder. The discovery that the components of complement are coded for within the major histocompatibility (MHC) locus (p. 160) means that the association of the deficiency of these components with specific HLA alleles could be due to linkage disequilibrium

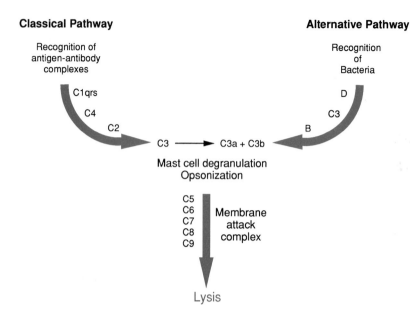

Classical Pathway

Recognition of
antigen-antibody
complexes

C1qrs
C4
C2

Alternative Pathway

Recognition
of
Bacteria

D
C3
B

C3 ⟶ C3a + C3b

Mast cell degranulation
Opsonization

C5
C6
C7
C8
C9

Membrane
attack
complex

Lysis

Fig. 12.7
Diagram of the classical and alternative pathways
of complement activation (adapted from Paul W E
(ed) 1993 Fundamental immunology. Raven Press,
New York).

(p. 101) rather than an HLA antigen disease association (p. 109), although disentangling the two mechanisms is difficult!

BLOOD GROUPS

Blood groups reflect the antigenic determinants on red cells and were one of the first areas in which an understanding of basic biology led to significant advances in clinical medicine. Our knowledge of the ABO and rhesus blood groups has resulted in safe blood transfusion and the prevention of rhesus haemolytic disease of the newborn.

THE ABO BLOOD GROUPS

The ABO blood groups were discovered by Landsteiner just after the turn of the century. The transfusion of red blood cells from certain persons to others, in some instances, resulted in rapid haemolysis, i.e. their blood was incompatible. Studies revealed there to be four major ABO blood groups: A, B, AB and O. Persons who are blood group A possess the antigen A on the surface of their red blood cells, persons of blood group B have antigen B, persons who are AB have A and B antigens whilst persons who are blood group O have neither. Persons of blood group A have naturally occurring anti-B antibodies in their blood, persons of blood group B have anti-A and persons of blood group O have both. The alleles at the ABO blood group locus for antigens A and B are inherited in a codominant manner but are both dominant to the gene for the O antigen (p. 80). There are, therefore, six possible genotypes. The homozygous and heterozygous state for antigens A and B (i.e. AA, AO,

BB, BO) can only be determined by family studies (Table 12.3).

Since individuals of blood group AB do not produce A or B antibodies they can receive a blood transfusion from individuals of all other ABO blood groups and are therefore referred to as *universal recipients*. On the other hand, since individuals of group O do not express either A or B antigens on their red cells they are referred to as *universal donors*. Antisera can differentiate two subgroups of A (A1 and A2), but this is of little practical importance as far as blood transfusions are concerned.

Molecular basis of ABO blood groups

Individuals with blood groups A, B and AB possess enzymes with glycosyltransferase activity which convert the basic blood group, which is known as the H antigen, into A or B antigens. The molecular basis for the ABO genotype has now been identified. The A and B genes differ in only a few single base substitutions which result in different A and B transferase activities. However the O gene results from a critical single base pair deletion which results in an inactive protein incapable of modifying the H antigen.

Table 12.3 ABO blood group phenotypes and genotypes

Red blood cells			React with antiserum	
Phenotype	Genotype	Antibodies	Anti–A	Anti–B
O	OO	anti–A, B	–	–
A	AA, AO	anti–B	+	–
B	BB, BO	anti–A	–	+
AB	AB	–	+	+

Secretor status

In the majority of persons, the ABO blood group antigens, in addition to being expressed on red blood cells, are secreted into various body fluids including saliva. This is controlled by two alleles at the *secretor locus*, secretor positive and secretor negative, the former being dominant to the latter. *Secretor status* is associated with a predisposition to peptic ulcer (p. 189). In addition, the secretor locus is linked to the locus for myotonic dystrophy. Family studies of secretor status, before the advent of DNA markers, were used to predict whether an asymptomatic person had inherited the gene for this disorder (p. 249).

RHESUS BLOOD GROUP

The rhesus (Rh) blood group system is based on serological testing and involves three sets of closely linked antigens, Cc, Dd and Ee. D is very strongly antigenic and persons are, for practical purposes, either Rh positive (possessing the D antigen) or Rh negative (lacking the D antigen).

Rhesus haemolytic disease of the newborn

A proportion of women who are Rh negative have an increased chance of having a child who will either die in utero or be born severely anaemic due to haemolysis. This occurs for the following reason. If Rh positive blood is given to persons who are Rh negative, the majority will develop anti-Rh antibodies. Such sensitisation occurs with very small quantities of blood and, once sensitised, further exposure results in the production of very high antibody titres.

In the case of an Rh negative mother carrying an Rh positive fetus, some of the red cells of the latter can enter the mother's circulation, for example after a miscarriage or at birth. This will induce the formation of Rh antibodies in the mother. In a subsequent pregnancy these can cross the placenta and enter the fetal circulation. This leads to haemolysis of the fetal red blood cells which can result either in fetal death, which is known as *erythroblastosis fetalis*, or a severe haemolytic anaemia of newborn infants which is called *haemolytic disease of the newborn*. Once a woman is sensitised there is a significantly greater risk that a child in a subsequent pregnancy, if Rh positive, will be more severely affected.

To avoid sensitising an Rh negative woman, Rh compatible blood must always be used in any blood transfusion. Furthermore, the development of sensitisation and therefore Rh incompatibility after delivery can be prevented by injecting Rh antibodies, so-called anti-D, into the mother so that any fetal cells which have found their way into the maternal circulation are destroyed before the mother is sensitised.

It is routine to screen all Rh negative women during pregnancy for the development of Rh antibodies. Despite these measures, however, a small proportion of women do become sensitised. If Rh antibodies appear, tests are then carried out to see if the fetus is affected. If so, then there is a delicate balance between early delivery, with the risks of prematurity and exchange transfusion, and treating the fetus in utero with blood transfusions.

Molecular basis

Recent biochemical evidence has shown there to be two types of Rh red cell membrane polypeptide. One corresponds to the D antigen and the other to the C and E series of antigens. Cloning of the genomic sequences responsible using Rh cDNA from reticulocytes has revealed that there are two genes coding for the Rh system, one for D & d and another for C & c and E & e. The D locus is present in most persons and codes for the major D antigen present in persons who are Rh positive. Rh negative individuals are homozygous for a deletion of the D gene. It is not, perhaps, surprising therefore that an antibody has never been raised to d!

Analysis of cDNA from reticulocytes in Rh negative persons, who were homozygous for dCe, dcE and dce, allowed identification of the genomic DNA sequences responsible for the different antigenic variants. This revealed that the antigenic variants are produced by alternative splicing of the mRNA transcript. The Ee polypeptide is a full length product of the CcEe gene, very similar in sequence to the D polypeptide. The E and e antigens differ by a point mutation in exon 5. The Cc polypeptides are, in contrast, products of a shorter length transcript of the same gene having either exons 4, 5 and 6 or 4, 5 and 8 spliced out. The difference between C and c is due to 4 amino acid differences in exons 1 and 2. These results simplify what was an apparently complex blood group system!

OTHER BLOOD GROUPS

There are approximately another 12 'common' blood group systems in humans, such as Duffy, Lewis, MN and S. These are usually only of concern in cross matching blood for persons who, because of repeated transfusions, have developed antibodies to one of these other blood group antigens. Until the advent of DNA fingerprinting (p. 56), they were used in linkage studies (p. 100) and paternity testing (p. 212).

TRANSPLANTATION GENETICS

With the use of *tissue-typing*, replacement of diseased organs by transplantation with healthy ones removed either from healthy living donors or from cadavers has become a routine part of clinical medicine. Except for corneal and bone grafts, the success of such transplants depends on the degree of antigenic similarity between the donor and recipient. The closer the similarity, the greater the likelihood that the transplanted organ or tissue, which is known as a *homograft*, will be accepted rather than rejected. Homograft rejection does not occur between identical twins or between non-identical twins where there has been mixing of the placental circulations before birth (p. 43). In all other instances, the antigenic similarity or *histocompatibility* of donor and recipient has to be assessed by testing the donor and recipient with suitable antisera or monoclonal antibodies for the major and minor histocompatibility antigens on donor and recipient tissues. As a general rule a recipient will reject a graft from any person who has antigens which the recipient lacks.

THE MAJOR HISTOCOMPATIBILITY HUMAN LEUCOCYTE ANTIGEN COMPLEX

The products of the genes of the major histocompatibility complex (MHC), named for its association with graft rejection, are involved in the immune response through the presentation of antigens to the T cell receptor. In humans, the MHC is known as the human leucocyte antigen or HLA system. This consists of a group of closely linked loci which includes what are known as the class I molecules (A, B, C, E, F and G) and the so-called class II molecules (D related or DR, DQ, DPA1, DPA2, DNA, DOB, DQB2 and DQA2).

The HLA system is highly polymorphic (Table 12.4). A virtually infinite number of phenotypes resulting from different combinations of the various alleles at these loci are theoretically possible. Two unrelated individuals are therefore very unlikely to have identical HLA phenotypes.

The close linkage of the HLA loci means that they tend to be inherited 'en bloc', the term *haplotype* being used to indicate the particular HLA alleles an individual carries on each of his two number 6 chromosomes. Thus any individual will have a 25% chance of having identical HLA antigens with a sib since there are only four possible combinations of the two paternal haplotypes (say P and Q) and the two maternal haplotypes (say R and S), i.e.

Table 12.5 Some HLA-associated diseases

Disease	HLA
Narcolepsy	DR2
Ankylosing spondylitis	B27
Chronic hepatitis	B8
Hodgkin's disease	B18
Haemochromatosis	A3
Insulin-dependent diabetes	DR3/4
Myasthenia gravis	B8, A2
Rheumatoid arthritis	DR4
Thyrotoxicosis	DR3
Pre-eclampsia	DR4

PR, PS, QR and QS. The sibs of a particular recipient are more likely to be antigenically similar than either of his parents, and the latter more than an unrelated person. For this reason, a brother or sister is frequently selected as a potential donor for organ or tissue transplantation.

Although crossing-over does occur within the HLA region, certain alleles tend to occur together more frequently than would be expected by chance, i.e. linkage disequilibrium (p. 101). An example is the association of the HLA antigens A1 and B8 in populations of Western European origin.

HLA polymorphisms and disease associations

A finding which helps to throw light on the pathogenesis of certain diseases is the demonstration of the association of specific diseases with certain HLA types (Table 12.5). The best documented is that between ankylosing spondylitis and HLA–B27. In the case of narcolepsy, a condition of unknown aetiology characterised by a periodic uncontrollable tendency to fall asleep, almost all affected individuals are HLA–DR2. The possession of a particular HLA antigen does not mean that an individual will necessarily develop the associated disease, merely that he or she has a greater relative risk of being affected than the general population (p. 109).

Explanations for the various HLA associated disease susceptibilities include close linkage to a susceptibility gene near the HLA complex, cross reactivity of antibodies to environmental antigens or pathogens with specific HLA antigens and abnormal recognition of 'self' antigens through defects in T cell receptors or antigen processing. At present, however, the mechanisms involved in most HLA disease associations are still not completely understood.

H–Y ANTIGEN

In a number of different animal species it was noted that tissue grafts from males were rejected by females of the same inbred strain. These *incompatibilities* were found to be due to a Y-linked (p. 85) histocompatibility antigen,

Table 12.4 Alleles at the HLA loci

HLA locus	Number of alleles
A	32
B	55
C	14
D	> 85

known as the *H–Y antigen*. The H–Y antigen seems, however, to play little part in transplantation in humans. Although the H–Y antigen seems to be important for testicular differentiation and function, its expression does not, however, necessarily correlate with the presence or absence of testicular tissue. The structural gene for the H–Y antigen in humans has been shown to be on chromosome 6 and it seems likely that there is a regulatory gene for the H–Y antigen on the Y chromosome. A separate sex-determining region of the Y chromosome (SRY) has been isolated which seems likely to be the testis-determining gene (p. 71).

ELEMENTS

1 The immune response in humans can be divided into two main types, cellular and humoral. The humoral response involves production of antibodies by mature B cells or plasma cells.

2 Antibodies are Y-shaped molecules and each is composed of two identical heavy (H) chains and two identical light (L) chains. The antibody molecule has two parts which differ in their function; two identical antigen binding sites (Fab) and a single binding site for complement (Fc).

3 There are five classes of antibody, IgA, IgD, IgE, IgG and IgM, each with a specific heavy chain. The light chain of any class of antibody can be made up of either kappa (κ) or lambda (λ) chains.

4 Each immunoglobulin light or heavy chain has a variable (V) region of approximately 110 amino acids at the amino terminal end. The carboxy terminal end consists of a constant (C) region of approximately 110 amino acids in the κ and λ light chains and three to four times that length in the heavy chain. Most of the amino acid sequence variation in both the light and heavy chains occurs within several small hypervariable regions. These are thought to be the sites of antigen binding.

5 The immunoglobulin chains are produced from combinations of separate groups of DNA segments. These consist of one from a variable number of DNA segments coding for the constant (C), variable (V) and joining (J) regions between the V and C regions for the κ and λ light chains and the various types of heavy chains. The heavy chains also contain a diversity (D) region located between the V and J regions. The total number of possible antibodies which could be produced by various combinations of these DNA segments accounts for the antibody diversity seen in man.

6 Complement consists of a series of inactive blood proteins which are sequentially activated in a cascade leading to phagocytosis of microorganisms. This can occur either through the classical pathway, being triggered by antibody binding to antigen, or the alternative pathway, with C3 being directly activated by invading microorganisms.

7 An understanding of the ABO and rhesus blood groups has resulted in safe blood transfusions and the prevention of rhesus haemolytic disease of the newborn.

8 The HLA system consists of a number of closely linked loci on chromosome 6. The many different alleles which can occur at each locus mean that a very large number of different combinations of these can result. The HLA loci are inherited 'en bloc' as a haplotype. The closer the match of HLA antigens between the donor and recipient in organ transplantation, the greater the likelihood of long-term survival of the homograft. Possession of certain HLA antigens is associated with an increased relative risk of developing specific diseases.

FURTHER READING

Bell J I, Todd J A, McDevitt H O 1989 The molecular basis of HLA-disease association. Adv Hum Genet 18: 1–41
Good review of the HLA disease associations.
Dreyer W J, Bennet J C 1965 The molecular basis of antibody formation: a paradox. Proc Nat Acad Sci USA 54: 864–869
The proposal of the generation of antibody diversity.
Hunkapiller T, Hood L 1989 Diversity of the immunoglobulin gene superfamily. Adv Immunol 44: 1–63
Good review of the structure of the immunoglobulin gene superfamily.
Lachmann P J, Peters K, Rosen F S, Walport M J 1993 Clinical aspects of immunology, 5th edn. Blackwell Scientific Publications, Oxford
A comprehensive 3 volume multi-author text covering both basic and clinical immunology.
Roitt I 1994 Essential immunology, 8th edn. Blackwell Scientific Publications, Oxford
Good basic immunology textbook.

CHAPTER 13

The genetics of cancer

Although our understanding of the genetic factors and cellular biology of cancer has advanced rapidly over the last decade, it is important to remember that there are also environmental causes.

ENVIRONMENTAL FACTORS

There are cancers in which environmental factors are of primary importance and heredity seems to play no part in causation. This is true of the 'industrial cancers' which result from prolonged exposure to carcinogenic chemicals. Examples include cancer of the skin in tar workers, cancer of the bladder in aniline dye workers, angiosarcoma of the liver in process workers making polyvinyl chloride (PVC), and cancer of the lung in asbestos workers.

In other cancers the distinction between genetic and environmental aetiological factors is not always obvious.

DIFFERENTIATING BETWEEN GENETIC AND ENVIRONMENTAL FACTORS IN CANCER

In the majority of human cancers there is no clear-cut mode of inheritance nor is there any clearly defined environmental cause. In certain cancers, such as breast and bowel cancer, genetic factors play an important, but not exclusive, role in the aetiology. Evidence to help differentiate environmental and genetic factors can come from a combination of epidemiologic, family and twin studies, disease associations, biochemical factors and animal studies.

EPIDEMIOLOGIC STUDIES

Breast cancer

Breast cancer is the most common cancer in women. Reproductive and menstrual histories are well recognised risk factors. Parous women have a lower risk of developing breast cancer than nulliparous women. In addition, the younger the age at which a woman has her first pregnancy, the lower her risk of developing breast cancer. Conversely, the later the age of onset of menstrual periods, the greater the risk of developing breast cancer.

The incidence of breast cancer varies greatly between different populations, being highest in women in North America and Western Europe and up to 8 times lower in women of Japanese and Chinese origin. While these differences could be attributed to genetic differences between these population groups, study of immigrant populations moving from an area with a low incidence to one with a high incidence has shown that the risk of developing breast cancer rises to that of the native population, supporting the view that breast cancer has a significant environmental component.

Gastric cancer

It has long been recognised that persons from the poorer socioeconomic groups have an increased risk of developing gastric cancer. Specific dietary and environmental substances, such as nitrates, have been suggested as being possible carcinogens. Gastric cancer also shows differences in incidence, being most common in Japanese and Chinese populations and up to 10 times less common in persons of Western European origin. Migration studies have shown that the risk of gastric cancer for immigrants from high risk populations does not fall to that of the native low risk population for 2 to 3 generations. It has been suggested that this could be due to exposure to environmental factors at an early age.

FAMILY STUDIES

Breast cancer

The lifetime risk for a woman in Western Europe to develop breast cancer is 1 in 12. Family studies have shown that the likelihood of a first-degree female relative of a woman with breast cancer developing breast cancer is between 1.8 and 3 times the risk for the general population. The risk varies depending on the age of onset in the proband, being greater the younger the age of onset in the proband (p. 174).

Gastric cancer

Similar studies in gastric cancer have shown that *first-degree relatives* of persons with cancer of the stomach have a 2 to 3 fold increased risk compared to the general population of developing gastric cancer. The increased risk of developing gastric cancer in near relatives is, however, relatively small suggesting that environmental factors are likely to be more important.

TWIN STUDIES

Concordance rates for breast cancer in twins are low for both types of twins, being only slightly greater in monozygotic female twins at 17% than 13% in dizygotic female twins, suggesting that environmental factors are more likely to be important than genetic factors. Twin studies in gastric cancer have failed to reveal increased concordance in monozygotic compared to dizygotic twins.

DISEASE ASSOCIATIONS

Blood groups are genetically determined and therefore association of a particular blood group with a disease suggests a significant genetic contribution to the aetiology. A large number of studies from a variety of countries have shown an association between blood group A and gastric cancer. It is estimated that persons with blood group A have a 20% increased risk over the general population for developing gastric cancer. In addition, it is also recognised that gastric cancer is associated with chronic gastritis and pernicious anaemia. Blood group A is associated with pernicious anaemia which is also closely associated with chronic gastritis. It appears, however, that pernicious anaemia has a separate association with gastric cancer. Persons with pernicious anaemia have a 3- to 6-fold increased risk of developing stomach cancer.

BIOCHEMICAL FACTORS

Biochemical factors can determine the susceptibility to environmental carcinogens. Examples include the association between slow acetylator status and a predisposition to bladder cancer (p. 143), as well as debrisoquine metaboliser status (p. 146) and glutathione S-transferase activity (p. 149) which influence the risk of developing lung cancer in smokers.

ANIMAL STUDIES

Certain inbred strains of mice have been developed which have a high chance of developing a particular type of tumour. The A (albino) Bittner strain is especially prone to develop tumours of the lung and breast; the C3H strain is particularly prone to develop breast tumours as well as tumours of the liver; the C58 strain is prone to develop leukaemia. Breeding experiments with mice have shown that cancer proneness is influenced by environmental factors. In strains with a high incidence of breast tumours, the frequency of these tumours is reduced by dietary restrictions and increased by high temperature.

VIRAL FACTORS

Bittner showed that the susceptibility to develop breast tumours in certain strains of mice depended on a combination of genetic factors as well as a 'milk agent'. In high incidence strains both genetic susceptibility and the milk agent are involved, but in some low incidence strains there is no milk agent. The milk agent has been shown to be a virus which is usually transmitted by the mother's milk but could also be transmitted by the father's sperm. By using foster-mothers from cancer-free strains to suckle newborn mice from strains with a high cancer susceptibility it is possible to reduce the incidence of breast cancer from 100% to less than 50%. Conversely, it is possible to increase the incidence in cancer-free strains by suckling the newborn mice with foster-mothers from high cancer-prone strains. Certain viruses are tumour-forming or *oncogenic* in humans.

Tumour viruses

A limited number of DNA tumour viruses are associated with certain types of human neoplasia (Table 13.1), while a variety of RNA viruses, or *retroviruses*, cause tumours

Table 13.1 Human DNA viruses implicated in carcinogenesis

Virus family	Type	Tumour
Papova	Papilloma (HPV)	Warts (plantar & genital), urogenital cancers (cervical, vulvar & penile), skin cancer
Herpes	Epstein–Barr (EBV)	Burkitt's lymphoma*, nasopharyngeal carcinoma, lymphomas in immunocompromised hosts
	Cytomegalovirus (CMV)	Kaposi's sarcoma
Hepadna	Hepatitis B (HBV)	Hepatocellular carcinoma*

*For full oncogenicity, 'co–carcinogens' are necessary, e.g. aflatoxin B_1 in hepatitis B associated hepatocellular carcinoma

Table 13.2 Oncogenic retroviruses, their hosts and associated tumours

Host	Virus	Tumour/disease
Chickens	Rous sarcoma virus	Sarcoma
	Avian leukosis virus	Avian leukaemia
Mice	Murine sarcoma virus	Sarcoma
	Murine leukaemia virus	Leukaemia
	Mouse mammary tumour virus	Breast cancer
Primates	Simian sarcoma virus	Sarcoma
	Gibbon ape leukaemia virus	Leukaemia
Humans	Human T-cell lymphotrophic viruses (HLTV)	T-cell leukaemia
	Human immunodeficiency virus type 1 (HIV-1)	Kaposi's sarcoma

in animals (Table 13.2). The study of the genetics and replicative processes of oncogenic retroviruses has revealed some of the cellular biological processes of carcinogenesis.

Retroviruses

In 1908 Ellerman and Bang showed that erythroid leukaemia in chickens was transmitted by a cell-free filtrate. At that time, however, leukaemia was regarded as a blood disease rather than a cancer and the significance of these observations was not realised. The work of Peyton Rous between 1910 and 1914, in contrast, attracted more interest. He showed that crude extracts of a tumour from a Plymouth Rock hen, inoculated into healthy chickens, resulted in the growth of new tumours.

The evidence for a viral aetiology in tumour formation in mammals followed over 30 years later, with Bittner's studies of the inheritance of breast cancer in an inbred strain of mice showing the so-called 'milk-agent'.

Viruses lack the genes necessary for autonomous replication. When viruses infect a cell, they replicate by taking over the biochemical machinery of the cell to manufacture the components of the progeny virions. Retroviruses, in which the genetic information is coded in RNA, contain an enzyme known as reverse transcriptase which makes a double stranded DNA copy of the viral RNA. This integrates into the host cell genome, allowing the appropriate proteins to be manufactured, resulting in repackaging of new progeny virions.

Until recently, naturally occurring retroviruses were thought to have only the three genes necessary to ensure replication, *gag*, encoding the structural proteins for the core antigens, *pol*, coding for reverse transcriptase, and *env*, the gene for the glycoprotein envelope proteins (Fig. 13.1). Study of the virus responsible for the transmissible tumour in chickens, the so-called Rous sarcoma virus, identified a fourth gene which results in *transformation* of cells in culture, a model for malignancy in vivo. This viral gene is known as an *oncogene*.

ONCOGENES

Oncogenes are known by three letter abbreviations which reflect their origin and/or the type of tumour with which they are associated (Table 13.3).

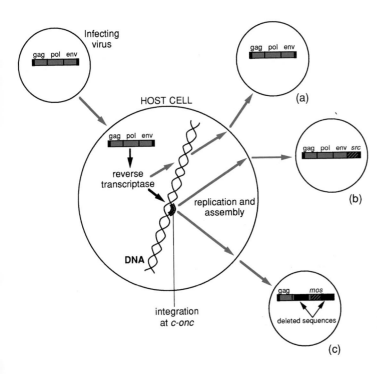

Fig. 13.1
Model for acquisition of transforming ability in retroviruses:
(a) Normal retroviral replication.
(b) The Rous sarcoma virus has integrated near a cellular oncogene. The transforming ability of this virus is due to the acquired homologue of the cellular oncogene, v-*src*.
(c) A defective transforming virus carries an oncogene similar to *src* but is defective in the structural genes, e.g. Moloney murine sarcoma virus which carries *mos*.

Table 13.3 Some transforming retroviruses, the species affected, the tumour formed and the oncogene responsible

Virus	Species	Virus induced tumour	Oncogene
Rous sarcoma	Chicken	Sarcoma	*src*
Avian erythroblastosis	Chicken	erythroleukaemia	*erb*–B
Avian myeloblastosis	Chicken	myeloblastic leukaemia	*myb*
Avian myelocytomatosis	Chicken	myelocytoma, sarcoma	*myc*
Abelson leukaemia	Mouse	pre-B cell leukaemia	*abl*
FBJ murine osteosarcoma	Mouse	osteosarcoma	*fos*
Moloney murine sarcoma	Mouse	sarcoma	*mos*
Harvey murine sarcoma	Rat	sarcoma	Ha–*ras*
Kirsten murine sarcoma	Rat	sarcoma	Ki–*ras*
Simian sarcoma	Monkey	sarcoma	*sis*

Studies have revealed the presence in normal mammalian cells of DNA sequences homologous to the viral oncogenes and these have been called *proto-oncogenes* or *cellular oncogenes*. It appears that the transforming viruses have acquired part of the host genome during integration into the host genome.

The terms proto-oncogene and cellular oncogene are often used interchangeably, although strictly speaking the term proto-oncogene is reserved for the normal gene and the term cellular oncogene, or c-*onc*, refers to a gene with oncogenic properties like the viral oncogenes, or v-*onc*.

RELATIONSHIP BETWEEN C-ONC AND V-ONC

Retroviral oncogenes are thought to form through errors in the replication of the retrovirus genome following their integration at random sites into the host DNA. The end result is a viral gene which is structurally similar to its cellular counterpart but is persistently different in its function. For example, the viral oncogene *sis* is almost identical to the gene for one chain of a growth factor known as the *platelet-derived growth factor* (PDGF) (p. 168). Cellular oncogenes are highly conserved in evolution. For example, DNA sequences of the *ras* oncogene are found as far apart in the evolutionary tree as yeast and humans.

CONVERSION OF PROTO-ONCOGENES TO CELLULAR ONCOGENES

Two models have been postulated for the conversion of proto-oncogenes to cellular oncogenes. The first is a quantitative one in which tumour formation is induced by an increase in the absolute amount of proto-oncogene product or by its production in inappropriate cell types. The second model supposes that the conversion from proto-oncogene to a transforming gene (c-*onc*) is a qualitative one, with changes in the nucleotide sequence being responsible for the acquisition of the new properties.

QUANTITATIVE MODEL OF ONCOGENE ACTION

Inappropriate amounts of oncogene products have been shown to be due to two mechanisms; insertional mutagenesis and gene amplification.

Insertional mutagenesis

The ability of a retrovirus to transform a cell without expressing the v-*onc* sequence was first noted during analysis of the bursal lymphomas caused by the transformation of B lymphocytes with the avian leukosis virus. When such a retrovirus integrates into the host genome in close proximity to a proto-oncogene, viral DNA sequences or *long terminal repeat* (LTR) sequences whose normal function is to regulate viral expression, have the potential to produce uncontrolled expression of the cellular gene. The resulting genetic disruption is called *insertional mutagenesis*.

In a number of experimentally induced tumours, the oncogenic retrovirus has been shown to be integrated into the cellular genome within or close to the c-*myc* gene, with the LTR of the virus acting as a promoter of gene expression. It has been suggested that activation of c-*myc* in this way could be a mechanism which leads to the development of Burkitt's lymphoma in humans, which is associated with infection with the Epstein–Barr virus.

Gene amplification

Proto-oncogenes can also be activated by making multiple copies of the gene or what is known as *gene amplification*, a mechanism known to have survival value when cells encounter environmental stress. For example, when leukaemic cells are exposed to the chemo-therapeutic agent methotrexate, the cells acquire resistance by making multiple copies of the gene for dihydrofolate reductase, the target enzyme for methotrexate.

Gene amplification can increase the number of copies of the oncogene per cell several fold to several hundred times, leading to greater amounts of the corresponding oncoprotein. In mammals the amplified sequence of DNA in tumour cells can be recognised by the presence of small extra chromosomes known as *double-minute chromosomes* or *homogeneously staining regions* of the chromosomes. These changes are seen in approximately 10% of tumours and are often present in the later rather than the initial stages of the malignant process.

Amplification of specific proto-oncogenes appears to be a feature of certain tumours and is frequently seen with the *myc* family of genes. For example, N-*myc* is amplified in approximately 30% of neuroblastomas but in advanced cases this figure rises to 50%, where gene amplification can be up to one thousand fold. Human small cell carcinomas of the lung also show amplification of c-*myc*, N-*myc*, and L-*myc*.

Amplification of c-*neu* or *erb*-B2 is a feature in 20% of breast carcinomas where it has been suggested that it correlates with a number of well established prognostic factors such as lymph node status, oestrogen and progestogen receptor status, tumour size and histological grade.

QUALITATIVE MODEL OF ONCOGENE ACTION

Proto-oncogenes can be converted into cellular oncogenes in two other ways, either through mutations in the coding sequence or by chromosomal translocations.

Mutation in coding sequence

The transformation of a well established cell line derived from mouse fibroblasts, called NIH 3T3, by DNA *transfection* from a human bladder carcinoma cell line, led to the discovery of a human DNA sequence homologous to the *ras* gene of the Harvey murine sarcoma virus. The human *ras* gene family consists of three closely related members, Ha-*ras*, Ki-*ras* and N-*ras*. The *ras* proteins are closely homologous to their viral counterparts and only differ markedly from one another near their carboxyl termini. Oncogenicity of the *ras* proto-oncogenes arises by point mutations in the nucleotide sequence.

Activating mutations in the *ras* gene have been detected in about 30% of human cancers but their incidence varies widely depending on the tumour origin. For instance, *ras* oncogenes are almost non-existent in carcinoma of the breast, but are seen in 25–30% of lung cancers, 50% of colonic cancers and 90% of pancreatic carcinomas. Activating mutations in the *ras* gene have also been detected in premalignant lesions, suggesting a role in initiation of the neoplastic process.

The involvement of *ras* genes in human cancers is not limited to their activation by point mutations as significant amplification of *ras* genes has been discovered in a variety of tumours, although the incidence of *ras* gene amplification in human neoplasia is no higher than 1–2%.

Chromosomal translocation

Chromosome aberrations are common in malignant cells which often show marked variation in chromosome number and structure. Certain chromosomes seemed to be especially involved and it was thought that these changes were secondary to the transformed state rather than causal. This attitude changed when evidence suggested that these translocations resulted in rearrangements within or adjacent to proto-oncogenes. It has been found that chromosomal translocations can alter the biochemical function or level of proto-oncogene activity. Chronic myeloid leukaemia is an example of the former, Burkitt's lymphoma an example of the latter.

Chronic myeloid leukaemia

In 1960, investigators in Philadelphia were the first to describe an abnormal chromosome in white blood cells from patients with chronic myeloid leukaemia. The abnormal chromosome, referred to as the Philadelphia, or Ph[1] chromosome, is an acquired abnormality found in blood or bone marrow cells but not found in other tissues from these patients. The Ph[1] is a tiny chromosome which is now known to be a chromosome 22 from which material from the long arm has been reciprocally translocated to and from the long arm of chromosome 9 (Fig. 13.2), i.e. t(9;22)(q34;q11). Occasionally the translocation is with another autosome. This chromosomal rearrangement is seen in 90% of persons with this form of leukaemia. This translocation has been found to transfer the cellular *abl* oncogene from chromosome 9 into a region of chromosome 22 known as the *break point cluster*, or *bcr*, region resulting in a *chimaeric* transcript derived from both the c-*abl* (70%) and the *bcr* genes.

Burkitt's lymphoma

An unusual form of neoplasia seen in children in Africa is a lymphoma which involves the jaw, known as Burkitt's lymphoma, so named after Dennis Burkitt who first described the condition in the late 1950s. Chromosomal analysis has revealed the majority (90%) of affected children to have a translocation of the c-*myc* gene from the long arm of chromosome 8 on to chromosome 14. Less commonly the c-*myc* gene is translocated to chromosome 2 or 22. The regions of chromosomes 14, 2 and 22 involved encode the genes for the immunoglobulin heavy chain and the kappa (κ) and lambda (λ) light chains respectively. As a consequence of these translocations c-*myc* comes under the influence of the regulatory sequences of the respective immunoglobulin gene and is over-expressed 10-fold or more.

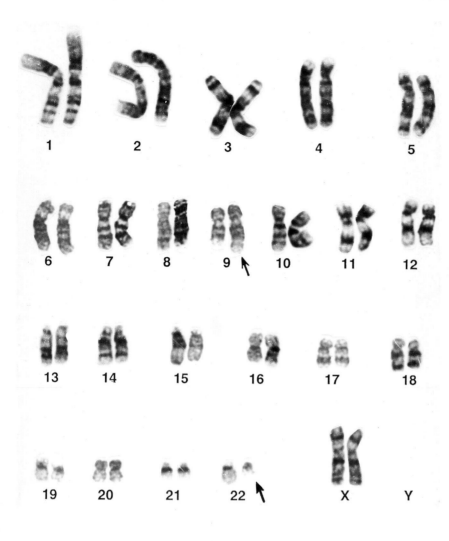

Fig. 13.2
Karyotype from a patient with chronic myeloid leukaemia, showing the chromosome 22 (arrowed) or Philadelphia chromosome which has material translocated to the long arm of one of the number 9 chromosomes (arrowed).

FUNCTION OF ONCOGENES

Cancers have characteristics which indicate, at the cellular level, loss of the normal mechanisms which control cellular proliferation and differentiation.

The cell cycle

The transition of a cell from G_0 to the start of the cell cycle (p. 30) is governed by substances called *growth factors*. Different types of cells require different growth factors to stimulate cell division. Two well known growth factors are *platelet derived growth factor* (PDGF) and *epidermal growth factor* (EGF). PDGF stimulates the proliferation of connective tissue cells while EGF stimulates a variety of cell types including epidermal cells. Growth factors stimulate cells to grow by binding to one of three types of specific growth factor receptor (Table 13.4) in a process known as *signal transduction*. Signal transduction is a complex multi-step pathway from the cell membrane, through the cytoplasm to the nucleus, with positive and negative feedback loops for accurate cell proliferation and differentiation (Fig. 13.3).

Table 13.4 Types of growth factor receptor and some examples of growth factors

Growth factor receptor type	Growth factor
GTP binding proteins	Thrombin, serotonin, angiotensin
Protein tyrosine kinase	Insulin, platelet and epidermal derived growth factors
Cytoplasmic tyrosinase kinase – linked haemopoietin receptors	Prolactin, erythropoietin

Types of oncogene

Oncogenes can be classified according to their cellular location and the function of their encoded oncoproteins in the signal transduction pathway (Table 13.5).

Growth factors

The best known oncogene which acts as a growth factor is the *sis* oncogene which encodes part of the biologically

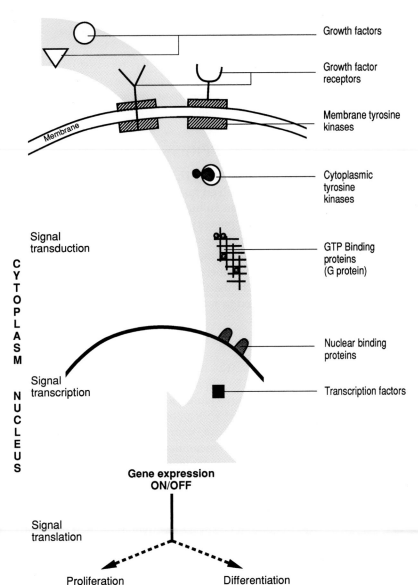

Growth factors

Growth factor
receptors

Membrane tyrosine
kinases

Membrane

Cytoplasmic
tyrosine
kinases

Signal
transduction

GTP Binding
proteins
(G protein)

C
Y
T
O
P
L
A
S
M

Nuclear binding
proteins

Signal
transcription

Transcription factors

N
U
C
L
E
U
S

**Gene expression
ON/OFF**

Signal
translation

Proliferation

Differentiation

Fig. 13.3
Simplified schema of the steps in signal
transduction and transcription from cell
surface to nucleus. The intracellular pathway
amplifies the signal by a cascade which
involves one or more of the steps.

active b chain of platelet derived growth factor. When
PDGF is added to non-tumourigenic, long term cell lines,
such as NIH 3T3, the cells are transformed and they
behave like neoplastic cells, i.e. their growth rate
increases. In vitro they lose contact inhibition and in vivo
they form tumours when injected into nude mice. Oncogene products showing homology to fibroblast growth
factors (FGF) include *hst* and *int*-2 which are amplified in
breast and oesophageal cancers and in malignant mela-
nomas.

Table 13.5 The functional classification of oncogenes

Growth factor	Growth factor receptors	GTP binding proteins	Post receptor tyrosine kinases	Cytoplasmic oncogenes	Nuclear oncogenes
sis (PDGF)	*erb-B*	N-*ras*	*src*	*mos*	*fos*
int (FGF-related)	*erb-B2*	Ha-*ras*	*abl*	A-*raf*	*jun*
hst (FGF-related)	*fms*	Ki-*ras*	*yes*	B-*raf*	*erb-A*
	kit		*fgr*		*myb*
	ros		*fes*		*myc*
	trk		*syn*		N-*myc*
	ret				L-*myc*
	sea				
	met				

Growth factor receptors

Many oncogenes encode proteins with tyrosine kinase activity or possess tyrosine kinase domains. Examples of receptors for tyrosine kinases include c-erb-B which encodes the epidermal growth factor (EGF) receptor and the related c-erb-B2 oncogene. C-erb-B2 is activated by amplification and is over expressed in cancers of the stomach, pancreas and ovary.

GTP binding proteins

GTP binding proteins are intracellular proteins associated with protein tyrosine kinases. The *ras* proteins are localised to the inner surface of the cell membrane. Mutant *ras* genes have a reduced capacity to terminate a growth stimulating signal, resulting in unrestrained growth.

Post receptor tyrosine kinases

Phosphorylation of the amino acid tyrosine is uncommon in normal cells. The genes whose products are capable of this phosphorylation are believed to be involved in the process of signal transduction. The *abl* oncogene has tyrosine kinase activity as does the *src* oncoprotein, which is responsible for the transforming properties of the Rous sarcoma virus.

Cytoplasmic oncogenes

A number of cytoplasmic gene products are recognised to be part of the signal transduction pathway. The *raf* gene product modulates the normal regulating cascade and may be directly responsible for transmitting a growth promoting signal to the nucleus.

Nuclear oncogenes

The oncogenes *fos*, *jun* and *erb*-A encode proteins that are specific transcription factors and regulate gene expression by activating or suppressing nearby DNA sequences. The function of c-*myc* and related genes remains uncertain but appears to be related to alterations in control of the cell cycle. The c-*myc* and c-*myb* oncoproteins stimulate cells to progress from the G_1 into the S phase of the cell cycle (p. 30). Their over production prevents cells from entering a prolonged resting phase, resulting in persistent cellular proliferation.

Apoptotic oncogenes

Cancer cells can accumulate either by increased growth and/or division or decreased cell death, which is known as *apoptosis*. The *bcl*-2 oncogene is the clearest example which leads to abnormal apoptosis.

CANCER GENETICS

While the study of oncogenes has revealed much about the cellular biology of malignancy, the study of hereditary cancer has revealed important concepts in what is known as *cancer genetics*.

TUMOUR SUPPRESSOR GENES

Studies, carried out by Harris and colleagues in the late 1960s which involved fusion of malignant cells with non-malignant cells in culture, resulted in the suppression of the malignant phenotype in the hybrid cells. The recurrence of the malignant phenotype with loss of certain chromosomes from the hybrid cells suggested that normal cells contain a gene(s) with tumour-suppressor activity which, if lost or inactive, can lead to malignancy. Such a gene is referred to as an *anti-oncogene*.

Retinoblastoma

Retinoblastoma (Rb) is a relatively rare, highly malignant cancer of the developing retinal cells (Fig. 13.4). It most commonly occurs before the age of 5 years but if treated early is associated with a good long-term outcome.

Retinoblastoma can occur either sporadically, so-called non-hereditary, or be familial, so-called hereditary, being inherited in an autosomal dominant manner. Non-hereditary cases usually affect only one eye, whereas hereditary cases can be either unilateral or bilateral or occur in more than one site, i.e. be multifocal. They also tend to occur at an earlier age than in the non-hereditary form.

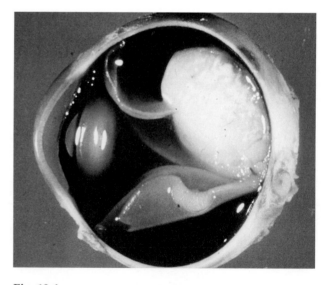

Fig. 13.4
Section of an eye showing a retinoblastoma in situ.

In 1971, Knudson carried out a statistical analysis of a large number of cases of both types of retinoblastoma and advanced a 'two-hit' hypothesis to explain the occurrence of this rare tumour in patients with and without a positive family history. He proposed that affected individuals with a positive family history had inherited one non-functional gene which was present in all the cells of the individual, or what is known as a *germ-line mutation*, with the second gene at the same locus becoming inactivated somatically in a developing retinal cell. This would explain the observation that in hereditary retinoblastoma the tumours can be bilateral and multifocal. In contrast, in the non-heritable or sporadic form, two inactivating *somatic mutations* would need to occur independently in the same retinoblast. This would explain the fact that tumours in these patients were often unilateral and unifocal and usually occurred at a later age than in the hereditary form.

Approximately 5% of children presenting with retinoblastoma have other physical abnormalities along with developmental concerns. Detailed cytogenetic analysis of blood samples from these children revealed some of them to have an interstitial deletion involving the long arm of one of their number 13 chromosome pair. Comparison of the regions deleted revealed a common 'smallest region of overlap' involving the sub-band 13q14 (Fig. 13.5).

The detection of a chromosomal region involved in the aetiology of these non-familial cases of retinoblastoma (p. 220) suggested that it could also be the locus involved in the dominant form of retinoblastoma. Family studies using a polymorphic enzyme, esterase D, which had previously been mapped to that region, rapidly confirmed linkage of the dominant hereditary form of retinoblastoma to that locus. Subsequent studies using DNA markers in this region confirmed this linkage and subsequently led to isolation of the retinoblastoma or Rb gene.

Loss of constitutional heterozygosity

Analyses of the DNA sequences in this region of chromosome 13 in the peripheral blood and in retinoblastoma tumour material of children who had inherited the gene for retinoblastoma showed them to have a loss of or a mutation in both alleles at the retinoblastoma locus in the tumour material or what is known as *loss of constitutional heterozygosity* (LOCH). An example of this is shown in Fig. 13.6 in which the mother transmits the retinoblastoma gene along with allele 2 at a closely linked marker locus. The father is homozygous for allele 1 at this same locus with the result that the child is constitutionally an obligate heterozygote at this locus. Analysis of the tumour tissue reveals apparent homozygosity for allele 2. In fact, there has been loss of the paternally derived allele 1 leading to loss of constitutional heterozygosity in the tumour material. This loss of heterozygosity is consistent with the 'two-hit' hypothesis leading to development of the malignancy as proposed by Knudson.

Loss of constitutional heterozygosity can occur as a result of loss of a chromosome through mitotic non-disjunction (p. 34), a deletion on the chromosome carrying the corresponding allele or a cross-over between the two homologous genes leading to homozygosity for the mutant allele.

Loss of heterozygosity has been observed in a number of other tumours (Table 13.6). One of the problems in identifying sites of loss of constitutional heterozygosity is the aneuploidy of many tumours which results in a significant degree of 'background' noise. Subsequent to the establishment of LOCH, linkage studies of familial cases can be carried out to determine if the familial cases are due to mutations at the same locus.

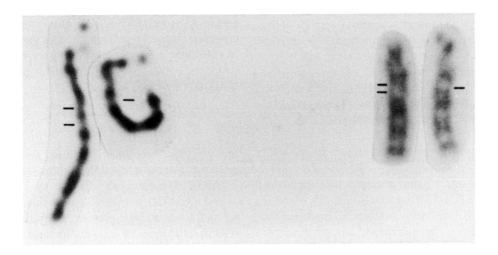

Fig. 13.5
Two sets of homologues of chromosome 13 from a patient with retinoblastoma showing an interstitial deletion of 13q14 in the right-hand homologue in each pair as indicated.

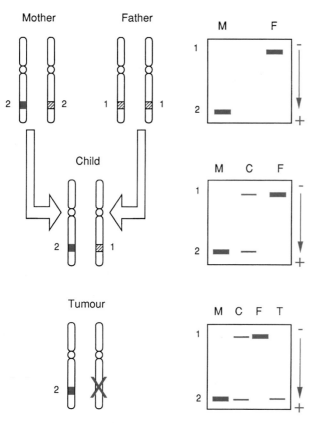

Fig. 13.6
Representation of loss of constitutional heterozygosity in the development of a tumour.

Table 13.6 Syndromes and cancers which show loss of heterozygosity and their chromosomal location

Syndrome or Cancer	Chromosomal localisation
Retinoblastoma	13q
Osteosarcoma	13q, 17p
Wilms' tumour	11p
Renal carcinoma	3p
von Hippel Lindau disease	3p
Bladder carcinoma	9q, 11p, 17p
Lung carcinoma	3p, 13q, 17p
Breast carcinoma	1q, 3p, 13q, 17p
Beckwith–Wiedemann syndrome	3p, 11p, 13q, 17p
Rhabdomyosarcoma	11p
Hepatoblastoma	11p
Hepatocellular carcinoma	11p
Gastric cancer	13q
Familial adenomatosis polyposis	5q
Colorectal carcinoma	5q, 17p, 18q
Neurofibromatosis 1 (NF–1, von Recklinghausen disease)	17q
Neurofibromatosis 2 (NF–2)	22q
Meningioma	22q
Multiple endocrine neoplasia type 1 (MEN–1)	11q
Insulinoma	11q
Thyroid medullary carcinoma	1p
Phaeochromocytoma	1p

Function of tumour suppressor genes

While familial retinoblastoma has classically been considered to be an autosomal dominant trait, this demonstration of the action of the retinoblastoma gene introduced the concept that it is, in fact, a recessive *tumour suppressor gene*. In other words, absence of the gene product in the homozygous state leads to the development of this particular tumour. The tumour suppressor activity of the retinoblastoma gene has been demonstrated in vitro in cancer cells.

In contrast to oncogenes, tumour suppressor genes are a class of cellular genes whose normal function is to suppress inappropriate cell proliferation. These genes are often lost, inactivated or mutated in neoplastic cells.

Rb gene

The Rb gene specifies a 4.7 kb transcript which encodes a nuclear protein, p105, which associates with DNA and is involved in the regulation of the cell cycle. Fortuitously, unrelated research on the mechanism of action of the E1A oncogene of human adenovirus, demonstrated that E1A oncoprotein forms a complex with p105 which is inhibited. As E1A is known to be a transcription regulator it is suggested that p105 is also involved in modulating the transcription of critical genes. The Rb gene product exists in a phosphorylated or unphosphorylated state. In its unphosphorylated state it is inactive in growth suppression. In its phosphorylated state it associates with an unidentified nuclear factor and suppresses growth.

The Rb gene product interacts with several viral oncoproteins, such as the transforming proteins of SV40 (large T antigen) and papilloma virus (E7 protein), thereby liberating cells from normal growth constraints.

These findings yield insight into the mechanisms of interaction between oncogenes and tumour suppressor genes. As research continues there could well be many other examples whereby oncogenes exert their influence by directly or indirectly inactivating the function of tumour suppressor gene encoded proteins or other proteins intimately involved in the cell cycle.

p53

The p53 protein was first identified as a host cell protein bound to T antigen, the dominant transforming oncogene of the DNA tumour virus SV40. After murine p53 was cloned it was shown to be able to co-operate with activated *ras* and act as an oncogene to transform primary rodent cells in vitro, even though the rodent cells expressed the wild type or normal p53. Subsequently, inactivation of p53 was frequently found in murine Friend virus induced erythroleukaemia cells, which led to the proposal that p53 is, in fact, a tumour suppressor gene.

Over 50% of bladder, breast, colon and lung cancers have been found to have p53 mutations which, although occurring in different codons, are clustered in highly conserved regions in exons 5 to 10. This is in contrast to p53 mutations in hepatocellular carcinoma which occur in a 'hot-spot' in codon 249. The base changes in this mutated codon, usually G to T, could be the result of an interaction with the carcinogen aflatoxin B_1 which is associated with liver cancer in China and South Africa, or with the hepatitis B virus which is also implicated as a co-factor in hepatomas. Interestingly, aflatoxin B_1, a ubiquitous food-contaminating aflatoxin in these areas, is a mutagen in many animal species and induces G to T substitutions in mutagenesis experiments. If an interaction between hepatitis B viral proteins and non-mutated p53 can be demonstrated, this will further support the role of this virus in the aetiology of hepatocellular carcinomas.

The p53 protein is a multimeric complex. Mutant p53 protein monomers are more stable than the normal p53 proteins and can form complexes with the normal wild type p53 acting in a *dominant-negative* manner to inactivate it. p53 has been coined the 'guardian of the genome' as it prevents progress through the cell cycle, allowing DNA damaged through normal 'wear and tear' to be repaired.

This provides evidence for a single 'hit' model for the inactivation of normal p53 as an acquired event in the common cancers (Table 13.6). Mutation of a single allele could be sufficient to induce neoplastic transformation even when one copy of the normal allele remains.

The Li–Fraumeni syndrome

As mutations in p53 appear to be a common event in the genesis of many cancers, an inherited or germ line mutation of p53 would be expected to have serious consequences. This hypothesis was substantiated with the discovery of such a defect in the Li–Fraumeni syndrome. Members of families with this rare syndrome (p. 175), which is inherited as an autosomal dominant trait are highly susceptible to a variety of early onset malignancies. These include sarcomas, adrenal carcinomas and breast cancer. Point mutations in highly conserved regions of the p53 gene (codons 245–258) were identified in the germ line of family members with tumour analysis revealing deletion of the normal allele.

'Deleted in colorectal cancer' (DCC)

Allele loss on chromosome 18q is seen in over 70% of colorectal carcinomas. The candidate gene for this region, called deleted in colorectal carcinoma, or DCC, has been identified and cloned and has a high degree of homology with the family of genes encoding cell adhesion molecules. The DCC gene is expressed in normal colonic mucosa but is either reduced or absent in colorectal carcinomas. As with p53, somatic mutations in the DCC gene

of the remaining allele occur in some cancers where gene expression is absent. With the known homology, this suggests that loss of DCC plays a role in cell–cell and cell–basement membrane interactions, features which are lost in overt malignancy.

Other human tumour suppressor genes

Polyposis coli and colon cancer

In humans, there is a rather rare condition known as polyposis coli, also known as familial adenomatous polyposis (FAP) and adenomatous polyposis coli (APC). In this disease the whole of the large bowel is lined with numerous polyps (Fig. 13.7). There is a high risk of carcinomatous change taking place in these polyps and without treatment more than 90% of affected persons would die from cancer of the bowel. Polyposis coli is inherited as an autosomal dominant trait.

The identification of an individual with FAP and a deletion of a particular region of the long arm of chromosome 5 (5q21) led to the demonstration of linkage of FAP to DNA markers in that region. Subsequent studies led to the isolation of the adenomatous polyposis coli gene. Analysis of the markers linked to polyposis coli in cancers from persons who have inherited the gene for this disorder has shown loss of constitutional heterozygosity, suggesting a similar mechanism of gene action in the development of this type of bowel cancer. In contrast, adenomas from patients with FAP rarely show allelic loss on 5q, a finding suggesting that in some cases loss of one tumour suppressor gene is sufficient to allow unrestrained growth in that cell through a threshold effect.

Studies in the common form of bowel cancer which is not inherited have shown similar loss of constitutional heterozygosity at 5q in the tumour material with the FAP gene being deleted in 30% and 60% of sporadically occurring adenomas and carcinomas of the colon. LOCH has also been reported at a number of different sites which include the regions 18q21–qter and 17pl2–13, with the latter region including the p53 gene, as well as another gene at 5q21 known as the *mutated in colorectal cancer* (MCC) gene. This suggests that the development of the common form of colon cancer is a multistep process.

THE MULTISTAGE PROCESS OF CARCINOGENESIS

Colorectal cancer

The majority of colorectal cancers are believed to develop from 'benign' adenomas. Conversely, only a small percentage of adenomas proceed to invasive cancer. Histologically, adenomatous polyps less than 1 cm in diameter rarely contain areas of carcinomatous changes, whereas the risk of carcinomatous change increases to 5–10% when the

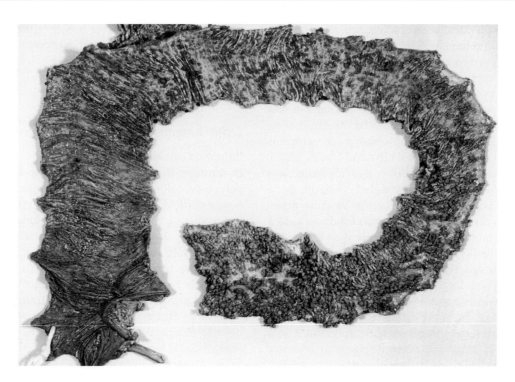

Fig. 13.7
Large bowel from a person with polyposis coli opened up to show multiple polyps throughout the colon (courtesy of Mr P Finan, Department of Surgery, General Infirmary, Leeds).

diameter of an adenoma reaches 2 cm. The transition from a small adenomatous polyp to an invasive cancer can take between 5 and 10 years. Adenomatous polyps less than 1 cm in diameter have mutations in the *ras* gene in less than 10% of cases. As the size of the polyp increases to between 1–2 cm the prevalence of *ras* gene mutations is in the region of 40%, rising to approximately 50% in colorectal cancers.

Similarly, allelic loss of chromosome 5 markers occurs in approximately 30% of adenomatous polyps and between 40% and 60% of carcinomas. Deletions on chromosome 17p containing the p53 gene, occur in more than 75% of carcinomas, but this is an uncommon finding in small or intermediate sized polyps. The region containing the DCC gene on 18q is deleted in about 10% of small adenomas, rising to almost 50% when the adenoma shows foci of invasive carcinoma and in over 70% of carcinomas.

It appears, therefore, that mutations of the *ras* and p53 genes and loss of heterozygosity for markers for the APC, DCC and MCC genes accumulate during the transition from a small 'benign' adenoma to carcinoma. Accumulation of alterations, rather than the number or order, appears to be more important in the development of carcinoma. More than one of these four alterations is seen in only 7% of small, early adenomas. Two or more such alterations are seen, with increasing frequency, when adenomas progress in size and show histological features of malignancy. Over 90% of carcinomas show two or more such alterations and approximately 40% show three.

Breast cancer

Family studies in breast cancer have shown that the risk of a woman developing breast cancer is greater the more affected female relatives she has and the earlier the age of presentation in these relatives. With breast cancer being as common as it is, it is possible to collect families with multiple affected females. Recent studies have shown that early-onset breast cancer (less than age 50 years) is linked to markers on the long arm of chromosome 17 (17q21) and behaves effectively like a dominant gene. Families with a later age of onset of breast cancer do not show linkage to this region, consistent with the aetiological heterogeneity one would expect from the epidemiological evidence. Nevertheless these findings are likely to provide important insights into the mechanism of the development of breast cancer not only in the early-onset group but possibly also for breast cancer in the general population.

The development of breast cancer also appears to be associated with multiple somatic mutations. A number of mutations have been identified, including amplification of *erb*-B1, *erb*-B2, *myc* and *int*-2 oncogenes as well as loss of heterozygosity for a number of chromosomes at a number of sites including 1q, 3p, 11p, 13q and 17p. In many tumours showing loss of heterozygosity, allelic loss occurs at 2 to 4 of the sites, again suggesting that the accumulation of alterations, rather than their order, is important in the evolution of breast cancer.

While the presence or absence of these mutations has

been used to try to predict survival or the disease free interval prior to relapse, there have been conflicting results. Lymph node status at the time of diagnosis is still a better predictor of the likely disease free interval and overall survival.

This type of model for cancer susceptibility is likely, of course, to be an over-simplification. For many of the common cancers, several tumour suppressor genes or oncogenes contribute to the development of a malignancy. It is also probable that the separation into the categories of oncogenes and tumour suppressor genes will not stand the test of time. In addition, the same inherited defect can produce different cancers at different sites in different individuals not just by chance, but because of the varying effects of a number of other genes as well as a variety of environmental agents.

FAMILIAL CANCER

It has been estimated that about 5% of colorectal and breast cancer arises as a result of an inherited cancer susceptibility gene. It is likely that, with the exception of cancers where there is an obvious external factor involved, a similar proportion of many other cancers are due to genetic factors.

Recognition of individuals with an inherited susceptibility to cancer usually relies on taking a careful family history to document the presence or absence of other family members with similar or related cancers. The malignancies which develop in susceptible individuals are often the same as those which occur in the population in general and only in rare instances are there other manifestations which give an indication of an underlying inherited cancer susceptibility. There are a number of other features which can suggest an inherited cancer susceptibility syndrome in a family (Table 13.7).

GENETIC BASIS OF FAMILIAL CANCER

Inherited cancer syndromes

While most cancers occur at a specific site, families have been described in which cancers occur at more than one site in an individual or at different sites in various members of the family more commonly than would be expected. These families are referred to as having a *familial cancer-predisposing syndrome*. The majority of the rare inherited familial cancer-predisposing syndromes currently recognised are dominantly inherited with offspring of affected individuals having a 50% chance of inheriting the gene and therefore being at increased risk of developing cancer (Table 13.8).

A number of different familial cancer-predisposing syndromes have been described, depending on the patterns of cancers seen. These include Lynch type I, in which

Table 13.7 Features suggestive of an inherited cancer susceptibility syndrome in a family

Several close (first or second degree) relatives with a common cancer
Several close relatives with related cancers, e.g. breast and ovary or bowel and endometrial
Two family members with the same rare cancer
An unusually early age of onset
Bilateral tumours in paired organs
Synchronous or successive tumours
Tumours in two different organ systems in one individual

family members are at risk for site-specific cancer of the colon, occurring most commonly right-sided, and cancer of the stomach, Lynch type II (sometimes, somewhat confusingly, known as the *cancer family syndrome*) in which family members are at risk of colon cancer, endometrial, breast and transitional cell cancers and the Li–Fraumeni syndrome, in which persons are at risk of developing soft-tissue sarcomas, breast cancer, brain tumours and leukaemia.

Persons with an inherited familial cancer-predisposing syndrome can develop a second tumour, either multifocal and/or bilateral, have an increased risk of developing a cancer at a relatively younger age than in persons with the sporadic form, and develop tumours at different sites in the body, although one type of cancer usually predominates.

These cancer groupings are not always distinct in an individual family. Only with time will it be clear how useful these groupings will be in understanding causation. Of particular interest, however, have been the reports of mutations in the p53 gene in a number of families with the Li–Fraumeni syndrome (p. 173).

Inherited susceptibility for the common cancers

The level of risk for persons with a family history of one of the *common cancers* such as bowel or breast cancer depends on a number of factors. These include the number of persons with cancer in the family, how closely related the person at risk is to the affected individuals and the age at which the affected family member(s) developed cancer. A few families with a large number of members affected with one of the common cancers are consistent with a dominantly inherited cancer susceptibility gene. In most instances there are only a few individuals with cancer in a family and there is doubt about whether a cancer susceptibility gene is responsible or not. In such an instance one relies on empirical data gained from epidemiological studies to provide risk estimates (Tables 13.9 and 13.10).

Table 13.8 Inherited familial cancer–predisposing syndromes, mode of inheritance, gene responsible and chromosomal site

Syndrome	Mode of inheritance*	Gene	Chromosomal site	Main cancer (s)
Breast and breast/ovary families	AD	BRCA1	17q	Breast, ovary
Dysplastic naevus syndrome (Familial atypical mole melanoma, FAMM)	AD	CMM1	1p	Melanoma
Hereditary non–polyposis colorectal cancer (HNPCC)				
Lynch I	AD	MSH2	18q	Colorectal
Lynch II	AD	LCF2	2p	Colorectal, endometrial, urinary tract, ovarian, gastric, small bowel, hepatobiliary, breast (?)
Familial adenomatous polyposis	AD	APC	5q	Colorectal, duodenal, thyroid
Familial juvenile polyposis	AD	?	?	Colorectal
Familial retinoblastoma	AD	RB1	13q	Retinoblastoma
Li–Fraumeni	AD	p53	17p	Sarcoma, breast, brain, leukaemia, adrenal cortex
Muir–Torre	AD	?	?	As Lynch II, plus sebaceous tumours, laryngeal
Multiple endocrine neoplasia (MEN) type 2a	AD	MEN2a	10q	Thyroid (medullary), phaeochromocytoma
Peutz–Jeghers	AD	?	?	Gastrointestinal, breast, uterus, ovary, testis
Turcot's	AR	?	?	Colorectal
von Hippel Lindau	AD	VHL	3p	CNS haemangioblastoma, renal, pancreatic, phaeochromocytoma

*AD = autosomal dominant, AR = autosomal recessive

Table 13.9 Lifetime risk of colorectal cancer for an individual according to the family history of colorectal cancer (from Houlston R S, Murday V, Harocopos C, Williams C B, Slack J 1990 Screening and genetic counselling for relatives of patients with colorectal cancer in a family screening clinic. Br Med J 301: 366–368)

Population risk	1 in 50
One first-degree relative affected	1 in 17
One first-degree relative & one second-degree relative affected	1 in 12
One relative aged under 45 affected	1 in 10
Two first-degree relatives affected	1 in 6
Three or more first-degree relatives affected	1 in 2

Table 13.10 Lifetime risk of breast cancer in females according to the family history of breast cancer

Population risk	1 in 12
Sister diagnosed 65–70 years of age	1 in 8
Sister diagnosed under 40 years of age	1 in 4
Two first-degree relatives affected under 40 years of age	1 in 3

SCREENING FOR FAMILIAL CANCER

Prevention or early detection of cancer is the ultimate goal of screening individuals at risk of familial cancer. The means by which prevention can be achieved include a change in lifestyle or diet, drug therapy and prophylactic surgery.

Screening of persons at risk for familial cancer is usually directed at detecting the phenotypic expression of the genotype, i.e. surveillance for a particular cancer or its precursor. Screening can also include diagnostic tests which indirectly reveal the genotype, i.e. evidence of the presence or absence of the gene, or what is, in effect, presymptomatic testing. For example, individuals at risk for familial adenomatous polyposis can be screened for evidence of the FAP gene by retinal examination looking for areas of _congenital hypertrophy of the retinal_ *pigment epithelium* or what is known as CHRPE. The finding of CHRPE increases the likelihood of the individual at risk being heterozygous for the FAP gene and therefore developing polyposis and malignancy.

Knowledge of the genotypic status of an individual at risk allows more efficient delivery of surveillance screening for the phenotypic expression, e.g. polyposis and consequently cancer of the bowel in persons with FAP, and avoids unnecessary surveillance of those identified as being at low risk. As more genes for cancer susceptibility are discovered there will be an increasing number of conditions for which DNA testing will enable presymptomatic determination of genotypic status (p. 248). Even though these developments will help to target screening resources more effectively, they will not eliminate the need for surveillance screening of heterozygotes.

Table 13.11 Suggested guidelines for screening persons at risk for the familial cancer-predisposing syndromes or for one of the common cancers

Condition *Cancer*	Screening test	Frequency	Starting age
Familial susceptibility for the common cancers			
Breast cancer			
Breast	Mammography	annual	35 (2 yearly from 50)
Breast/Ovary			
Breast	Mammography	annual	35 (2 yearly from 50)
Ovary	US/Doppler	annual	25
Familial cancer-predisposing syndromes			
Familial adenomatous polyposis	Retinal examination (CHRPE)*		Childhood
Colorectal	Sigmoid/colonoscopy*+	annual	12
Duodenal	Gastroscopy	3 yearly	20
Thyroid (women)	None/US?	annual	20
HNPCC–Lynch I			
Colorectal	Colonoscopy	3–5 yearly	35
HNPCC–Lynch II			
Colorectal	Colonoscopy	3–5 yearly	35
Endometrial	US	annual	35
Ovary	US	annual	25
Renal tract	US	annual	35
Gastric	Gastroscopy	1–2 yearly	35
Small bowel	None		
Hepatobiliary	None		
Breast	Mammography	annual	35 (2 yearly from 50)
Li–Fraumeni			
Breast	Mammography	annual	35? (2 yearly from 50)
Sarcoma	None		
Brain	None		
Leukaemia	None		
Adrenal cortex	None		
Multiple endocrine neoplasia type 2	Pentagastrin stimulation test*	10 years of age	
Medullary thyroid	US	?	10
Phaeochromocytoma	Urinary VMA	annual	10
Parathyroid adenoma	Ca^{2+}, PO_4, PTH	annual	10
von Hippel Lindau			
Retinal angioma	Retinal examination*	annual	5
Haemangioblastoma	CNS CT/MRI	3 yearly	15 (5 yearly from 40 years)
Phaeochromocytoma	Urinary VMA	annual	10
Renal	Abdominal CT	3 yearly	20
	Abdominal US	annual	20

*Test to detect heterozygous state
+In individuals found to be affected, annual colonoscopy prior to colectomy and lifelong 4–6 monthly surveillance of the rectal stump, after subtotal colectomy

US = ultrasound, CHRPE = congenital hypertrophy of the retinal pigmentary epithelium, CT = computed tomography, MRI = magnetic resonance imaging, PTH = parathyroid hormone, VMA = vanillyl mandelic acid

While the potential for prevention of cancer through screening persons in this high risk group is considerable, the impact on the overall rate of cancer will be small as only a minority of the cases of cancer in the general population are due to a genetic susceptibility.

Familial cancer-predisposing syndromes

Many familial cancer-predisposing syndromes are inherited as autosomal dominant traits which are fully penetrant with the consequent risk for heterozygotes of developing cancer approaching 100%. This level of risk means that more invasive means of screening, more frequent implementation and earlier initiation of protocols are justified than would be acceptable for the population in general (Table 13.11).

Inherited susceptibility for the common cancers

Screening for the common cancers due to inherited susceptibility has only relatively recently been established and by its very nature involves a long term undertaking for the individual at risk as well as his/her physician or surgeon. It is important to emphasise that the natural enthusiasm for screening needs to be balanced with the paucity of hard data in many instances on the relative benefits and risks. Screening protocols are often based on current opinion rather than on formal evaluation (Table 13.12).

Who should be screened?

In the case of the rare dominantly inherited single gene familial cancer-predisposing syndromes such as FAP, those who should be screened can be identified on a simple Mendelian basis. For persons with a family history of the common cancers, such as bowel or breast cancer, the risk levels at which screening is recommended and below which screening is not likely to be of benefit will vary. At each extreme of risk the decision is usually straightforward, but with intermediate risks there will be doubt as to relative benefits and risks of screening.

What age and how often?

Cancer in persons with a family cancer syndrome tends to occur at a relatively earlier age than in the population in general and screening programmes must reflect this. With the exception of familial adenomatous polyposis, in which it is recommended that sigmoidoscopy to detect rectal polyps should start in the teenage years, most cancer screening programmes do not start until age 25 years or later. The age band during which the risk to develop cancer for most susceptibilities is greatest is

Table 13.12 Requirements of a screening test for persons at risk for a familial cancer-predisposing syndrome or at increased risk for the common cancers

The test should detect a malignant or premalignant condition at a stage prior to it producing symptoms with high sensitivity and specificity

The treatment of persons detected by screening should improve the prognosis

The benefits of early detection should outweigh potential harm from the screening test

The test should preferably be non-invasive since most at risk individuals require long-term surveillance

Adequate provision for pre-screening counselling and follow-up should be available

from 35 to 50 years but, because cancer can still develop in those at risk at a later age, screening is usually continued thereafter. In some families the age of onset of cancer can be especially young and it is recommended that screening of persons at risk in these families is begun five years before the age of onset in the earliest affected member of the family.

The recommended interval between repeating screening procedures should be determined from the natural history of the particular cancer. The development of colorectal cancer from an adenoma is believed to occur over a number of years and as a result it is thought that 5-year screening intervals will suffice. If, however, a polyp is found, then the interval between screening procedures is usually brought down to three years. Breast cancer is not detectable in a premalignant stage and early diagnosis is critical if there is to be a good prognosis. Annual mammography for females at high risk is therefore recommended from age 35.

What sites should be screened?

Having decided who is at risk within a family, one has to judge which types of cancer are most likely to occur and which systems of the body should be screened.

Familial cancer-predisposing syndromes

This can be a very difficult problem with some of the family cancer syndromes, such as the Lynch type I and II syndromes, in which a person at risk can develop cancer at a number of different sites. Screening for every possible cancer which could occur would mean frequent investigation by a variety of different specialists. This would result in an unwieldy protocol. Persons at risk for Lynch type I and II should have regular colonoscopy while females at risk for Lynch type II should also be offered pelvic screening for gynaecological malignancies. Some of the other cancers which can occur in persons at risk for Lynch type II, such as stomach cancer, are not seen in every family and so screening is usually restricted to persons from those families in which at least one member has had that particular malignancy. In persons at risk for the Li–Fraumeni syndrome, a wide spectrum of cancers can occur. The available screening protocol is, as yet, of unproven benefit with the possible exception of regular mammography.

Inherited susceptibility for the common cancers

Colorectal cancer

Colorectal carcinoma holds the greatest promise for prevention by screening. Endoscopy provides a sensitive and specific means of examination of the colorectal mucosa and polypectomy can be carried out with relative ease so that screening, diagnosis and treatment can take place concurrently. While colonoscopy is the preferred screening method, it does require a skilled operator and, as it is an invasive procedure, it has a consequent but small morbidity.

Failure to visualise the right side of the colon with colonoscopy necessitates a barium enema to view this region, particularly in persons at risk for the *hereditary nonpolyposis colorectal cancer* (HNPCC) syndrome, in which proximal right-sided involvement commonly occurs. For persons with a moderately increased risk of developing colorectal cancer, the majority of cancers occur in the distal colon and at a relatively later age. Flexible sigmoidoscopy, which is much less invasive than colonoscopy, provides an adequate screening tool for persons in this risk group and can be employed from the age of 50 years.

Breast cancer

National screening of women aged 50 years and over for breast cancer by regular mammography has become established as a result of studies demonstrating improved survival. For women identified as having an increased risk of developing breast cancer because of their family history, there is conflicting evidence for the relative benefit of screening. It is argued that the radiation exposure associated with annual mammography could be detrimental if started at an earlier age, leading to an increased risk of breast cancer through the screening when carried out over a long period of time. This is of particular concern in families with the Li–Fraumeni syndrome because p53 mutations have been shown experimentally to impair the repair of DNA damaged by X-irradiation. The present view is, however, that there is a greater relative benefit than risk in identifying and treating breast cancer in women from this high risk group.

Mammography is usually only offered to women at increased risk of breast cancer after the age of 35 years, since interpretation of mammograms is difficult before this age due to the density of the breasts. As a con-

sequence women at increased risk of developing breast cancer should be taught breast self-examination and undergo regular clinical examination.

Ovarian cancer

Ovarian cancer in the early stages is frequently asymptomatic and often incurable by the time a woman presents with symptoms. Early diagnosis of ovarian cancer in individuals at high risk is vital, with prophylactic oophorectomy being the only logical, if radical, alternative. The position of the ovaries within the pelvis makes screening difficult. Ultrasound imaging provides the most sensitive means of screening. Transvaginal scanning is more sensitive than conventional transabdominal scanning, and the use of colour doppler blood flow imaging further enhances screening of women at increased risk. If a suspicious feature is seen on scanning and confirmed on further investigation, then laparoscopy or a laparotomy is usually required to confirm the diagnosis. Screening should be carried out annually as interval cancers can develop if screening is carried out less frequently.

WHAT TREATMENT IS APPROPRIATE ?

Surgical intervention for persons at risk for one of the familial cancer-predisposing syndromes, or for persons with a high risk due to an inherited susceptibility for one of the common cancers, is a well accepted option. In a number of the familial cancer-predisposing syndromes and for persons at high risk for one of the common cancers, alternative non-surgical treatments are under evaluation. These include the use of the non-steroidal anti-inflammatory sulindac for persons at risk for FAP and tamoxifen in women at risk for breast cancer (Table 13.13).

Table 13.13 Conditions in which prophylactic surgery is an accepted treatment and treatments which are under evaluation as an option for the familial cancer-predisposing syndromes or individuals at increased risk for the common cancers

Disorder	Treatment
Accepted treatment	
Familial adenomatous polyposis	Total colectomy
Ovarian cancer families	Oophorectomy
Breast cancer families	Bilateral mastectomy
MEN2	Total thyroidectomy
Under evaluation	
Familial adenomatous polyposis	Non-digestible starch – to delay onset of polyposis
	Sulindac – to reduce rectal and duodenal adenomas
Breast cancer families	Tamoxifen – to prevent development of breast cancer

ELEMENTS

1 Cancer has both genetic and environmental causes.

2 Genetic and environmental factors in the aetiology of cancer can be differentiated by epidemiologic, family and twin studies and by analysis of disease, biochemical and viral associations.

3 Studies of tumour viruses have revealed genes present in humans known as oncogenes which are involved in carcinogenesis by altering cellular control mechanisms.

4 Study of rare dominantly inherited tumours in humans, such as retinoblastoma, has led to the identification of tumour suppressor genes consistent with the hypothesis that the development of cancer involves a minimum of two 'hits'. Persons at risk of familial cancer inherit the first 'hit' in the germ cell, the second 'hit' occurring in somatic cells in mitosis. In persons with sporadically occurring cancer both 'hits' occur in somatic cells.

5 5% of the common cancers, such as breast and bowel cancer, arise as a result of an inherited cancer susceptibility. Familial susceptibility for cancer can occur as an inherited susceptibility for a single type of cancer or for a number of different types of cancer as part of a familial cancer-predisposing syndrome.

6 Persons at risk of an inherited cancer susceptibility can be screened for associated features of a familial cancer-predisposing syndrome or for particular cancers.

FURTHER READING

Harris H, Miller O J, Klein G, Worst P, Tachibam T 1969 Suppression of malignancy by cell fusion. Nature 350: 377–378
Studies which eventually led to the concept of tumour suppressor genes.
Hodgson S V, Maher E R 1993 A practical guide to human cancer genetics. Cambridge University Press, Cambridge
An up-to-date text covering the developing field of human cancer genetics.
King R A, Rotter J I, Motulsky A G (eds) 1992 The genetic basis of common diseases. Oxford University Press
Six chapters of this text cover the basic biology, epidemiology and familial aspects of cancer.
Knudson A G 1971 Mutation and cancer: statistical study of retinoblastoma. Proc Nat'l Acad Sci USA 68: 820–823
Proposal of the 'two hit' hypothesis for the development of retinoblastoma.
Li F P, Fraumeni J F 1969 Soft tissue sarcomas, breast cancer, and other neoplasms: a familial syndrome? Ann Int Med 71: 747–752
The original description of the Li–Fraumeni syndrome.
Lynch H T 1967 'Cancer families': adenocarcinomas (endometrial and colon carcinoma) and multiple primary malignant neoplasms. Rec Results Cancer Res 12: 125–142
The description of the cancer family syndrome now known as Lynch II.

CHAPTER 14

Genetic factors in common diseases

Medical genetics usually concentrates on the study of unifactorial chromosomal and single gene disorders. Diseases, such as stroke, coronary artery disease, diabetes and cancer are responsible, however, for the majority of the morbidity and mortality in developed countries. They are also likely to be of greater importance in the future with the elderly accounting for an increasing proportion of the population. These diseases, known as the *common diseases*, do not usually show a simple pattern of inheritance. The contributing genetic factors are often multiple and complex, interacting with environmental factors. In fact, it is uncommon for heredity or environment to be entirely responsible for a particular disorder or disease. In most cases both genetic and environmental factors are usually responsible, although sometimes one can appear more important than the other (Fig. 14.1).

At one extreme are diseases such as Duchenne muscular dystrophy which are exclusively genetic in origin and the environment seems to play no direct part in aetiology. At the other extreme are infectious diseases which are almost entirely the result of environmental factors. Between these two extremes are conditions such as diabetes mellitus, hypertension, coronary artery disease,

peptic ulcer, schizophrenia, the common cancers and congenital abnormalities, in which both genetic and environmental factors are involved.

GENETIC SUSCEPTIBILITY TO COMMON DISEASE

For many of the common diseases a small but significant proportion of cases are due to single gene causes but the major proportion of the genetic basis of common diseases can be considered to be due to an inherited predisposition or *genetic susceptibility*. These diseases result from a complex interaction of the effects of multiple different genes, or what is known as *polygenic inheritance*, with environmental factors and influences, in what is known as *multifactorial inheritance* (p. 106).

TYPES AND MECHANISMS OF GENETIC SUSCEPTIBILITY

Genetic susceptibility can involve susceptibility to a particular disease through single gene inheritance of an

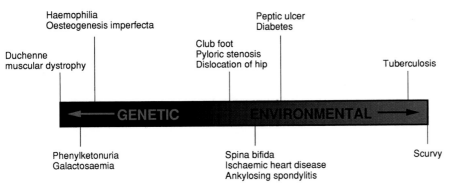

Fig. 14.1
Human disease represented as being on a spectrum ranging from those which are largely environmental in causation to those which are entirely genetic.

abnormal gene product involved in a particular metabolic pathway, e.g. early coronary artery disease due to familial hypercholesterolaemia (p. 134). In this instance, the genetic susceptibility is the main determinant of the development of the disease but it can be modified by alteration of the environment, e.g. reduction in dietary cholesterol and avoidance of other risk factors such as obesity, lack of exercise and smoking.

Inheritance of a single gene susceptibility does not necessarily lead to development of a disease. For some diseases exposure to specific environmental factors will be the main determinant in the development of the disease, e.g. smoking or occupational exposures in the development of pulmonary emphysema in persons with α_1-antitrypsin deficiency (p. 140).

In other instances the mechanism of the genetic susceptibility is less clear. This can involve inheritance of a single gene polymorphism (p. 97) which leads to differences in susceptibility to a disease, e.g. acetaldehyde dehydrogenase activity and alcoholism (p. 147). In addition, inherited single gene polymorphisms appear to determine the response to, as yet, undefined environmental factors, e.g. the HLA antigens of the major histocompatibility complex and specific disease associations (p. 160), e.g. insulin–dependent diabetes, rheumatoid arthritis and coeliac disease. Lastly, genetic susceptibility can determine differences in responses to therapy, e.g. isoniazid inactivation status in the treatment of tuberculosis (p. 145).

APPROACHES TO DEMONSTRATE GENETIC SUSCEPTIBILITY TO COMMON DISEASES

In attempting to understand the genetics of a particular condition, the investigator can approach the problem in a number of ways (Table 14.1). These can include studying the incidence of the disease among relatives, i.e. family studies, comparing the incidence in identical and non-identical twins, determining the effect of environmental changes, e.g. adoption studies, comparing prevalence and incidence in various different population groups and the effects of immigration and studying the

Table 14.1 Types of genetic approach to the common diseases

Family studies
Twin studies
Adoption studies
Population studies
Immigration studies
Polymorphism associations
Biochemical studies
Animal models

association of the disease with various other characteristics, such as the blood groups or biochemical factors. In addition, study can be made of the pathological components of the disease in relatives, e.g. serum lipids among the relatives of patients with coronary artery disease. Study of diseases in animals which are analogous to diseases which occur in humans can also be helpful. Before considering the use of these different approaches in a number of the common diseases, specific aspects of some of these approaches will be discussed in more detail.

Family studies

A genetic susceptibility to a disease can be suggested by the finding of a higher frequency of a family history of the disease in relatives than in the general population. The proportion of affected relatives of a specific relationship, e.g. first-degree, second-degree, etc., provides information for empiric recurrence risks in genetic counselling (p. 259). Familial aggregation does not, however, prove a genetic susceptibility since families share a common environment. The frequency of the disease in spouses, who share the same environment but who will usually have a different genetic background, can be used as a control, particularly for possible environmental factors in adult life.

Twin studies

If both members of a pair of identical twins have the same trait this does not prove that the trait is hereditary. Since twins tend to share the same environment it is possible they will be exposed to the same environmental factors. For example, if one of a twin pair contracts a contagious disease such as impetigo, it is likely that the other twin will also become affected. This problem can be partly resolved by comparing differences between non-identical or dizygotic (DZ) and identical or monozygotic (MZ) twin pairs.

Both members of a pair of twins are said to be *concordant* when either both are affected or neither is affected. The term *discordant* is used when only one member of a pair of twins is affected. Both types of twins will have a tendency to share the same environment but, whereas identical twins have identical genotypes, non-identical twins are no more similar genetically than brothers and sisters. If a disease is entirely genetically determined then, barring such rare events as chromosome non-disjunction or a new mutation occurring in one twin, both members of a pair of identical twins will be similarly affected but non-identical twins can differ. If a disease is entirely due to environmental factors, then concordance rates will be very much the same whether they are identical or non-identical.

Although all twins tend to share the same environment, it is probable that this is more likely in identical twins than in non-identical twins. Similarities between identical twins can therefore reflect their shared environment as much as their identical genotypes. One way of getting round this difficulty is to study differences between identical twins who are reared apart from an early age. If a particular disease is entirely genetically determined then, if one identical twin is affected, the other will also be affected even if they have been brought up in different environments. It is rare, however, for identical twins to be separated from early childhood and so only a limited number of studies on such individuals exist. In one study of identical twins reared separately, the data clearly showed that each pair of twins differed little in height but differed considerably in weight. These observations suggest that heredity could play a bigger part in determining stature than it does in determining weight.

Adoption studies

Another approach for separating genetic from environmental factors is to compare the frequency of a disease in individuals who remain with their biological parents and in those who are adopted. Adopted individuals take their genes with them to a new environment. If the frequency of a disease in the adopted individuals is similar to the biological parents, then genetic factors are likely to be more important. If, conversely, the frequency of the disease is similar in the adopted individuals to that of the adoptive parents, then environmental factors are likely to be more important.

Population and immigration studies

Differences in the incidence of a particular disease in different population groups suggest the possibility of genetic factors being important but could also be explained by differences in environmental factors. Studies of immigrant groups moving from a population group with a low incidence of a disease to one with a high incidence, in which the incidence of the disease in the immigrant group rises would suggest that environmental factors are more important. Conversely, maintenance of a low incidence of the disease in the immigrant group would suggest that genetic factors are more important.

DIABETES MELLITUS

There are two main forms of diabetes mellitus which are clinically distinct. One form which accounts for 5–10% of diabetes has a peak age of onset in adolescence and can only be controlled by regular injection of insulin. This is referred to as type 1 or insulin-dependent diabetes (IDDM). The second more common and less severe form usually affects older persons and often responds to simple dietary restriction of carbohydrate intake although some patients require medication and, on occasion, insulin. This is known as type 2 or non-insulin-dependent diabetes mellitus (NIDDM).

In addition, 1–2% of persons with diabetes develop non-insulin-dependent diabetes in their early 20's and are recognised to have what is known as maturity onset diabetes of the young (MODY). Lastly, 1–3% of women develop glucose intolerance during pregnancy. This is known as gestational diabetes. This abnormal glucose tolerance usually reverts to normal after the pregnancy, although 50–75% of these women go on to develop diabetes later in life.

Diabetes can also occur secondary to a variety of other genetic and non-genetic disorders. For example, it is well recognised that individuals with the autosomal dominant muscle disorder myotonic dystrophy (p. 249) have an increased risk of developing diabetes. Diabetes mellitus is therefore aetiologically heterogeneous.

EVIDENCE FOR GENETIC FACTORS

While there are animal models of diabetes which are inherited and population and immigration studies suggest that genetic factors are important in diabetes, the evidence that diabetes mellitus is in part genetically determined comes mainly from twin and family studies.

Twin studies

A number of surveys have shown that between 45% and 96% of identical twins are concordant for diabetes whereas between only 3% and 37% of non-identical twins are concordant. In some studies, however, only some of the twin pairs had completed their life spans. The concordance rates are likely to have been higher if all the twins had been followed till death. More recent twin studies in which the concordance rates for insulin dependent and non-insulin-dependent diabetes have been looked at separately have shown concordance rates for the former to be in the region of 50% while for the latter they have been in excess of 90%. These data indicate that genetic factors are important in both forms of diabetes. The fact that a significant proportion of the identical twins were discordant for IDDM suggests that environmental influences are also involved. The very high concordance of MZ twins for NIDDM suggests that the primary determining factor is genetic although a suitable diabetogenic diet could be necessary for the susceptibility to be expressed.

Family studies

Between 25% and 50% of diabetics have a family history of diabetes as opposed to less than 15% in the general population. A variety of formal family studies have shown a prevalence of diabetes in relatives which ranges from 10–30% in the relatives of diabetics compared to between 1% and 6% in relatives of non-diabetics (Table 14.2).

The diagnostic criteria for diabetes used in the different studies have not always been the same, ranging from frank clinical diabetes through formal glucose tolerance tests to random blood sugars. In addition, while some studies looked at risks in relatives dependent on the type or age of onset of the diabetes in the proband, many of the studies considered all ages of onset and different types of diabetes lumped together. These factors can account, to some extent, for the differences seen in the percentage of affected relatives in the various studies.

ASSOCIATED RISK FACTORS

Persons with IDDM are recognised to have an increased risk of developing autoimmune disorders such as auto-immune thyroiditis, pernicious anaemia and Addison's disease. A significant proportion of persons with IDDM also develop pancreatic islet cell antibodies. Not surprisingly, perhaps, IDDM has been found to be associated with specific HLA antigens, with 95% of persons with IDDM having the HLA DR3 and/or DR4 antigens.

Table 14.2 Population and recurrence risks for NIDDM and IDDM (from Rotter J I, Vadhein C M, Rimoin D L Diabetes mellitus, Chapter 21 in King, Rotter & Motulsky)

Group	%
NIDDM	
Population	4–5 (ages 20–74)
First-degree relatives	10–15
IDDM	
Population	0.2
1 high risk allele (DR3 or DR4)	0.25
HLA DR3/3 or HLA DR4/4	0.75
HLA DR3/4	2.5
Relatives	
Siblings	7
No antigens shared	1
1 antigen shared	5
2 antigens shared	16
2 antigens shared – DR3/4	20–25
Offspring	4
Offspring of affected female	2–2.5
Offspring of affected male	5

Siblings with IDDM have HLA haplotypes (p. 160) in common more frequently than expected by chance. An individual with either of the DR3 or DR4 HLA antigens has a slightly increased risk of developing IDDM compared to the general population (Table 14.2). The presence of either of these two antigens in siblings of an individual with IDDM increases their chance of developing diabetes significantly and if a sibling has both of the high risk antigens the risk is greatly increased! The reported peak of onset of IDDM in the autumn and winter seasons along with the autoimmune observations have suggested a possible viral aetiology in genetically susceptible individuals.

While a number of genes have been suggested as candidate susceptibility genes for both forms of diabetes, none has, as yet, been shown to have a major effect in determining a genetic predisposition to diabetes.

MODELS OF INHERITANCE

If diabetes were due to a recessive allele (d) and an affected person (dd) had two unaffected parents, the parents must have the genotype Dd and it would be expected that, on average, 25% of their offspring would be affected. If one parent of an affected individual is a diabetic then the mating must be dd x Dd and 50% of their offspring should be affected. Finally, if both parents are affected then all their offspring should be affected. The ratios of affected offspring in these three types of mating would therefore be 1/4:1/2:1 or 1:2:4. Some studies have obtained results which agree with these expected ratios based on these assumptions. It must be pointed out, however, that from the data obtained in family studies it can be estimated that about 5% of the general population must be homozygous for this gene! Surveys have shown that only about 1% of the population has diabetes. Therefore if diabetes mellitus is due to a recessive gene, then the gene cannot be fully penetrant and only about 20% of those who are presumed to be homozygous actually have the disease. Some investigators who support the idea that diabetes mellitus is due to a recessive gene have suggested that the severe childhood form of the disease represents the homozygous state, whereas non-insulin dependent diabetes represents the heterozygous state. Family studies do not, however, support this proposal. Similar attempts to fit the family data to an autosomal dominant gene exhibiting reduced penetrance have not met with obvious success. Suggestions of mixed models of dominant and recessive genes have also been made.

It seems most likely that the aetiology of genetic susceptibility to diabetes is very heterogeneous and that no one simple genetic explanation will fit all the facts.

MATURITY ONSET DIABETES OF THE YOUNG

The initial description of MODY resulted in reports of a number of families consistent with autosomal dominant inheritance. Further studies have indicated that only a proportion of families are consistent with it being due to a dominant gene. There are a few reports of associated risk factors for MODY. The initial reports of chlorpropamide-alcohol induced flushing (p. 147) as a marker for MODY have not been substantiated in most families.

Linkage studies in MODY families with what could be considered obvious candidate genes, such as the insulin, insulin receptor and the glucose transport protein genes, have been negative. Linkage of MODY to markers on the long arm of chromosome 20 near the adenosine deaminase gene has been demonstrated but approximately one-half of MODY families have been shown not to be linked to this locus. Subsequent linkage studies showed a significant proportion of this latter group were linked to the glucokinase gene on chromosome 7. These two types have been called type I and II MODY respectively.

GESTATIONAL DIABETES

While it was originally suggested that gestational diabetes was a pre-type 2 or non-insulin dependent form of diabetes, it appears to be genetically heterogeneous, showing association with HLA antigens DR3 and DR4, pancreatic islet cell antibodies and autoimmune disorders.

PREDISPOSITION TO DIABETIC COMPLICATIONS

Persons with diabetes are at risk of developing complications in a number of systems, specifically the kidneys, the retina and large blood vessels in the form of early coronary artery and peripheral vascular disease. While the development of complications in these systems primarily relates to the duration and control of the diabetes, there is preliminary evidence to suggest that there could be specific genetic factors determining the predisposition to these complications. It is, however, difficult to differentiate this susceptibility for specific complications from the susceptibility to the diabetes itself.

HYPERTENSION

Various studies have shown that between 10% to 25% of the population is hypertensive but the prevalence is age dependent with up to 40% of 75–79 year olds being hypertensive. Hypertension leads to an increased morbidity and mortality through a greater risk of stroke, coronary artery and renal disease. There is substantial evidence that treatment of hypertension prevents these risks.

Persons with hypertension fall into two groups. In one the onset is usually in early adult life and is a consequence of another disorder such as kidney disease or abnormalities of certain endocrine glands. This is referred to as secondary hypertension. In the second more common group, hypertension usually begins in middle age and there is no recognised cause. This is known as essential hypertension. The following discussion is concerned with only essential hypertension.

GENETIC FACTORS IN HYPERTENSION

Family and twin studies have shown that hypertension is familial (Table 14.3) and that blood pressure correlates with the degree of relationship (Table 14.4) suggesting the importance of genetic factors in the aetiology in hypertension. In addition, there are differences in the prevalence of hypertension between populations, hypertension being more common in persons of Afro-Caribbean origin and less common in Eskimos, Australian Aborigines and Central and South American Indians.

Environmental factors, such as high sodium levels in the diet, obesity, alcohol intake and reduced exercise, are recognised as being associated with an increased risk of hypertension. Hypertension is also more prevalent in persons from poorer socio-economic groups. Studies of adopted children have shown lower correlation of their

Table 14.3 Recurrence risks for hypertension (from Burke W & Motulsky A G Hypertension, Chapter 10 in King, Rotter & Motulsky)

Group	%
Population	5
2 Normotensive parents	4
1 Hypertensive parent	8–28
2 Hypertensive parents	25–45

Table 14.4 Coefficient of correlation for blood pressure in various relatives (from Burke W & Motulsky A G Hypertension, Chapter 10 in King, Rotter & Motulsky

Group	Correlation coefficient
Siblings	0.12–0.34
Parent/child	0.12–0.37
Dizygotic twins	0.25–0.27
Monozygotic twins	0.55–0.72

blood pressure with their biological parents than with children remaining with their biological parents. In addition, migration studies involving persons moving from a population with a low prevalence to one with a high prevalence of hypertension have shown that the immigrant group acquires the prevalence of hypertension of their new population group during the course of 1 to 2 generations. This suggests that environmental factors are also of major importance in the aetiology of hypertension.

MODELS OF INHERITANCE

If blood pressure measurements are made on a large enough number of persons, the results are normally distributed and show no evidence of any bimodality. Hypertension could therefore be considered to represent one extreme of the normal distribution curve and to be due to the action of many genes which interact with the environment and have an effect on factors such as pulse rate and calibre of blood vessels. This would be consistent with a multifactorial or polygenic basis.

Another school of thought considers that essential hypertension could be due to a common dominant gene. It is argued that if essential hypertension is a disorder of middle age resulting from the action of a dominant gene, it would be expected that the sibs of hypertensive patients would segregate into two groups: those who inherit the disorder and those who do not. Analysis of blood pressure readings from sibs of persons known to have hypertension, excluding as far as possible cases of secondary hypertension by choosing all cases from the age group 45–60, showed that the blood pressure values of the sibs were not normally distributed but had a bimodal distribution with two peaks corresponding to systolic blood pressures of 130 and 160 mm Hg (Fig. 14.2). This suggested that those with systolic blood pressure values around 130 mm Hg had inherited the normal gene whereas those with systolic blood pressure values around 160 mm Hg had inherited the gene for hypertension.

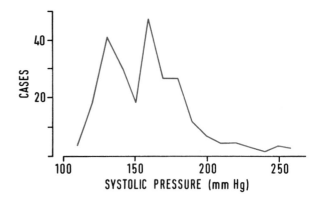

Fig. 14.2
Distribution of systolic blood pressures in 252 sibs of persons aged 45–60 with hypertension (after Platt R 1959 Lancet ii: 57, with permission).

Further early evidence in favour of a single gene model involved a study of blood pressure of 302 symptomless London busmen aged 45–60. The blood pressure readings of these men were normally distributed. When the same men were classified according to the longevity of their parents, however, quite a different result was obtained. The busmen were divided according to the age at which their parent(s) died, into those whose parents died in middle age (40–64) and those whose parents survived past the age of 65. It was argued that essential hypertension, especially if untreated, frequently leads to death in middle age and that this would give a crude subdivision into two groups more or less likely to be hypertensive. They found that the systolic blood pressure values of busmen whose parents had lived to 65 or over were normally distributed (Fig. 14.3). However, in the group of busmen whose parents died in middle age, the systolic blood pressure values showed a bimodal distribution with one peak at 140 and another at 175 mm Hg.

Much of the controversy between these two schools of thought concerning the hereditary nature of hypertension revolves around the definition of bimodality. Critics of the single gene theory claim that what others have

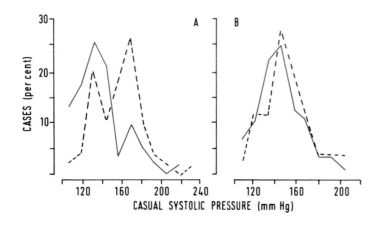

Fig. 14.3
Distribution of casual systolic blood pressures in bus drivers aged 45–54 (continuous line) and 55–60 (interrupted line). (A) One or both parents died in middle age; (B) Both parents living to old age (after Morrison S L, Morris J M 1959 Lancet ii: 865, with permission).

interpreted as bimodality are merely irregularities in the distribution curve which are of no significance. It is argued that with small sample sizes the distribution curve of any variable can show small dips and irregularities. If a large enough sample is taken then the resultant distribution curve would be less likely to show any irregularities.

BIOCHEMICAL STUDIES

Biochemical studies support the possibility of a common autosomal dominant gene being responsible for hypertension. In some persons with hypertension there is defective extrusion of sodium from red cells because of an abnormality in the enzymatically controlled sodium–potassium cotransport in the red cell membrane. This membrane abnormality results in an increased intracellular sodium and has been proposed as a major biochemical determinant of hypertension on the basis that this could reflect a generalised membrane abnormality in vessel walls. Family studies have shown that this membrane abnormality appears to be inherited in an autosomal dominant manner.

Dietary salt has long been recognised as a contributory factor in hypertension and a salt-free diet has been used in the treatment of hypertension. In communities which use little salt the incidence of hypertension is less than, for example, among the Japanese who eat large amounts of salty foods. Individuals with hypertension can eat little salt and, conversely, some people eat large amounts of salt yet remain normotensive. This could be explained as follows. If an individual does not have the membrane abnormality then salt can be taken with impunity, but individuals with the abnormality should perhaps restrict their dietary salt as a prophylaxis.

Another red cell ion transport assay has been developed known as the sodium–lithium countertransport system. This involves loading red blood cells with lithium and measuring the rate of efflux of lithium from the red cells in high and low sodium concentrations. Increased sodium–lithium countertransport correlates positively with hypertension. Studies of the correlation of sodium–lithium countertransport in different types of biological relatives of hypertensives are compatible with a genetic rather than an environmental basis. Segregation analysis testing different models of inheritance suggests that sodium–lithium countertransport is compatible with a recessive gene of major effect on a polygenic background.

Studies in North American individuals of Afro–Caribbean origin suggest that differences in sodium–lithium countertransport are not as important a factor in that population as in other population groups even though they are twice as likely to develop hypertension as North Americans of Caucasian origin. This emphasises the importance of possible differences between various population groups in genetic susceptibility.

A third assay known as the ouabaine sensitive sodium–potassium ATPase system has been investigated as a possible indicator of genetic susceptibility. Although attempts to correlate the findings from these various assay systems have not been straightforward, it is probably fair to say that these findings provide supportive evidence for the role of a single gene of major importance in determining predisposition to essential hypertension.

OTHER RISK FACTORS

Women who develop pre-eclampsia in pregnancy were thought to have an increased risk of hypertension after the pregnancy. Strict definition of pre-eclampsia, which involves oedema and proteinuria as well as hypertension, has shown that many women did, in fact, have a pre-existing predisposition to hypertension which was incidentally revealed by pregnancy.

While the renin-angiotensin-aldosterone system is integrally involved in the biological control of hypertension, inherited polymorphisms in these factors have not, as yet, shown any obvious consistent correlations with hypertension in families. Differences in renin levels and possible differences in the response to certain antihypertensives in various population groups suggest that this could, however, be an important area for future study.

CORONARY ARTERY DISEASE

Coronary artery disease is the major cause of death in many of the developed countries of the world. It is due to *atherosclerosis*, which involves deposition of lipid in the walls of the blood vessels with consequent narrowing of the coronary arteries. Thickening and reduction of compliance of the vascular wall is known as *arteriosclerosis*. The exact cellular and biochemical mechanism by which the focal accumulation of lipid occurs is still not clear and it could occur as part of the normal 'wear and tear' process. It is clear, however, from a number of lines of evidence that genetic factors are important in the aetiology of coronary artery disease.

EPIDEMIOLOGY

The incidence of coronary artery disease varies greatly between different population groups, being one-sixth as common in Japan as in many western countries. These differences can, in part, be attributed to well known environmental risk factors. Support for this comes from the results of migration studies which show that persons moving from populations with a low risk of coronary artery disease to areas with a high risk, acquire the higher risk of their new population group within 10 to 20 years.

Coronary artery disease is more common in males than in females, although after the menopause, the risk for females increases and approaches that of males within 10 to 15 years.

FAMILY AND TWIN STUDIES

The familial nature of coronary artery disease has been recognised since the early part of this century. The risk to a first-degree relative of a person with premature coronary artery disease, defined as occurring before age 55 in males and age 65 in females, varies between 2 and 7 times that for the general population (Table 14.5). Twin studies of concordance for coronary artery disease vary from 15% to 25% for dizygotic twins and from 39% to 48% for monozygotic twins. Although these figures support the involvement of genetic factors, the low concordance rate for monozygotic twins clearly suggests that environmental factors are also important.

GENETIC MODELS

Coronary artery disease can occur secondary to other diseases, e.g. diabetes mellitus and hypertension. However, in the majority of persons presenting with coronary artery disease, it is not inherited in any simple way and is not associated with any other disease process. While the most likely explanation is that it is determined on a polygenic or multifactorial basis, family studies of the hyperlipidaemias, such as familial hypercholesterolaemia, are consistent with a single gene being a major factor determining genetic susceptibility within some families. In other hyperlipidaemias, such as type III hyperlipoproteinaemia, certain polymorphic variants of the apolipoprotein, apo E, appear to be an important interacting determinant of predisposition to early coronary artery

disease. In the majority of persons the risk of coronary artery disease is multifactorial in origin.

RISK FACTORS

A variety of different genetic and environmental risk factors have been identified which predispose to early onset of the atherosclerotic process. Well publicised environmental risk factors include exercise, dietary cholesterol and smoking. The metabolic pathways by which the body absorbs, synthesises, transports and catabolises dietary and endogenous lipids is, suffice to say, complex. A number of inherited polymorphisms of the apolipoproteins of the plasma lipoproteins involved in the transport of lipids have been found to be associated with an increased risk of coronary artery disease.

Apo E is a major protein constituent of two of the classes of plasma lipoprotein involved in the transport and metabolism of lipids. It binds with the low-density lipoprotein receptors on cell surfaces which are responsible for cholesterol uptake by the cell. Polymorphic variants of apo E have been shown to be associated with elevated cholesterol levels and an increased risk of early coronary artery disease.

Lp(a) is a glycoprotein which binds to apo B. Apo B is the principal apolipoprotein constituent of low density lipoprotein, the major lipoprotein involved in cholesterol transport. Lp(a) is highly polymorphic and also shows variation in levels of up to 1000 fold in the population. Elevated Lp(a) levels are associated with elevated plasma cholesterol levels and an increased risk of early coronary artery disease. Of interest is that Lp(a) has sequence homology with one of the fibrinolytic enzymes, plasminogen, and could be involved in the link between atherosclerosis and thrombosis.

Some of the inherited disorders of lipid metabolism are associated with an increased risk of early coronary artery disease. The best known example of a dominantly inherited disorder of lipid metabolism is familial hypercholesterolaemia. Familial hypercholesterolaemia is associated with a significantly increased risk of early coronary artery disease and is inherited as an autosomal dominant disorder. It has been estimated that about 1 person in 500 in the general population, and about 1 in 20 persons presenting with early coronary artery disease, are heterozygous for familial hypercholesterolaemia. Molecular studies in familial hypercholesterolaemia have revealed that it is due to a variety of defects in the number, function or processing of the low density lipoprotein (LDL) receptors on the cell surface (p. 134).

Probably the most common disorder of lipid metabolism associated with an increased risk of early coronary artery disease is familial combined hyperlipidaemia in which there are both elevated triglyceride and cholesterol levels. This is present in 1% of the population and,

Table 14.5 Recurrence risks for premature coronary artery disease (data from Slack J, Evans K A 1966 The increased risk of death from ischaemic heart disease in first degree relatives of 121 men and 96 women with ischaemic heart disease. J Med Genet 3:239–257)

Proband	Relative risk
Male (< 55 years)	
Brother	5
Sister	2.5
Female (< 65 years)	
Sibs	7

although some family studies suggest it to be inherited as an autosomal dominant disorder, this is not proven.

PEPTIC ULCER

Peptic ulceration is of two kinds, gastric and duodenal, depending on whether the ulceration involves the lining of the stomach or the duodenum. In an individual it is not always possible to say whether the ulcer is in the stomach or the duodenum without a full clinical investigation which can include gastroscopy or X-ray examination. For this reason, in many studies the two conditions are often considered together. This is probably not justified for it is possible that, as in the case of diabetes mellitus, they are two different diseases with different aetiologies. In the past, gastric ulcer, for example, was more common in persons from the poorer socio-economic groups whereas duodenal ulcer was more frequent in persons from the more affluent socio-economic groups, which suggested that different environmental factors were involved in the aetiology of the two conditions.

EPIDEMIOLOGY

Historically, the frequency of peptic ulceration appeared to peak in the period 1930 to 1965 and has stabilised over the last two to three decades. It is estimated that 2% to 10% of the population will develop peptic ulceration during the course of their lifetime. The prevalence of peptic ulceration at any point of time is just over 1% for duodenal ulceration and approximately 0.25% for gastric ulceration. The prevalence and mortality associated with peptic ulceration can vary up to 10 fold or more between different population groups. Migration studies of persons moving from areas of low to high prevalence have shown that the immigrant group rapidly acquires the higher prevalence of their new population group.

A number of environmental factors including smoking, stress and alcohol intake are associated with peptic ulceration. Recent interest has been shown in a possible infective cause with the recognition of chronic gastritis due to *Helicobacter pylori* possibly being associated with peptic ulceration.

Peptic ulceration has previously been found to be twice as common in males as females but recently the sex ratio has become approximately equal, possibly due to changes in smoking habits and work related stress as a consequence of more women entering the workforce.

FAMILY AND TWIN STUDIES

Gastric and duodenal ulcers are twice as common among first-degree relatives of affected persons as in the general population. In addition, the type of ulcer tends to be the same in the affected relative. It could be argued that the increased risk in close relatives merely reflects a common family environment. The results of an extensive study in twins showed that, of 29 identical twin pairs selected because one twin was affected with peptic ulceration, in 12 pairs the other twin was also affected. However, in the non-identical twin pairs of the same sex, only 10 out of 46 were both affected. Other studies have shown similar results, namely that the concordance in identical twins is roughly twice that seen in non-identical twins, suggesting the operation of genetic factors. However, since the concordance in identical twins is nowhere near 100% in any of the studies, environmental factors must also play an important part in aetiology.

ASSOCIATED RISK FACTORS

A variety of different risk factors have been reported as possibly being associated with peptic ulceration.

ABO blood group

In a large number of studies carried out in a variety of different population groups an increased proportion of persons with peptic ulceration have been found to have blood group O (Fig. 14.4). These findings do not mean that all persons with blood group O will develop a duodenal ulcer but merely that their risk of having a duodenal ulcer is greater than in persons with other blood groups. It has been calculated that persons with blood group O are about 30% more likely to develop duodenal ulceration than persons with blood groups A, B or AB.

Gastric ulcer is also associated with blood group O but the association is not as strong as in the case of duodenal

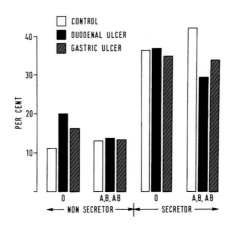

Fig. 14.4
Distribution of different blood groups and secretory types in a control population and in patients with duodenal ulcer (1000 patients) and gastric ulcer (251 patients) (data from Clarke C A 1961 Blood groups and disease. Prog Med Genet 1: 81–119, with permission).

ulcer. The finding of the association of blood group O and duodenal ulcer in different population groups from North America, Europe and Japan means that the association cannot simply be due to the studies having been limited to a particular group of people with a high frequency of blood group O and a coincidentally high susceptibility to duodenal ulcer. The manner in which the blood group association is aetiologically linked with peptic ulceration is not known.

Secretor status

Peptic ulceration is also associated with the secretor status for the ABO blood group system (p. 158). It has been found that duodenal ulcers, and gastric ulcers to a lesser extent, are more common in persons who are non-secretors than in persons who are secretors (Fig. 14.4). In fact, secretor status appears to be more important than a person's blood group in determining the likelihood of developing a peptic ulcer, with persons who are non-secretors being 50% more likely to develop peptic ulceration than the general population. The two factors together have a multiplicative effect, with persons who are non-secretors and blood group O having 2.5 times the risk of developing peptic ulceration compared to the general population.

These finding suggest that peptic ulceration could involve lack of some substance which, in secretors and persons with blood groups other than O, protects the mucosal lining from ulceration. This cannot be the entire answer because of all cases of peptic ulcer, only about 25% are blood group O and non-secretors.

Pepsinogen

The pepsinogens, pepsinogen I and II, are the inactive precursors of the proteolytic enzyme pepsin. These are synthesised by the chief cells of the gastric mucosa and released into the circulation and gastric lumen. Increased serum pepsinogen I levels have been reported in association with duodenal ulceration. It is thought that this could possibly reflect an increased secretory capacity for acid and pepsin by the gastric mucosa.

Other risk factors

Other polymorphisms have been reported as possibly being associated with an increased relative risk of developing peptic ulceration (Table 14.6). The variablility of these findings in the limited number of studies carried out in some instances, along with the difficulty of disentangling possible interactions between these factors, requires further investigation.

MODELS OF INHERITANCE

Peptic ulceration can occur as a frequent feature of certain rare single gene disorders. One example is the

Table 14.6 Relative risks with various associated genetic factors in peptic ulceration (from Peptic ulcer disease by Rotter J I, Shohat T, Petersen G M, Chapter 13 in King, Rotter and Motulsky)

Genetic marker	Allele	Relative risk
ABO blood group	O	1.3
Secretor status	Non-secretor	1.5
Rhesus blood group	Rh^+	1.1
α_1-antitrypsin	Deficiency	1.4–3.0
Pepsinogen	Increased urinary pepsinogen I	2.4
HLA complex	B5, B12, Bw35, Bw49	2.1–2.9

autosomal dominant disorder multiple endocrine neoplasia type I, in which there is a risk of developing pituitary, parathyroid and pancreatic adenomas. Other inherited disorders, such as cystic fibrosis (p. 235) and α_1-antitrypsin deficiency (p. 140), are also reported as being associated with an increased risk of peptic ulceration.

However, most evidence points towards peptic ulceration being an aetiologically heterogeneous disorder which shows multifactorial inheritance. Well recognised environmental factors include smoking and certain drugs such as phenylbutazone. Evidence for a genetic contribution comes from family and twin studies as well as physiological markers such as blood group, secretor status, gastric emptying time, basal and maximal acid secretion levels and variation in mucosal and immunological factors.

SCHIZOPHRENIA

Schizophrenia is a psychotic illness with an onset usually in early adult life. It is characterised by personality and emotional changes associated with a withdrawal from reality accompanied by hallucinations and delusions.

EPIDEMIOLOGY

Schizophrenia is a principal cause of chronic mental illness. There is a 1% lifetime risk for a person to develop schizophrenia and at any one time approximately 0.2% of the population is affected.

EVIDENCE FOR GENETIC FACTORS

The nature and extent of the genetic contribution to schizophrenia is not clear. This is partly because of past and continuing controversy concerning the definition of schizophrenia and the term schizoid. The latter term refers to the schizophrenia-like traits often seen in relatives of schizophrenics. The problem arises because clinical criteria to distinguish schizoid from normal personality are lacking. For the sake of simplicity we can regard the term schizoid as referring to a person with the fundamental symptoms of schizophrenia but in a milder form. It has been estimated that roughly 4% of the general population have schizophrenia or a schizoid personality disorder.

Family and twin studies

The results of several studies of the prevalence of schizophrenia and schizoid disorder among the relatives of schizophrenics are summarised in Table 14.7.

If the two conditions are considered together, then almost 90% of identical *co-twins* have one or other of these disorders, as do approximately 50% of first-degree relatives. What interpretation can be put on these results? The simplest would be that schizophrenia and schizoid disorders are both inherited as an autosomal dominant trait with almost complete penetrance. The idea that schizophrenia and schizoid disorders represent a single genetic disease is supported by their clinical similarity and the fact that both occur with almost equal frequency in identical co-twins of schizophrenics. If the two conditions are considered together, then the proportion of affected first-degree relatives fits well with the hypothesis of autosomal dominant inheritance, with 50% of first-degree relatives of an affected individual and 75% of the offspring of two affected individuals being affected. However, the proportion of more distant relatives

being affected does not fit this mode of inheritance so well.

Adoption studies

Other evidence which provides compelling support for genetic factors in the causation of schizophrenia is provided by the results of adoption studies. The nature of schizophrenia can result in disruption of the family, with children being placed with adoptive parents. Any differences in the frequency of schizophrenia between individuals adopted away from their biological parents and their siblings can help to separate genetic and environmental influences.

In one study of 47 offspring of schizophrenic mothers, 5 developed schizophrenia compared to none of 50 offspring of age- and sex-matched control mothers. Another study looked at the prevalence of schizophrenia in the relatives of adoptees who were schizophrenic as compared to matched control adoptees who were not schizophrenic. This showed a five-fold increase in the prevalence of schizophrenia in the biological relatives of the schizophrenic adoptees compared to biological relatives of the control adoptees, the prevalence in the latter group being the same as that seen in the adoptive relatives in both groups. These observations, along with studies which have shown similar concordance rates of schizophrenia in identical twin offspring born to a schizophrenic parent, whether reared together or separated at birth, provide compelling evidence that genetic factors are important in the causation of schizophrenia.

Table 14.7 Proportions (%) of first-degree relatives of individuals with schizophrenia who are similarly affected or have a schizoid disorder (from Heston LL 1970 The genetics of schizophrenia and schizoid disease. Science, NY 167:249–256)

Relatives	Proportion (%) of relatives		
	Schizophrenia*	Schizoid	Total schizophrenia + schizoid
Identical twins	46	41	87
Offspring (of 1 schizophrenic)	16	33	49
Sibs	14	32	46
Parents	9	35	44
Offspring (of 2 schizophrenics)	34	32	66
General population	1	3	4

* age corrected

MOLECULAR STUDIES

The report of a proband and his maternal uncle with schizophrenia, who both had an unbalanced translocation leading to partial trisomy for part of the long arm of chromosome 5, led molecular geneticists to carry out linkage studies in schizophrenia. The results so far, however, have been conflicting. In several Icelandic and two English families with schizophrenia there was evidence supporting linkage of schizophrenia to DNA markers on the long arm of chromosome 5, but studies in Swedish and Scottish families have not been able to confirm these findings.

The design of studies to detect linkage in disorders which are likely to be genetically heterogeneous presents difficult problems (p. 110). These include the difficulty of identifying a gene with a major effect, and also the need for very sophisticated statistical tests, if reliable and reproducible results are to be obtained. It could be, of course, that the apparently conflicting results in schizophrenia are a reflection of genetic heterogeneity as well as different major predisposing loci in different populations. Whatever the explanation, there is no doubt that genetic factors are likely to be important in schizophrenia.

POSSIBLE SELECTIVE ADVANTAGE

The high prevalence of schizophrenia in the general population must mean that, if the condition is due to a single gene, the mutation rate must be unusually high, which is most unlikely, or that there is a selective advantage to the heterozygote as such a deleterious disorder would tend to be eliminated by natural selection. It has been demonstrated that schizophrenics have a higher than normal resistance to traumatic or surgical shock, to allergies in general and to a number of pharmacologically active substances such as histamine and insulin. It has been suggested that, in the past, resistance to mass epidemics of diseases like smallpox and the plague could have been a contributing factor to the prevalence of schizophrenia. This is, however, speculative at present and there is no compelling supportive evidence for this hypothesis.

MODELS OF INHERITANCE

Schizophrenia has been associated with a number of complex traits such as body build and intelligence. It is also clear from twin studies and other findings that environmental factors play an important part in the aetiology of schizophrenia. The prevalence of schizophrenia among close relatives could partly be due to sharing of a common environment but most investigators consider that schizophrenia is, in fact, determined in a multifactorial manner, the genetic contribution being on a polygenic basis.

ELEMENTS

1 Both genetic and environmental factors are involved in the aetiology of many of the common diseases affecting humans. The genetic factors can be considered to be due to an inherited predisposition or genetic susceptibility.

2 The genetic contribution in a particular condition can be assessed by studying the incidence of disease in relatives, comparing concordance rates in identical and non-identical twins, studying differences between populations and the effects of immigration, studying the effects of adoption, biochemical studies, evaluating any possible association with other inherited factors and studying animal models.

3 For common disorders such as diabetes mellitus, hypertension, coronary artery disease, peptic ulcer, schizophrenia, the common cancers and the common congenital abnormalities, a multifactorial mode of inheritance is most likely. However it is also becoming clear that many of these conditions are heterogeneous, i.e due to a variety of genetic and environmental factors.

4 Prevention of the common diseases involves determining causative environmental agents as well as identifying those individuals who are genetically susceptible to such agents.

FURTHER READING

Heston L L 1966 Psychiatric disorders in foster home reared children of schizophrenic mothers. Br J Psychiat 112: 819–825
A classic paper demonstrating genetic factors in the aetiology of schizophrenia.
King R A, Rotter J I, Motulsky A G (eds) 1992 The genetic basis of common diseases. Oxford University Press, Oxford
An excellent multi-author text covering the principles of analysis with an extensive review of the genetic basis of the common diseases plus an exhaustive reference list.

CHAPTER 15

Genetics and congenital abnormalities

The formation of a human being involves an extremely complicated and as yet very poorly understood interaction of genetic and environmental factors. Given the extraordinary complexity of this process it is not surprising that it can go wrong. Nor is it surprising that in many congenital abnormalities genetic factors can clearly be implicated. In this chapter we shall consider the overall impact of abnormalities in morphogenesis by reviewing:

1. The incidence of abnormalities in morphogenesis at various stages from conception onwards.
2. Their nature and the ways in which they can be classified.
3. Their causes, when known, with particular emphasis on the role of genetics.

INCIDENCE

SPONTANEOUS FIRST TRIMESTER PREGNANCY LOSS

At least 15% of all recognised pregnancies end in spontaneous miscarriage before 12 weeks gestation. Even if material from the abortus can be obtained it is often very difficult to establish why a pregnancy loss has occurred. However, careful study of large numbers of aborted embryos has shown that gross structural abnormalities are present in between 80% and 85%. These abnormalities vary from complete absence of an embryo in the developing pregnancy sac, or what is known as a 'blighted ovum', to a very distorted body shape, or a specific abnormality in a single body system.

Chromosome abnormalities such as trisomy, monosomy and triploidy are found in 50% of all spontaneous abortions. This incidence rises to 60% when a gross structural abnormality is present (p. 215).

CONGENITAL ABNORMALITIES AND PERINATAL MORTALITY

Perinatal mortality figures include all infants who are stillborn after 28 weeks gestation plus all babies who die during the first week of life. Studies undertaken in several centres in Europe and North America have shown that between 25% and 30% of all perinatal deaths occur as a result of a serious structural abnormality. In 80% of these cases genetic factors can be implicated, with a recurrence risk to future pregnancies equal to 1% or greater. The relative contribution of structural abnormalities to perinatal mortality is lower in less well developed countries where environmental factors play a much greater role.

NEWBORN INFANTS

Surveys of birth defects in newborn infants have been undertaken in many parts of the world. Usually these have reviewed the incidence of both major and minor anomalies. A major anomaly is defined as one which has an adverse outcome on either the function or social acceptability of the individual (Table 15.1). In contrast minor abnormalities are of neither medical nor cosmetic

Table 15.1 Examples of major congenital structural abnormalities

System and abnormality	Incidence per 1000 births
Cardiovascular	10
Ventricular septal defect	2.5
Atrial septal defect	1
Patent ductus arteriosus	1
Fallot's tetralogy	1
Central nervous system	10
Anencephaly	1
Hydrocephaly	1
Microcephaly	1
Lumbo-sacral spina bifida	2
Gastro-intestinal	4
Cleft lip/palate	1.5
Diaphragmatic hernia	0.5
Oesophageal atresia	0.3
Imperforate anus	0.2
Limb	2
Transverse amputation	0.2
Urogenital	4
Bilateral renal agenesis	2
Polycystic kidneys (infantile)	0.02
Bladder exstrophy	0.03

Table 15.2 Examples of minor congenital structural abnormalities

Pre-auricular pit or tag
Epicanthic folds
Lacrimal duct stenosis
Brushfield spots in the iris
Lip pits
Single palmar crease
Fifth finger clinodactyly
Syndactyly between second and third toes
Supernumerary nipple
Umbilical hernia
Hydrocele
Sacral pit or dimple

Table 15.3 The incidence of structural abnormalities

	Incidence (%)
Spontaneous miscarriages	
First trimester	80–85
Second trimester	25
All babies	
Major abnormality	
Apparent at birth	2–3
Apparent later	2
Minor abnormality	10
Deaths in perinatal period	25
Deaths in first year of life	25
Deaths from 1 to 9 years	20
Deaths from 10 to 14 years	7.5

importance (Table 15.2).

These surveys have consistently shown that between 2% and 3% of all babies have at least one major abnormality apparent at birth. The true incidence, taking into account abnormalities such as brain malformations which present later in life, is probably close to 5%. Minor abnormalities are found in approximately 10% of all newborn babies.

The long-term outlook for a baby with a major abnormality obviously depends on the nature of the specific defect and whether it can be treated successfully. Taken together as a group the overall prognosis is relatively poor with 25% dying in early infancy, 25% having subsequent mental or physical disability and only the remaining 50% having a fair to good outlook after treatment.

CHILDHOOD MORTALITY

Congenital abnormalities make a significant contribution to mortality throughout childhood. During the first year of life approximately 25% of all deaths are due to major structural abnormalities. This figure falls to 20% between the ages of 1 and 10 years and to around 7.5% for children aged between 10 and 15 years.

Taking into account the incidence of major and minor abnormalities noted in newborn surveys and the high incidence of defects observed in early spontaneous miscarriages, it is evident that at least 15% of all human conceptions are structurally abnormal (Table 15.3). It is probable that genetic factors are involved in the causation of at least 50% of all structural abnormalities.

DEFINITIONS AND CLASSIFICATION OF BIRTH DEFECTS

So far in this chapter the terms 'congenital abnormality' and 'birth defect' have been used in a general sense to describe all types of structural abnormality which can occur in an embryo, fetus or newborn infant. Whilst these terms are perfectly acceptable for the purpose of

lumping together all these abnormalities when studying their overall incidence, they do not provide any insight into possible underlying mechanisms. More specific definitions have been devised which have the added advantage of providing a combined clinical and aetiological classification.

MALFORMATION

A *malformation* is a primary structural defect of an organ or part of an organ which results from an inherent abnormality in development. This used to be known as a *primary* or *intrinsic* malformation. The presence of a malformation implies that the early development of a particular tissue or organ has been arrested or misdirected. Common examples of malformations include congenital heart abnormalities such as ventricular or atrial septal defects, cleft lip and/or palate (p. 108), and neural tube defects such as anencephaly or lumbo-sacral myelomeningocele (Fig. 15.1). Most malformations involving only a single organ show multifactorial inheritance, implying an interaction of many genes with an adverse environment (p. 105).

DISRUPTION

The term *disruption* refers to abnormal structure of an organ or tissue as a result of external factors disturbing the normal developmental process. This used to be known as a secondary or *extrinsic* malformation. Extrinsic factors which can disrupt normal development include ischaemia, infection and trauma. An example of a disruption is the effect seen on limb development when a strand or band of amnion becomes entwined around a baby's forearm or digits (Fig. 15.2). By definition a disruption is not genetic although occasionally genetic factors can predispose to disruptive events. For example a small proportion of amniotic bands are caused by an

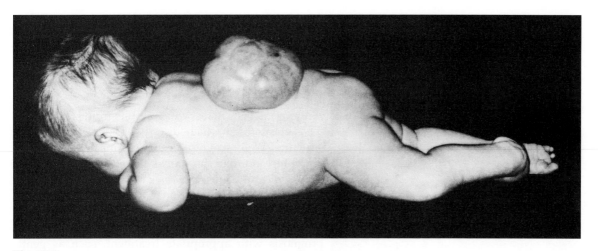

Fig. 15.1
Child with a large thoraco-lumbar myelomeningocele consisting of protruding spinal cord covered by meninges.

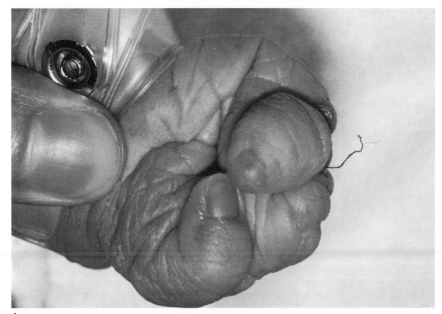

A

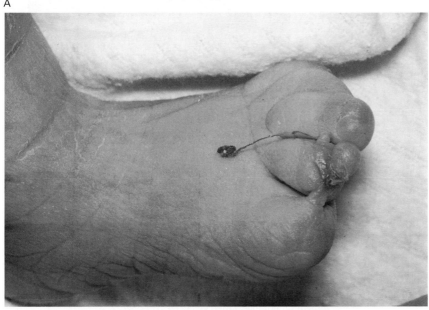

B

Fig. 15.2
(A) Hand and (B) foot of a baby with digital amputations due to amniotic bands. Residual strands of amnion can be seen (courtesy of Dr Una MacFadyen, Leicester Royal Infirmary).

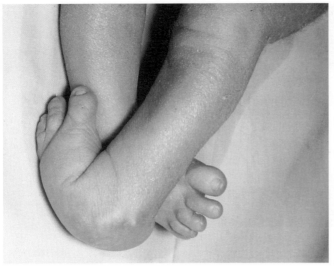

Fig. 15.3
The lower limbs of a baby with talipes equinovarus.

underlying, genetically determined defect in collagen which weakens the amnion making it more liable to tear or rupture.

DEFORMATION

A *deformation* is a defect which results from an abnormal mechanical force which distorts an otherwise normal structure. Well recognised examples include dislocation of the hip and mild 'positional' talipes ('club foot'), both of which can be caused by lack of amniotic fluid (oligo-hydramnios) or intra-uterine crowding due to twinning or a structurally abnormal uterus (Fig. 15.3). Deformations usually occur late in pregnancy and convey a good prognosis with appropriate treatment, such as gentle splinting for talipes, as the underlying organ is fundamentally normal in structure.

DYSPLASIA

A *dysplasia* is an abnormal organisation of cells into tissue. Usually the effects will be seen in all parts of the

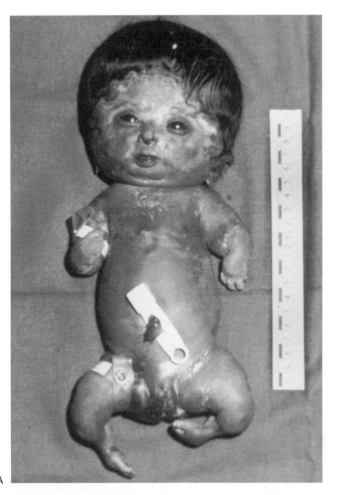

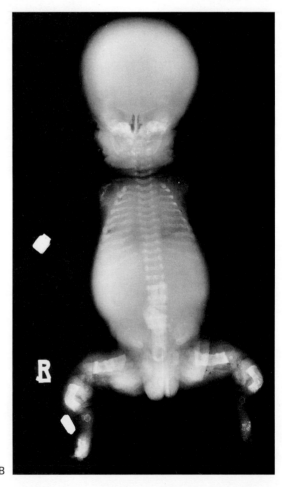

A   B

Fig. 15.4
(A) Stillborn infant with a lethal form of osteogenesis imperfecta. (B) X-ray of the infant showing crumpled long bones and thickened ribs. These appearances are due to multiple intra-uterine fractures (reproduced with permission from Young I D, Thompson E M, Hall C M, Pembrey M E 1987 Osteogenesis imperfecta type IIA. Evidence for dominant inheritance. J Med Genet 24: 386–389).

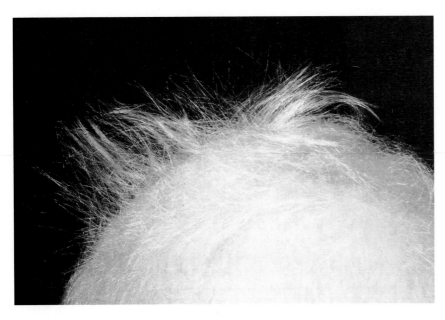

Fig. 15.5
Appearance of the hair in a child with ectodermal dysplasia.

body in which that particular tissue is present. For example, in a skeletal dysplasia such as osteogenesis imperfecta, almost all parts of the skeleton are affected (Fig. 15.4). Similarly, in an ectodermal dysplasia, widely dispersed tissues of ectodermal origin such as hair, teeth and nails are involved (Fig. 15.5). Most dysplasias are caused by single gene defects and are associated with high recurrence risks for siblings and/or offspring.

SEQUENCE

The most logical and easily understood pattern of multiple abnormalities is the concept of a *sequence*. This describes the findings which occur as a consequence of a cascade of events initiated by a single primary factor.

This can often be a single organ malformation. In the 'Potter' sequence, chronic leakage of amniotic fluid or defective urinary output results in oligohydramnios (Fig. 15.6). This, in turn, leads to fetal compression, resulting in squashed facial features, dislocation of the hips, talipes and usually life-threatening pulmonary hypoplasia (Fig. 15.7).

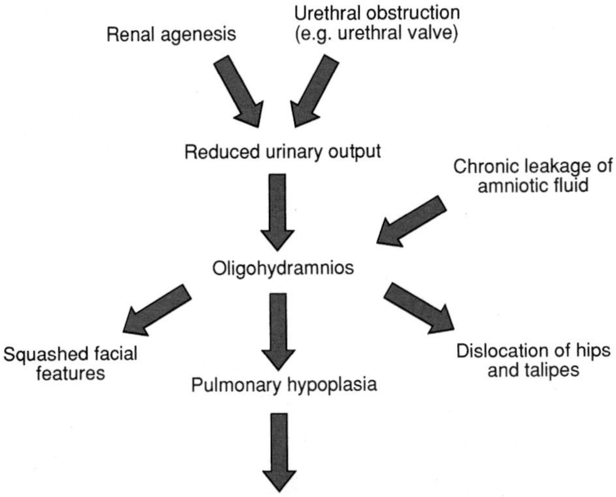

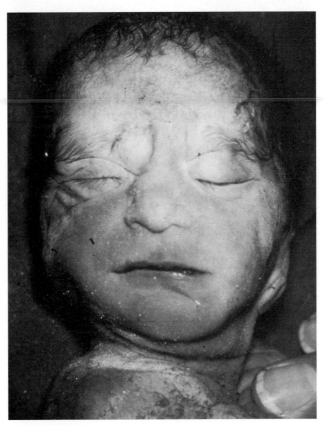

Fig. 15.7
Facial appearance of a baby with bilateral renal agenesis. Note the squashed appearance with lines under the eyes.

Renal agenesis → Urethral obstruction (e.g. urethral valve)

↓ ↓

Reduced urinary output

Chronic leakage of amniotic fluid

↓

Oligohydramnios

↙ ↓ ↘

Squashed facial features — Pulmonary hypoplasia — Dislocation of hips and talipes

↓

Death

Fig. 15.6
The 'Potter' sequence showing the cascade of events leading to and resulting from oligohydramnios (reduced volume of amniotic fluid).

SYNDROME

In practice the term *syndrome* is used very loosely (e.g. the amniotic band 'syndrome'), but in theory it should be reserved for consistent patterns of abnormalities for which there will often be a known underlying cause. These underlying causes can include chromosome abnormalities, as in Down's syndrome, or single gene defects, as in Meckel's syndrome, which is characterised by polydactyly, an encephalocele and polycystic kidneys (Fig. 15.8).

Several thousand multiple malformation syndromes are now recognised. This field of study is known as *dysmorphology*. The diagnosis of individual syndromes has been greatly helped by the development of computerised databases. It is possible to obtain a list of differential diagnoses by providing the computer with details of key abnormal clinical features. Even with the help of this extremely valuable diagnostic tool, there are many *dysmorphic* children for whom no diagnosis can be reached.

ASSOCIATION

The term *association* has been introduced in recognition of the fact that certain malformations tend to occur together more often than would be expected by chance, yet this non-random association of abnormalities cannot be explained on the basis of a sequence or a syndrome. The main differences from a syndrome are the lack of consistency of abnormalities from one case to another and absence of a satisfactory underlying explanation. The names of associations are often acronyms devised by juggling the first letters of the organs or systems most commonly involved. For example the VATER association features <u>V</u>ertebral, <u>A</u>nal, <u>T</u>racheo-<u>E</u>sophageal and <u>R</u>enal abnormalities. Associations are associated with a low risk of recurrence and are, therefore, not usually genetic in origin even though the underlying cause is generally unknown.

It is recognised that this classification of birth defects is not perfect. It will be readily apparent that it is far from being either fully comprehensive or mutually exclusive. For example, bladder outflow obstruction caused

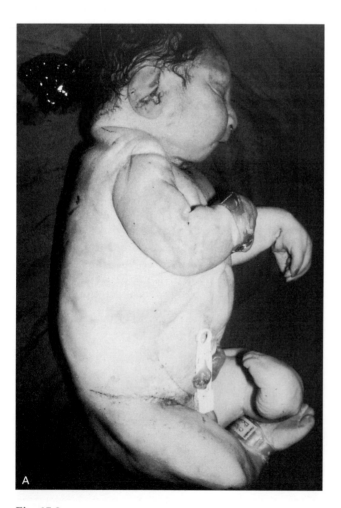

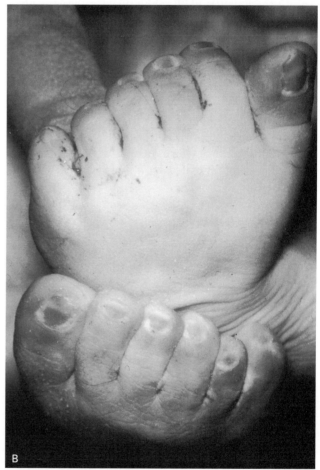

Fig. 15.8
A baby with Meckel's syndrome. Note in: (A) The occipital encephalocele. (B) The polydactyly involving both feet (reproduced, with permission from Young I D, Rickett A B, Clarke M 1985 High incidence of Meckel's syndrome in Gujurati Indians. J Med Genet 22: 301–304).

by a *malformation* such as a urethral valve will result in the oligohydramnios or Potter *sequence* leading to *deformations* such as dislocation of the hip and talipes. To complicate matters further, the absence of both kidneys, which will result in the same sequence of events, is widely referred to as Potter's *syndrome*. Despite this semantic confusion, adherence to this classification is important as an aid to understanding and ensuring that correct information is given about possible recurrence risks (p. 259).

AETIOLOGY

There are many recognised causes of congenital abnormalities although it is notable that in up to 50% of all cases no clear explanation can be established (Table 15.4).

GENETIC

Chromosome abnormalities

These account for approximately 6% of all recognised congenital abnormalities. As a general rule any perceptible degree of autosomal imbalance, such as duplication, deletion, trisomy or monosomy, will result in severe structural and developmental abnormality. If very severe this can lead to early spontaneous miscarriage. Common chromosome syndromes are described in detail in Chapter 17.

Single gene defects

These account for approximately 7.5% of all congenital abnormalities. Some of these are isolated, i.e. they involve only one organ or system (Table 15.5). Other single gene defects result in multiple congenital abnormality syn-

Table 15.5 Congenital abnormalities which may be caused by single gene defects

Isolated

Central nervous system	Inheritance	
Hydrocephalus	XR	
Megalencephaly	AD	
Microcephaly	AD/AR	

Ocular		
Aniridia	AD	
Cataracts	AD/AR	
Microphthalmia	AD/AR	

Limb		
Brachydactyly	AD	
Ectrodactyly	AD	
Polydactyly	AD	

Other		
Infantile polycystic kidneys	AR	

Syndromes

Syndrome	Inheritance	Abnormalities
Apert	AD	Craniosynostosis, syndactyly
EEC	AD	Ectodermal dysplasia, ectrodactyly, cleft lip/palate
Meckel	AR	Encephalocoele, polydactyly, polycystic kidneys
Roberts	AR	Cleft lip/palate, phocomelia
van der Woude	AD	Cleft lip/palate, lip pits

AD – autosomal dominant, AR – autosomal recessive, XR – sex-linked recessive

dromes involving many organs or systems which do not have any obvious underlying embryological relationship. For example, ectrodactyly (Fig. 15.9) in isolation can show autosomal dominant inheritance. It can also occur as one manifestation of the EEC syndrome (Ectodermal dysplasia, Ectrodactyly and Cleft lip/palate), which also shows autosomal dominant inheritance. There is abundant evidence from the study of dysmorphology that several different mutations, allelic or non-allelic, can cause similar if not identical malformations.

The importance of identifying birth defects which show single gene inheritance is two-fold. From the family's point of view it is essential that correct counselling is available so that close relatives can be alerted to possible risks. From the academic point of view, the identification of a molecular defect causing an isolated or syndromal abnormality in a particular organ, can provide a clue as to the locus of a susceptibility gene for other malformations affecting the same organ which show multifactorial inheritance. For example, the DiGeorge syndrome, in which thymic aplasia is associated with cardiac abnormalities, has been shown to be due to a microdeletion of

Table 15.4 Causes of congenital abnormalities

Genetic	
Chromosomal	6%
Single gene	7.5%
Multifactorial	20–30%
Subtotal	30–40%
Environmental	
Drugs and chemicals	2%
Infections	2%
Maternal illness	2%
Physical agents	1%
Subtotal	5–10%
Unknown	50%
TOTAL	100%

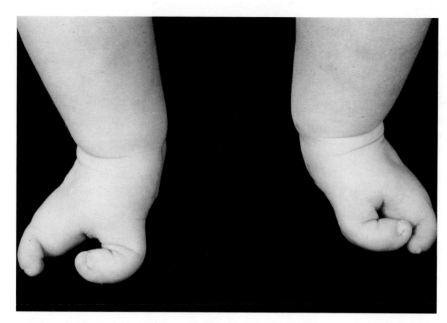

Fig. 15.9
Appearance of the feet in a child with ectrodactyly.

chromosome 22q11. In several families showing clustering of isolated apparently multifactorial cardiac abnormalities similar molecular defects have been identified (pp. 155, 221).

Multifactorial inheritance

Multifactorial inheritance accounts for the majority of congenital abnormalities in which genetic factors can be clearly implicated. These include most isolated ('non-syndromal') malformations involving the heart, central nervous system and kidneys (Table 15.6). For many of these conditions empiric risks have been derived (p. 259) based on large family studies, so that it is usually possible to provide the parents of an affected child with a clear indication of the likelihood that a future child will be similarly affected. Risks to the offspring of patients who were themselves treated successfully in childhood are becoming available. These are usually similar to the risk figures which apply to siblings as would be predicted by the multifactorial model (p. 108).

Neural tube defects

Neural tube defects, such as spina bifida and anencephaly, illustrate many of the underlying principles of multifactorial inheritance and emphasise the importance of trying to identify possible adverse environmental factors. These conditions result from defective closure of the developing neural tube during the first month of embryonic life. A defect occurring at the upper end of the developing neural tube results in either anencephaly or an encephalo-

Table 15.6 Isolated (non-syndromal) malformations which may show multifactorial inheritance

Cardiac
Atrial septal defect
Fallot's tetraology
Patent ductus arteriosus
Ventricular septal defect

Central nervous system
Anencephaly
Encephalocele
Spina bifida

Genito-urinary
Hypospadias
Renal agenesis
Renal dysgenesis

Other
Cleft lip/palate
Congenital dislocation of hips
Talipes

cele (Fig. 15.10). A defect occurring at the lower end of the developing neural tube leads to a spinal lesion such as a lumbo-sacral myelocele or meningomyelocele (Fig. 15.1). Most neural tube defects have serious consequences. Anencephaly is not compatible with survival for more than a few hours after birth. Large lumbo-sacral lesions usually cause partial or complete paralysis of the lower limbs with impaired bladder and bowel continence.

The empiric recurrence risks to first degree relatives (siblings and offspring) vary according to the local population incidence and are as high as 4–5% in areas where neural tube defects are common. No specific neural tube defect genes have been identified but it is known that the

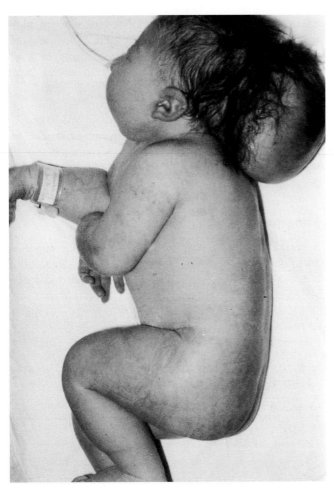

Fig. 15.10
A baby with a large occipital encephalocele.

ENVIRONMENTAL FACTORS

An agent which can cause a birth defect by interfering with normal embryonic or foetal development is known as a *teratogen*. Many teratogens have been identified and exhaustive tests are now undertaken before any new drug is approved for use by pregnant women. The potential effects of any particular teratogen will usually depend on the dosage and timing at which it is administered during the pregnancy and the susceptibility of both the mother and her unborn baby.

An agent which conveys a high risk of teratogenesis, such as rubella or thalidomide, will usually be identified relatively easily. Unfortunately, it can be much more difficult to detect a low grade teratogen which causes an abnormality in only a small proportion of cases. This is because of the relatively high background incidence of congenital abnormalities and also because many pregnant women take medication at some time in pregnancy, often for an ill-defined 'flu-like' infection. Despite extensive study controversy still surrounds the use of a number of drugs in pregnancy. The antinausea drug Debendox has been the subject of litigation in the United States despite the absence of firm evidence to support a definite teratogenic effect.

Drugs and chemicals

Drugs and chemicals which have a proven teratogenic effect in humans are listed in Table 15.7. Overall these account for approximately 2% of all congenital abnormalities.

incidence in the United Kingdom is highest in people of Celtic origin. If such individuals move from their country of origin to another part of the world, the incidence of neural tube defects in their offspring declines but remains higher than amongst the indigenous population. These observations suggest that there is a relatively high incidence of adverse susceptibility genes in the Celtic populations.

Environmental factors have also been identified. These include poor socio-economic status and multiparity. Firm evidence has emerged that periconceptional multivitamin supplementation significantly reduces the risk of recurrence when a woman has had one affected child. A large multicentre study has shown that folic acid is likely to be the effective constituent of multivitamin preparations. In the United Kingdom all women who have had a child with a neural tube defect are offered folic acid supplementation in all future pregnancies, and it is now recommended that low dose folic acid should be given to all women in pregnancy regardless of whether or not they have a family history of neural tube defects.

Table 15.7 Drugs with a proven teratogenic effect in humans

Drug	Effects
Alcohol	Cardiac defects, microcephaly, characteristic facies
Chloroquine	Chorioretinitis, deafness
Diethylstilboestrol	Uterine malformations, vaginal adenocarcinoma
Lithium	Cardiac defects (Ebstein's anomaly)
Phenytoin	Cardiac defects, cleft palate, digital hypoplasia
Retinoids	Ear and eye defects, hydrocephaly
Streptomycin	Deafness
Tetracycline	Dental enamel hypoplasia
Thalidomide	Phocomelia, cardiac and ear abnormalities
Valproic acid	Neural tube defects, characteristic facies
Warfarin	Nasal hypoplasia, stippled epiphyses

The thalidomide tragedy

Thalidomide was used widely in Europe during the years 1958 to 1962 as a sedative. In 1961 an association with severe limb anomalies in babies whose mothers had taken the drug during the first trimester was recognised and the drug was subsequently withdrawn. It has been estimated that during this short period over 10 000 babies were damaged by this drug. Review of these babies' records indicated that the critical period for fetal damage was between 20 and 35 days from conception, i.e. 34 to 50 days after the beginning of the last menstrual period.

The most characteristic abnormality caused by thalidomide was phocomelia (Fig. 15.11). This is the name given to a limb which is malformed due to absence of some or all of the long bones, with retention of digits giving a 'flipper' or 'seal-like' appearance. Other external abnormalities included ear defects, microphthalmia and cleft lip/palate. It is less well known that about 40% of 'thalidomide babies' died in early infancy as a result of severe internal abnormalities affecting the heart, kidneys and gastro-intestinal tract.

The thalidomide tragedy focused attention on the importance of avoiding all drugs in pregnancy as far as is possible, unless absolute safety has been established. Drug manufacturers undertake extensive research trials before releasing a drug for general use and invariably urge caution about the use of any new drug in pregnancy. Monitoring systems have been set up in most Western countries so that it is unlikely that an 'epidemic' on the scale of the thalidomide tragedy could ever happen again.

The fetal alcohol syndrome

Children born to mothers who have consistently consumed large quantities of alcohol during pregnancy tend to show a distinctive facial appearance with short palpebral fissures (eye apertures) and a long smooth philtrum (upper lip). They also show mild developmental delay and are often hyperactive and clumsy in later childhood. This condition is referred to as the fetal alcohol syndrome.

There is uncertainty about the level of alcohol consumption which is 'safe' in pregnancy and there is evidence that even mild to moderate ingestion can be harmful. Generally it is advised that all women should try to abstain from alcohol completely throughout pregnancy.

Maternal infections

Several infectious agents can interfere with embryogenesis and fetal development (Table 15.8). The developing brain, eyes and ears are particularly susceptible to damage by infection.

Table 15.8 Infectious teratogenic agents

Infection	Effects
Viruses	
Cytomegalovirus	Chorioretinitis, deafness, microcephaly
Herpes simplex	Microcephaly, microphthalmia
Rubella	Microcephaly, cataracts, retinitis, cardiac defects
Varicella zoster	Microcephaly, chorioretinitis, skin defects
Bacteria	
Syphilis	hydrocephalus, osteitis, rhinitis
Parasites	
Toxoplasmosis	hydrocephalus, microcephaly, cataracts, chorioretinitis, deafness

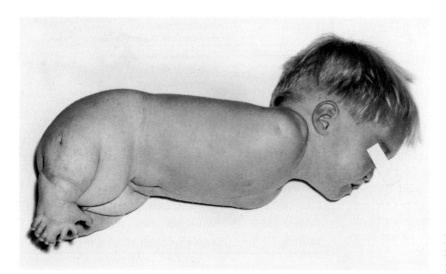

Fig. 15.11
A child with upper limb amelia, lower limb phocomelia and polydactyly of the toes due to thalidomide (courtesy of Emeritus Professor R.W. Smithells, University of Leeds).

Rubella

The rubella virus, which damages between 15% and 25% of all babies infected during the first trimester, also causes cardiovascular malformations such as patent ductus arteriosus and peripheral pulmonary artery stenosis. Congenital rubella infection can be prevented by the widespread use of immunisation programmes based on administration of either the measles, mumps, rubella (MMR) vaccine in early childhood or the rubella vaccine alone to young adult women.

Cytomegalovirus

At present no immunisation is available against the cytomegalovirus (CMV) and naturally occurring infection does not always produce long-term immunity. The risk of abnormality is greatest if infection occurs during the first trimester. Overall this virus causes damage in only 5% of infected pregnancies.

Toxoplasmosis

Maternal infection with the parasite causing toxoplasmosis conveys a risk of 20% that the fetus will be infected during the first trimester rising to 75% in the second and third trimesters. Vaccines against toxoplasmosis are not available.

If a woman is exposed to any of these infectious agents during pregnancy then an attempt can be made to establish whether the fetus has been infected by sampling fetal blood to look for specific IgM antibodies. Fetal blood analysis can also reveal generalised evidence of infection such as abnormal liver function and thrombocytopaenia.

There is some evidence to suggest that maternal infection with listeriosis can cause a miscarriage and a definite association has been established between maternal infection with this agent and neonatal meningitis. Maternal infection with parvovirus can cause severe anaemia in the fetus resulting in *hydrops fetalis* and pregnancy loss.

Physical agents

Women who have had babies with congenital abnormalities are understandably anxious that exposure to agents such as radiowaves, ultrasound and magnetic fields could have caused their babies' problems. Unfortunately, it is difficult to prove or disprove any of these possibilities as exposure to these agents is almost universal.

However there is evidence that two physical agents can have teratogenic effects.

Ionising radiation

Heavy doses of ionising radiation, far in excess of those used in routine diagnostic radiography, can cause microcephaly and ocular defects. The most sensitive time of exposure is from 2 to 5 weeks after conception. Ionising radiation can also have mutagenic (p. 19) and carcinogenic effects, and although risks with low dose diagnostic procedures are minimal, radiography should always be avoided during pregnancy if at all possible.

Prolonged hyperthermia

It is suggested that prolonged hyperthermia in early pregnancy can cause microcephaly and microphthalmia as well as neuronal migration defects. Consequently it is recommended that care should be taken to avoid excessive use of hot baths and saunas during the first trimester.

Maternal illness

Diabetes mellitus

Maternal insulin dependent diabetes mellitus is associated with a two- to three-fold increase in the incidence of congenital abnormalities in offspring. Malformations which occur most commonly in such infants include congenital heart disease, neural tube defects, sacral agenesis, femoral hypoplasia and sirenomelia ('mermaidism'). The likelihood of an abnormality is inversely related to the quality of the control of the mother's blood glucose levels during early pregnancy. This can be assessed by regular monitoring of blood glucose and glycosylated haemoglobin levels. Non-insulin dependent diabetes and gestational diabetes do not convey an increased risk of congenital malformations in offspring.

Phenylketonuria

The other main maternal metabolic condition which conveys a risk to offspring is untreated phenylketonuria (p. 129). A high serum level of phenylalanine in a pregnant woman with phenylketonuria who is not on a special diet will almost invariably result in serious damage to the fetus with the incidence of mental retardation close to 100%. Structural abnormalities can include microcephaly and congenital heart defects. All women with phenylketonuria should be strongly advised to adhere to a strict low phenylalanine diet both before and during pregnancy.

Maternal epilepsy

There has been considerable interest in whether or not maternal epilepsy leads to congenital abnormalities. There have been a number of studies of this problem and it seems that maternal epilepsy itself is not associated with an increased risk of congenital abnormalities. Treatment of the mother with one of the anticonvulsants can, however, be associated with teratogenic effects on the fetus. Phenytoin is associated with a risk of cleft lip and/or palate of about 1–2%, while with sodium valproate there is a risk of anencephaly and spina bifida of about 2%. Of course, risks to the fetus have to be weighed against the dangers of stopping treatment and risking seizures during pregnancy. Medical advice, at present, is that if the patient has been seizure-free for at least 2 years she can be offered withdrawal of anticonvulsant treatment before proceeding with a pregnancy. If therapy is essential, then single drug treatment is preferred, since a combination of several anticonvulsants appears to carry a greater risk of fetal abnormality.

UNKNOWN

In up to 50% of all congenital abnormalities no clear cause can be established. This applies to many relatively common conditions such as isolated diaphragmatic hernia, tracheo-oesophageal fistula, anal atresia and single limb reduction defects. For an isolated limb defect, such as absence of a hand, it is reasonable to postulate that loss of vascular supply at a critical time during the development of the limb bud leads to developmental arrest with formation of only vestigial digits. It is much more difficult to envisage how vascular occlusion could result in an abnormality such as oesophageal atresia with an associated tracheo-oesophageal fistula.

Whilst it is obviously frustrating for the parents of a child with one of these abnormalities that no factual explanation can be given, they can at least be reassured that the empiric risk of recurrence for siblings is very low. It is worth noting that this does not necessarily mean that genetic factors are irrelevant. Some 'unexplained' malformations and syndromes could well be due to new dominant mutations (p. 79), submicroscopic microdeletions (p. 219) or uniparental disomy (p. 88). All of these would convey negligible recurrence risks to future siblings. There is optimism that molecular techniques will provide at least some of the answers to the many unresolved issues surrounding the causes of the many congenital malformations which at present cannot be explained.

ELEMENTS

1 Congenital abnormalities are apparent at birth in 1 in 40 of all newborn infants. They account for 20–25% of all deaths occurring during the perinatal period and childhood up to the age of 10 years.

2 Terms such as malformation, deformation, dysplasia and syndrome can be clearly defined and should be used advisedly. Most isolated malformations show multifactorial inheritance, whereas most dysplasias have a single gene aetiology. Deformations and associations are usually not genetic.

3 Genetic factors contribute to at least 40% of all congenital abnormalities with the major contribution being made by malformations showing multifactorial inheritance. The importance of recognising environmental factors, i.e. teratogens, lies in the potential for their prevention.

FURTHER READING

Aase J 1990 Diagnostic dysmorphology. Plenum Medical Book Company, London
A detailed text of the art and science of dysmorphology.
Carter C O 1965 The inheritance of common congenital malformations. Prog Med Genet 4: 59–83
One of the early reviews of the inheritance of the common congenital malformations.
Graham J M, 1988 Smith's recognizable patterns of human deformation, 2nd edn. Saunders, Philadelphia
An illustrated guide to human deformations and how they are caused.
Jones K L, 1988 Smith's recognisable patterns of human malformation, 4th edn. Saunders, Philadelphia
The standard paediatric text-book guide to syndromes.
Kalter H, Warkany J 1983 Congenital malformations. (In two parts.) New England Journal of Medicine 308: 424–431, 491–497
A detailed review of the known causes of congenital malformations.
Smithells R W, Newman C G H 1992 Recognition of thalidomide defects. Journal of Medical Genetics 29: 716–723
A comprehensive account of the spectrum of abnormalities caused by thalidomide.
Spranger J, Benirschke K, Hall J G et al 1982 Errors of morphogenesis: concepts and terms. Recommendations of an international working group. Journal of Pediatrics 100: 160–165
A short paper providing a classification and clarification of the terms used in describing birth defects.

SECTION C
CLINICAL GENETICS

CHAPTER 16

Genetic counselling

Any couple who have had a child with a serious abnormality must inevitably reflect on why this has happened and whether any child(ren) they choose to have in future could be similarly affected. Individuals who have a family history of a serious disorder are likely to be equally concerned that they could either develop the disorder or transmit it to future generations. Realisation of the needs of such individuals and couples and awareness of the importance of providing them with accurate and appropriate information has led to the widespread introduction of genetic counselling clinics, with the establishment of clinical genetics as a recognised medical specialty.

DEFINITION

Since the first introduction of genetic counselling services approximately 40 years ago many attempts have been made to devise a satisfactory and all-embracing definition. A theme common to all is the concept of *genetic counselling* being a communication process which addresses an individual's concerns relating to the development and/or transmission of a hereditary disorder.

An individual who seeks genetic counselling is known as a *consultand*. During the genetic counselling process it is widely agreed that the counsellor should try to ensure that the consultand is provided with information which enables him or her to understand:

1. The medical diagnosis and its implications in terms of prognosis and possible treatment.
2. The mode of inheritance of the disorder and the risk of developing and/or transmitting it.
3. The choices or options available for dealing with the risks.

It is also agreed that genetic counselling should include a strong communicative and supportive element, so that those who seek information are able to reach their own fully informed decisions without undue pressure or stress (Table 16.1).

Table 16.1   Steps in genetic counselling

Diagnosis – based on history, examination and investigations
Risk assessment
Communication
Discussion of options
Long-term contact and support

ESTABLISHING THE DIAGNOSIS

The most crucial step in any genetic consultation is that of establishing the diagnosis. If this is incorrect, then inappropriate and totally misleading information could be given with potentially tragic consequences.

Reaching a diagnosis in clinical genetics usually involves the three fundamental steps of any medical consultation, i.e. taking a history, carrying out an examination and undertaking appropriate investigations. Often information about the consultand's family history will have been obtained by a skilled genetics nurse or counsellor as part of a pre-clinic home visit. Further information about the consultand's family and personal medical history often emerges at the clinic visit, when a full examination can be undertaken and appropriate investigations initiated. These can include chromosome and molecular studies as well as referral on to specialists in other fields such as neurology and ophthalmology.

It cannot be over-emphasised that genetic counselling should only be undertaken when facilities exist to ensure that an accurate diagnosis can be made.

Even when a firm diagnosis has been made, problems can arise if the disorder in question shows aetiological heterogeneity. Common examples include deafness and non-specific mental retardation, both of which can be caused by either environmental or genetic factors. In these situations empiric risks can be used (p. 259) although these are not as satisfactory as risks based on a precise and specific diagnosis.

A disorder is said to show *genetic heterogeneity* if it can be caused by more than one genetic mechanism (p. 81). Many such disorders are recognised and counselling can

Table 16.2 Hereditary disorders which can show different patterns of inheritance

Disorder	Inheritance patterns
Cerebellar ataxia	AD, AR
Charcot–Marie–Tooth disease (HMSN)	AD, AR, XR
Congenital cataract	AD, AR, XR
Ehlers–Danlos syndrome	AD, AR, XR
Ichthyosis	AD, AR, XR
Microcephaly	AD, AR
Polycystic kidney disease	AD, AR
Retinitis pigmentosa	AD, AR, XR
Sensori-neural deafness	AD, AR, XR

AD – autosomal dominant
AR – autosomal recessive
XR – sex-linked recessive

be extremely difficult if the heterogeneity extends to different modes of inheritance. Commonly encountered examples include the various forms of Ehlers–Danlos syndrome (Plate 13), Charcot–Marie–Tooth disease and retinitis pigmentosa, all of which can show autosomal dominant, autosomal recessive and sex-linked recessive inheritance (Table 16.2). Fortunately, progress in molecular genetics is providing solutions to some of these problems. For example, the most common form of Charcot–Marie–Tooth disease, which is also known as hereditary motor and sensory neuropathy type I (HMSN I) (Fig. 16.1), has been shown to result from a small duplication on the short arm of chromosome 17. If this is found to be present in a consultand or a family relative, then accurate counselling can be undertaken.

CALCULATING AND PRESENTING THE RISK

In some counselling situations, calculation of the recurrence risk is relatively straightforward and requires little more than a reasonable knowledge of Mendelian inheritance. However, many factors such as delayed age of onset, reduced penetrance and the use of linked DNA markers can result in the calculation becoming much more complex. The theoretical aspects of risk calculation are considered in more detail later (p. 253).

The provision of a recurrence risk does not simply involve conveying a stark risk figure in isolation. It is very important that information which is provided is understood and that parents are given as much background information as possible to help them reach their own decision. As a working rule of thumb, recurrence risks should be quantified, qualified and placed in context.

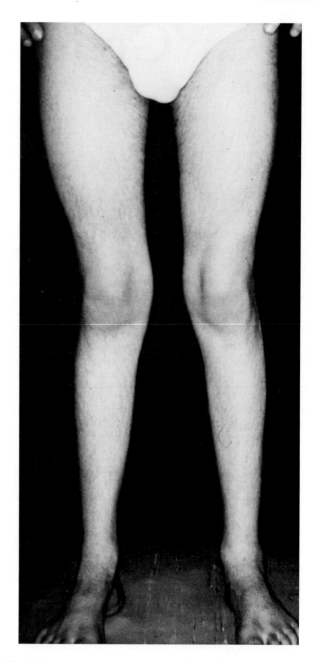

Fig. 16.1
Lower limbs of a male with hereditary motor and sensory neuropathy showing severe muscle wasting below the knees.

QUANTIFICATION – THE NUMERICAL VALUE OF A RISK

Most prospective parents will be familiar to some degree with the concept of risks, but experience indicates that a risk of 1 in 4 can easily be misinterpreted or remembered as 4 to 1, 1 in 40 or even 14%. An equally alarming but entirely understandable misconception is that this risk applies only to every fourth child, so that having had an affected child there should be no problems with the next three children! It is therefore vital to emphasise that the risk applies to **each** child, and that chance does not have a memory. The most often quoted analogy is that of the tossed coin which cannot be expected to remember whether it came down heads or tails at the last throw and cannot therefore be expected to know what it should do at the next throw.

It is also important that genetic counsellors should not be seen exclusively as prophets of doom. Continuing the penny analogy, the good side of the coin should also be emphasised. For example a couple faced with a probability of 1 in 25 that their next baby will have a neural tube defect should be reminded that there are 24 chances out of 25 that their next baby will not be affected.

QUALIFICATION – THE NATURE OF A RISK

Several studies have indicated that the factor which most influences parents when deciding whether or not to have another child is the nature of the long-term burden associated with a risk rather than its precise numerical value. Therefore a 'high' risk of 1 in 2 for a trivial problem such as an extra digit (polydactyly) will deter very few parents. In contrast a 'low' risk of 1 in 25 for a disabling condition such as a neural tube defect can have a very significant deterrent effect. Other factors, such as whether a condition can be successfully treated, whether it is associated with pain and suffering, and whether prenatal diagnosis is available, will all be relevant to the decision making process.

PLACING RISKS IN CONTEXT

Prospective parents seen at a genetic counselling clinic should be provided with information which enables them to put their risks in context so as to be able to decide for themselves whether a risk is 'high' or 'low'. For example, it can be helpful to point out that approximately 1 in 40 of all babies has a congenital malformation or handicapping disorder. Therefore an additional quoted risk of 1 in 50, whilst initially alarming, on reflection can be looked upon as low. As an arbitrary guide, risks of 1 in 10 or greater tend to be regarded as high, 1 in 20 or less as low, and intermediate values as moderate.

DISCUSSING THE OPTIONS

Having established the diagnosis and discussed the risk of occurrence or recurrence, the counsellor is obliged to ensure that the consultands are provided with all the information necessary for them to arrive at their own informed decision. This information will include details of all the choices open to them, which often will involve a lengthy discussion of reproductive options. This can include consideration of alternative approaches to conception such as artificial insemination by donor (AID) and, increasingly, the use of donor ova, as well as a review of the techniques, limitations and risks associated with methods available for prenatal diagnosis (p. 201).

These are issues which should be broached with great care and sensitivity. For some couples the prospect of prenatal diagnosis followed by selective termination of pregnancy is unacceptable, whereas others can see this as the less difficult of two difficult choices, and their only means of ensuring that any children they have will be healthy. Whatever the personal views of the counsellor, the consultands are entitled to knowledge of those prenatal diagnostic procedures which are both technically feasible and legally permissible.

COMMUNICATION AND SUPPORT

Although it should, by now, be self-obvious, the ability to communicate is essential in genetic counselling. Communication is a two-way process. Not only does the counsellor provide information, but he or she also has to be receptive to the fears and aspirations, expressed or unexpressed, of the consultand. Information must be presented in a clear, sympathetic and appropriate manner.

Often an individual or couple will be extremely upset when first made aware of a genetic diagnosis. Everyone involved in genetic counselling needs to remember that the delivery of potentially distressing information cannot be carried out in isolation. Genetic counsellors need to take into account the complex psychological and emotional factors which can influence the counselling dialogue. The setting should be agreeable, private and quiet with ample time for discussion and questions. When possible, technical terms should be avoided or, if used, fully explained. Questions should be answered openly and honestly, and if information is lacking it is certainly not a fault or sign of weakness to admit that this is so. Most couples respect and recognise the truth, and some parents of children whose condition cannot be diagnosed derive a curious pleasure from knowing that their child appears to be unique and has bamboozled the medical profession (unfortunately this is not particularly difficult!).

Despite all these measures, a counselling session can be so intense and intimidating that the amount and accuracy of information retained on follow-up at a later date is very disappointing. For this reason a letter summarising the topics discussed at a counselling session is often sent to the family. In addition, they can be contacted at a later date by a member of the counselling team with an offer of a home visit providing an opportunity for clarification of any confusing issues and for further questions to be answered.

It would be unfair to simply convey information of a distressing nature without providing an offer of continued dialogue and long-term support. Most counselling centres offer long-term informal contact mediated by genetic nurses and counsellors who are familiar with the family and their problems. Support is particularly important for prospective parents at high risk when they embark upon a pregnancy which involves specific prenatal diagnostic investigations. Genetic registers (p. 274) provide a particularly useful means of ensuring that effective contact is maintained with such couples.

GENETIC COUNSELLING – DIRECTIVE OR NON-DIRECTIVE?

It has already been emphasised that genetic counselling involves primarily the provision of information. Its ultimate goal is to ensure that an individual or couple can reach their own decision based on full information about risks and options. There is universal agreement that genetic counselling should be **non-coercive** with no attempt being made to direct the consultand along a particular course of action. In the same spirit the genetic counsellor should also strive to be **non-judgmental**, even if a decision is reached which seems ill-advised or is contrary to the counsellor's own beliefs.

Genetic counsellors are often asked what they themselves would do if placed in the consultand's position. Generally it is unwise to be drawn into expressing an opinion, although it is reasonable to suggest that consideration be given to the consequences of each possible course of action, whilst emphasising that an irreversible reproductive decision should not be made in haste. Ultimately it is the consultands and not the counsellors who have to live with the consequences of their decision.

OUTCOMES IN GENETIC COUNSELLING

It is difficult to devise careful studies of the outcomes in genetic counselling as these can be influenced by numerous variables including socio-economic status, religious and ethnic background, the nature of the risks involved and whether prenatal diagnosis and/or effective treatment are available. Nevertheless, many studies have been undertaken to try to determine the effectiveness of genetic counselling in providing better understanding and its impact on subsequent reproductive decisions.

In general these studies have shown that most patients who have attended a genetic counselling clinic have a reasonable recall of the information given, particularly if this was reinforced by a personal letter or follow-up visit. It is disappointing, however, that as many as 30% of counsellees have difficulty in recalling a precise risk figure, although it is not particularly surprising that many have struggled with the concepts of probability and risk. A recent study has shown that almost one third of women counselled because of a family history of Duchenne muscular dystrophy did not have an accurate recollection of their carrier risk and in many instances these women confused their carrier risk with the risk of having an affected baby.

Studies which have focused on the subsequent reproductive behaviour of couples who have received genetic counselling have shown that approximately 50% have been influenced to some extent. Factors which have been shown to be important are the severity of the disorder, the parents' desire to have children and whether prenatal diagnosis or treatment are available. There is evidence that skilled genetic counselling is particularly appreciated during 'crisis' situations, such as the incidental discovery of a sex chromosome abnormality at amniocentesis. In this situation less than 50% of parents of unborn children with Klinefelter's syndrome (p. 222) or Turner's syndrome (p. 222) opt for termination of pregnancy when counselled objectively using information from prospective studies of children ascertained in an unbiased way through newborn surveys.

SPECIAL PROBLEMS IN GENETIC COUNSELLING

CONSANGUINITY AND INCEST

A *consanguineous* marriage is one between blood relatives who have at least one common ancestor no more remote than a great-great-grandparent. A union between first-degree relatives (brother–sister or parent–child) is referred to as being *incestuous*. Marriage between first-degree relatives is forbidden in almost every culture. Marriage between second-degree relatives (Table 16.3) is also illegal in many countries, although uncle–niece marriage is common in parts of India.

Several extensive studies have shown that among the offspring of consanguineous marriages there is an increase in both morbidity and mortality, with an increased incidence of congenital structural abnormalities and conditions which present later, such as deafness and mental retardation. Fortunately the overall risks are usually relatively small so that most consanguineous couples can be offered reassurance that they do not run a particularly high risk of having a handicapped child.

Based on the study of children born to consanguineous parents it has been estimated that most individuals carry

Table 16.3 Genetic relationship between relatives and risk of abnormality in their offspring

Genetic relationship of partners	Proportion of shared genes	Risk of abnormality in offspring
First degree parent–child brother–sister	1/2	50%
Second degree uncle–niece aunt–nephew double first cousins	1/4	5–10%
Third degree first cousins	1/8	3–5%

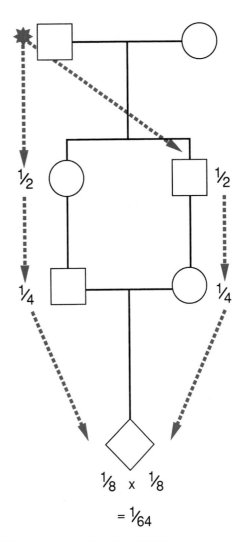

Fig. 16.2
Shows the probability that the first child of first cousins will be homozygous for the deleterious allele (*) carried by the common great-grandfather. A similar risk of 1 in 64 will apply to the deleterious allele belonging to the common great-grandmother giving a total risk of 1 in 32.

between two and six lethal recessive mutations plus one autosomal recessive mutation for a harmful but viable disorder. As most prospective consanguineous parents are concerned primarily with the risk that they will have a handicapped child, it is customary to estimate this risk on the assumption that each common ancestor carried one deleterious recessive mutation.

Therefore, for first cousins, the probability that their first child will be homozygous for their common grand-father's deleterious gene will be 1 in 64 (Fig. 16.2). Similarly, the risk that this child will be homozygous for the common grand-mother's recessive gene will also be 1 in 64. This gives a total probability that the child will be homozygous for one of the grand-parent's deleterious genes of 1 in 32. This risk should be added to the general population risk of 1 in 40 that any baby will have a major congenital abnormality (p. 193), to give an overall risk of approximately 1 in 20 that a child born to first cousin parents will be either malformed or handicapped in some way. Risks due to consanguinity for more distant relatives are much lower.

For consanguineous marriages there is also a slightly increased risk that a child will have a multifactorial dis-order, such as one of the common congenital malfor-mations. In practice this risk is usually very small. In contrast a close family history of an autosomal recessive disorder can convey a relatively high risk that a consanguineous couple will have an affected child. For example, if the sibling of someone with an autosomal recessive disorder marries a first cousin, the risk that their first baby will be affected equals 1 in 24 (p. 257).

Incestuous relationships are associated with a high risk of abnormality in offspring with only half the children of such unions being entirely healthy (Table 16.4).

ADOPTION AND GENETIC DISORDERS

The issue of adoption can arise in several situations relating to genetics. Firstly, parents at high risk of having a child with a serious abnormality often express interest in adopting rather than run the risk of having an affected baby. In genetic terms this is a perfectly reasonable option, although in practice the number of couples wishing to adopt far exceeds the number of babies and children available for adoption.

Table 16.4 Frequencies of the 3 main types of abnormalities in the children of incestuous relationships

Mental retardation	25%
Autosomal recessive disorder	10–15%
Congenital malformation	10%

The physician with a knowledge of genetics can also be called upon to try to determine whether a child who is being placed for adoption will develop a genetic disorder. For the offspring of consanguineous or incestuous matings, risks can be given as outlined previously (Table 16.3). Adoption societies sometimes also wish to place a child with a family history of a particular hereditary disorder. This raises the difficult ethical dilemma of predictive testing in childhood for conditions showing onset in adult life (p. 289). Increasingly it is felt that such testing should not be undertaken unless this will be of direct medical benefit to the child. In practice, even when a child is actually affected by a genetic disorder, suitable adoptive parents can usually be found.

DISPUTED PATERNITY

This presents a difficult problem for which the help of a clinical geneticist is sometimes sought. Until recently paternity could never be proved with absolute certainty, although it could be disproved or excluded in two ways. If a child was found to possess a blood group or other polymorphism not present in either the mother or the putative father, then paternity could be confidently excluded. For example, if the mother and putative father both lacked blood group B, but this was present in the child, then the putative father could be excluded.

Similarly, if a child lacked a marker which the putative father would have had to transmit to all of his children, then once again paternity could be excluded. As an example, a putative father with blood group AB could not have a child with blood group O.

Until recently attempts to confirm paternity were based on analysis of several different polymorphic systems such as blood groups, isoenzymes and HLA haplotypes. The results of these studies can be consistent with paternity but cannot give absolute proof of it. Depending on the number of polymorphic systems analysed and their frequencies in the general population, it is possible to calculate the relative probability that a particular male is the father as compared with any male taken at random from the general population.

The limitations of these approaches have been overcome by the development of genetic fingerprinting using minisatellite repeat sequence probes (p. 56). The pattern of DNA fragments generated by these probes is so highly polymorphic that the restriction map obtained is unique to each individual, with the exception of identical twins (Fig. 16.3). If DNA from the child and the mother

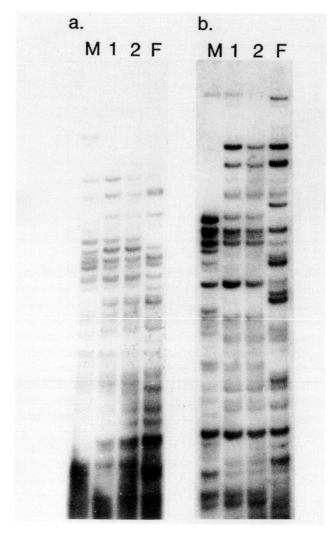

Fig. 16.3
Genetic fingerprint obtained using two mini-satellite probes with DNA from a mother (M), father (F) and their twins (1 and 2). The twins have an identical set of bands and each band in the twins originates from one of the parents. Reproduced with permission from the American Journal of Medical Genetics. (Courtesy of Dr Raymond Dalgleish and Professor Sir Alec Jeffreys, University of Leicester, reproduced from Young I D, Dalgleish R, Mackay E H, MacFadyen U M 1988 Discordant expression of the G syndrome in monozygotic twins. Am J Med Genet 29: 863–869. Reprinted by permission of John Wiley & Sons, Inc.)

is analysed then the bands inherited from the biological father can be analysed and compared with those present in DNA from the putative father(s). If these match, this gives an extremely high mathematical probability that the putative and biological fathers are the same individual.

ELEMENTS

1 Genetic counselling can be defined as a communication process which deals with the risk of developing or transmitting a genetic disorder.

2 The three most important steps in genetic counselling are the establishment of a diagnosis, estimation of a recurrence risk and communication of relevant information in a sympathetic manner.

3 Genetic counselling should be non-directive and the genetic counsellor should be non-judgmental. The goal of genetic counselling is to provide accurate information which enables counsellees to make their own fully informed decisions.

4 Marriage between blood relatives conveys an increased risk of an autosomal recessive disorder in future offspring. The probability that first cousins will have a child with an autosomal recessive disorder is approximately 3%, although this risk can be greater if there is a family history of an autosomal recessive disorder.

5 The most sensitive technique for paternity testing is genetic fingerprinting. Other polymorphic systems can disprove paternity but cannot confirm with a high statistical probability that a particular male is the biological father.

FURTHER READING

Emery A E H, Pullen I (eds) 1984 Psychological aspects of genetic counselling. Academic Press, London
A multiauthor guide to the psychosocial aspects of genetic counselling.

Evers-Kiebooms G, van den Berghe H 1979 Impact of genetic counselling: a review of published follow-up studies. Clinical Genetics 15: 465–474
A review of nine studies undertaken between 1970 and 1979 to assess the impact of genetic counselling. The authors emphasise the difficulties of designing adequate studies.

Frets P G, Niermeijer M F 1990 Reproductive planning after genetic counselling: a perspective from the last decade. Clinical Genetics 38: 295–306
A review of studies undertaken between 1980 and 1989 to determine which factors are most important in influencing reproductive decisions.

Harper P S 1993 Practical genetic counselling, 4th edn. Butterworth Heinemann, Oxford
An extremely useful practical guide to all aspects of genetic counselling.

Jeffreys A J, Brookfield J F Y, Semeonoff R 1985 Positive identification of an immigration test-case using human DNA fingerprints. Nature 317: 818–819
A neat demonstration of the value of genetic fingerprinting in analysing alleged family relationships.

CHAPTER 17

Chromosome disorders

INTRODUCTION

The development of a reliable technique for chromosome analysis in 1956 soon led to the discovery that several previously described conditions were due to an abnormality in chromosome number. Within three years the causes of Down's syndrome (47,XX/XY, +21), Klinefelter's syndrome (47,XXY) and Turner's syndrome (45,X) had been established. Shortly afterwards other autosomal trisomy syndromes were recognised and gradually over the ensuing years many other multiple malformation syndromes were described in which there was loss or gain of chromosome material.

To date well over 100 chromosome syndromes have been reported. Whilst on an individual basis many of these are rare, together they make a major contribution to human morbidity and mortality. Chromosome abnormalities are now known to account for a large proportion of spontaneous pregnancy loss and childhood disability and can also contribute to the genesis of a significant proportion of malignancy in both childhood and adult life as a consequence of acquired somatic chromosome aberrations (p. 167).

In Chapter 3 the basic principles of chromosome structure and function were described. Details of chromosome behaviour during cell division were also provided along with a theoretical account of the range of chromosome abnormalities and how these can both arise and be transmitted in families. In this chapter the medical aspects of chromosome abnormalities will be considered and common disorders due to specific chromosome aberrations will be described.

INCIDENCE OF CHROMOSOME ABNORMALITIES

There is good reason to believe that chromosome abnormalities account for the loss of a very high proportion of all human conceptions. Between 15% and 20% of all recognised pregnancies end in spontaneous miscarriage and many more zygotes and embryos are so abnormal that survival beyond the first few days or weeks of pregnancy is not possible. Given that approximately 50% of all spontaneous miscarriages have a chromosome abnormality (Table 17.1), it is likely that the incidence of chromosome abnormalities at conception is at least as high as 20%.

From conception onwards the incidence of chromosome abnormalities falls rapidly. By birth it has fallen to a level of 0.5–1%, although the total is much higher (5%) if only stillborn infants are considered. Table 17.2 lists the incidence figures for chromosome abnormalities based on newborn surveys. It is notable that amongst the commonly recognised aneuploidy syndromes there is also a high proportion of spontaneous pregnancy loss (Table 17.3). This has been confirmed by comparison of the incidence of conditions such as Down's syndrome at the time of chorion villus sampling (10–11 weeks), amniocentesis (16 weeks) and birth (Fig. 17.1).

Table 17.1 Chromosome abnormalities in spontaneous abortions (percentage figures relate to total of chromosomally abnormal abortuses)

Abnormality		Incidence (%)
Trisomy	13	2
	16	15
	18	3
	21	5
	other	25
Monosomy X		20
Triploidy		15
Tetraploidy		5
Other		10

Table 17.2 Incidence of chromosome abnormalities in the newborn

Abnormality		Incidence per 10 000 births
Autosomal		
Trisomy	13	2
	18	3
	21	15
Sex chromosomes		
Female births		
	45,X	1
	47,XXX	10
Male births		
	47,XXY	10
	47,XYY	10
Other unbalanced including rearrangements		10
Balanced rearrangements		30
Total		≃ 90

Table 17.3 Spontaneous pregnancy loss in commonly recognised aneuploidy syndromes

Disorder	Proportion undergoing spontaneous pregnancy loss (%)
Trisomy 13	95
Trisomy 18	95
Trisomy 21	80
Monosomy X	98

DISORDERS OF THE AUTOSOMES

DOWN'S SYNDROME (TRISOMY 21)

This condition derives its name from Dr Langdon Down who first described it in the Clinical Lecture Reports of the London Hospital in 1866. The chromosomal basis of Down's syndrome was not established until 1959 by Lejeune and his colleagues in Paris.

Table 17.4 Incidence of Down's syndrome in relation to maternal age

Maternal age at delivery in years	Incidence of Down's syndrome
20	1 in 1500
25	1 in 1350
30	1 in 900
35	1 in 400
36	1 in 300
37	1 in 250
38	1 in 200
39	1 in 150
40	1 in 100
41	1 in 85
42	1 in 65
43	1 in 50
44	1 in 40
45	1 in 30

(Adapted from Cuckle HS, Wald NJ, Thompson SG 1987 Estimating a woman's risk of having a pregnancy associated with Down's syndrome using her age and serum alpha-fetoprotein level. Br J Ob Gynae 94: 387–402)

Incidence

The overall incidence at birth is approximately 1 in 650 to 1 in 700. There is a strong association between the incidence of Down's syndrome and advancing maternal age (Table 17.4).

Clinical features

These are summarised in Table 17.5. The most common findings in the newborn period are general lethargy and severe hypotonia. Usually the facial characteristics of upward sloping palpebral fissures, small ears and protruding tongue (Fig. 17.2) prompt rapid suspicion of the diagnosis, although this can be delayed in very small or premature babies. Single palmar creases are found in 50% of Down's syndrome children (Fig. 17.3) in contrast to 2–3% of the general population.

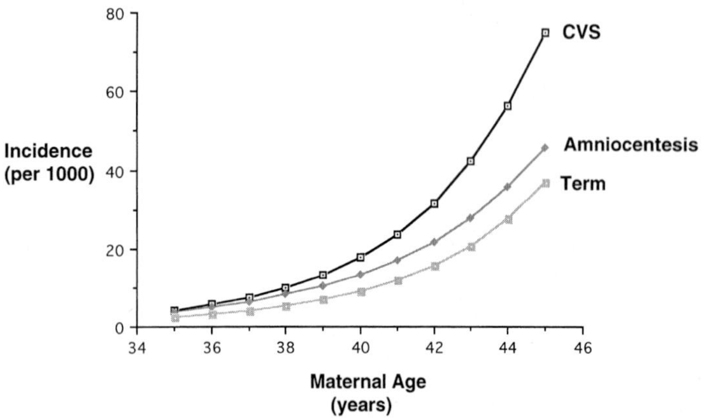

Fig. 17.1
Approximate incidence of trisomy 21 at the time of chorion villus sampling (10–11 weeks), amniocentesis (16 weeks) and delivery (data from Hook E B, Cross P K, Jackson L, Pergament E, Brambati B 1988 Maternal age-specific rates of 47, +21 and other cytogenetic abnormalities diagnosed in the first trimester of pregnancy in chorionic villus biopsy specimens. Am J Hum Genet 42: 797–807 and Cuckle H S, Wald N J, Thompson S G 1987 Estimating a woman's risk of having a pregnancy associated with Down's syndrome using her age and serum alpha-fetoprotein level. Br J Ob Gynae 94: 387–402).

Table 17.5   Common findings in Down's syndrome

Newborn period
Hypotonia, sleepy, excess nuchal skin

Craniofacial
Brachycephaly, epicanthic folds, protruding tongue, small ears, upward sloping palpebral fissures

Limbs
Single palmar crease, small middle phalanx of 5th finger, wide gap between first and second toes

Cardiac
Atrial and ventricular septal defect, common atrioventricular canal, patent ductus arteriosus

Other
Anal atresia, duodenal atresia, short stature, strabismus

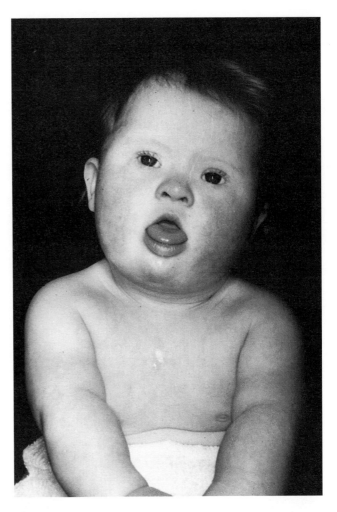

Fig. 17.2
A child with Down's syndrome.

Natural history

Affected children show a broad range of intellectual ability with IQ scores ranging from 25 to 75. Social skills are relatively well advanced and most children with Down's syndrome are happy and very affectionate. Adult height is usually around 150 cm, and in the absence of a severe cardiac anomaly, which leads to early death in 15–20% of cases, life expectancy is good. Most affected adults develop Alzheimer's disease in later life, possibly because of a gene dosage effect as the locus for the amyloid precursor protein gene is on chromosome 21. This gene has been implicated in some familial cases of Alzheimer's disease (p. 109).

Chromosome findings

These are listed in Table 17.6. In cases due to trisomy 21, the additional chromosome is maternal in origin in over

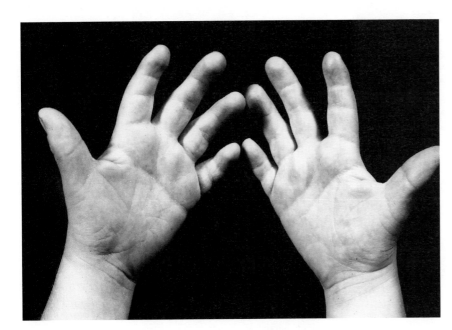

Fig. 17.3
The hands of an adult with Down's syndrome. Note the single palmar crease in the left hand plus bilateral short curved fifth fingers (clinodactyly).

Table 17.6 Chromosome abnormalities in Down's syndrome

Trisomy	95%
Translocation	3%
Mosaicism	2%

90% of cases, and DNA studies have shown that this usually arises as a result of non-disjunction in maternal meiosis I. Robertsonian translocations (p. 38) account for approximately 3% of all cases, in roughly one third of which one of the parents is found to be a balanced carrier. Children with mosaicism are usually less severely affected than in the full syndrome.

Recurrence risk

For straightforward trisomy 21 the recurrence risk is related to maternal age and is usually of the order of 1/200 to 1/100. In translocation cases similar figures apply if neither parent is a carrier. In familial translocation cases, the recurrence risks vary from around 1–3% for male carriers up to 10–15% for female carriers, with the exception of very rare carriers of a 21q21q translocation for whom the recurrence risk is 100% (p. 39).

Prenatal diagnosis can be offered based on analysis of chorionic villi or cultured amniotic cells. Prenatal screening programmes are being introduced based on the so-called triple test of maternal serum at 16 weeks gestation (p. 270).

TRISOMY 13 (PATAU'S SYNDROME) AND TRISOMY 18 (EDWARDS' SYNDROME)

These very severe conditions were first described in 1960 and share many features in common (Figs. 17.4 and 17.5). They show incidence figures of 1 in 5000 and 1 in

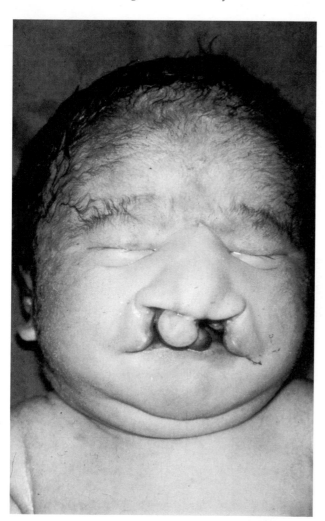

Fig. 17.4
Facial view of a child with trisomy 13 showing severe bilateral cleft lip and palate.

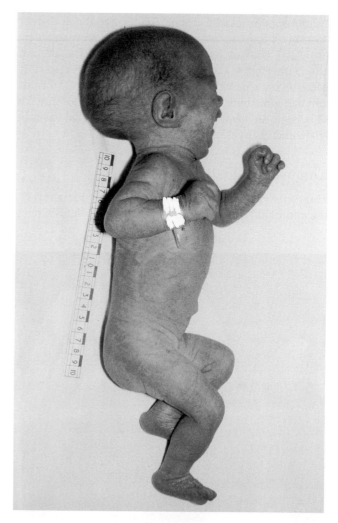

Fig. 17.5
A baby with trisomy 18. Note the prominent occiput and tightly clenched hands.

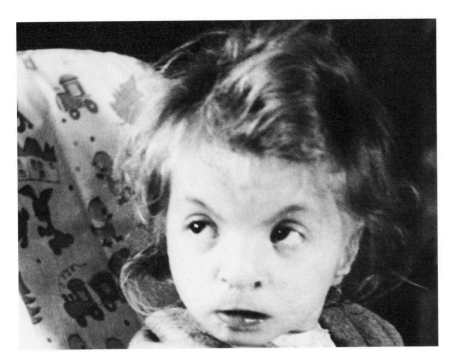

Fig. 17.6
Facial view of a 3-year-old child with the Wolf–Hirschhorn syndrome.

3000 respectively and convey a universally gloomy prognosis with most affected infants dying during the first few weeks of life. In the unusual event of long-term survival there is severe mental retardation. Cardiac abnormalities occur in at least 90% of all cases.

Usually chromosome analysis reveals straightforward trisomy. Both of these disorders show an association between increasing incidence and advanced maternal age, and in both the additional chromosome is usually of maternal origin (Table 3.3). Approximately 10% of cases are due to mosaicism or unbalanced rearrangements, particularly Robertsonian translocations in cases of Patau's syndrome.

CHROMOSOME DELETION SYNDROMES

Microscopically visible deletions of the terminal portions of chromosomes 4 and 5 cause the Wolf–Hirschhorn (4p) (Fig. 17.6) and cri-du-chat (5p-) (Fig. 17.7) syndromes respectively. In both conditions there is severe mental retardation, often in association with failure to thrive. The cri-du-chat syndrome derives its name from the characteristic cat-like cry of affected neonates which results from underdevelopment of the larynx. Both conditions are very rare with estimated incidences of approximately 1 in 50 000 births.

MICRODELETION SYNDROMES

Through a combination of high resolution prometaphase banding (p. 27) and FISH (p. 28), an increasing number

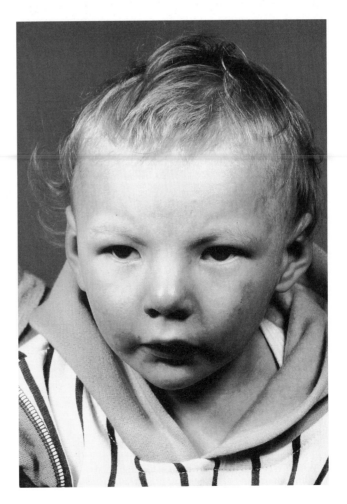

Fig. 17.7
Facial view of a 2-year-old boy with the cri-du-chat syndrome.

of syndromes are being shown to be due to submicroscopic or 'micro-' deletions. Some of these microdeletions involve loss of only a few genes at closely adjacent loci, resulting in what are known as *contiguous gene syndromes*. For example, several boys with Duchenne muscular dystrophy (DMD) have been described who also have other X-linked disorders such as retinitis pigmentosa and glycerol kinase deficiency (p. 62). The loci for these disorders are known to be very close to the DMD locus on Xp21.

In several other microdeletion syndromes it is likely that more than a few loci are involved. Examples are given in Table 17.7. Even when considered together these conditions are rare, but improvements in molecular technology are likely to show that microdeletion syndromes are more common than is realised. Many malformations and syndromes have been described for which there is as yet no recognised cause (p. 204).

Lessons from microdeletion syndromes

Retinoblastoma

The first clue to the location of the gene for retinoblastoma was provided by the discovery that approximately 5% of children presenting with retinoblastoma had other abnormalities including mental retardation. In several of these children a constitutional interstitial deletion of a region of the long arm of chromosome 13 was identified. The smallest region of overlap was 13q14 which was subsequently found to be the position of the disease locus for the autosomal dominant form of retinoblastoma leading to the cloning of the gene and identification of the gene product (pp. 170, 172).

Wilms' tumour

A proportion of children who develop the rare kidney neoplasm known as Wilms' tumour (or hypernephroma)

Table 17.7   Microdeletion syndromes

Syndrome	Chromosome
Williams	7
Langer–Giedion	8
WAGR*	11
Angelman	15
Prader–Willi	15
Rubinstein Taybi	16
Miller–Dieker	17
Smith–Magennis	17
DiGeorge	22
Shprintzen	22

*WAGR = Wilms' tumour, Aniridia, Genitourinary malformations and Retardation of growth and development

also have Aniridia (an absent iris), Genital abnormalities and Retardation of growth and development, or what is called the WAGR syndrome. Chromosomal analysis of these children has shown a number to have an interstitial deletion of a particular region of the short arm of one of their chromosomes 11. Molecular studies have led to the isolation of what is known as the Wilms' tumour 1 (WT1) gene. Mutations in the WT1 gene have been shown in dysmorphic syndromes with birth defects which are developmentally related (p. 69).

The familial cases of autosomal dominant Wilms' tumour have been shown not to be linked to this locus and the ocurrence of Wilms' tumour in children with the rare overgrowth syndrome known as the Beckwith–Wiedemann syndrome has been associated with a deletion and imprinting (p. 88) of a separate locus on the short arm of chromosome 11.

These types of observation illustrate that the discovery of a microdeletion in a child with multiple problems which include a single gene disorder or embryonal tumour can provide a vital clue as to the position of the relevant disease locus.

The Angelman and Prader–Willi syndromes

Recent developments in these disorders have generated particular interest. Children with Angelman's syndrome (Fig. 6.19) show inappropriate laughter with convulsions, poor coordination (ataxia) and mental retardation. Children with the Prader–Willi syndrome (Fig. 6.18) are extremely floppy (hypotonic) in early infancy and develop quite marked obesity with mild to moderate mental retardation in later years. A large proportion of children with both of these disorders show a microdeletion involving the proximal part of the long arm of chromosome 15q (15q11–12).

It is now known that if the deletion occurs de novo on the paternally inherited number 15 chromosome the child will have the Prader–Willi syndrome. In contrast, a deletion occurring at the same region on the maternally inherited number 15 chromosome causes Angelman's syndrome. Non-deletion cases also exist and are often due to uniparental disomy (p. 88), with both number 15 chromosomes being paternal in origin in Angelman's syndrome and maternal in origin in the Prader–Willi syndrome. Thus loss of a critical region from a paternal number 15 chromosome causes the Prader–Willi syndrome. Loss of an identical or similar region from a maternally inherited number 15 chromosome causes Angelman's syndrome. These observations are fundamental to the concept of imprinting (p. 88) and illustrate how new technological developments coupled with clinical observation have helped shed new light on underlying genetic mechanisms.

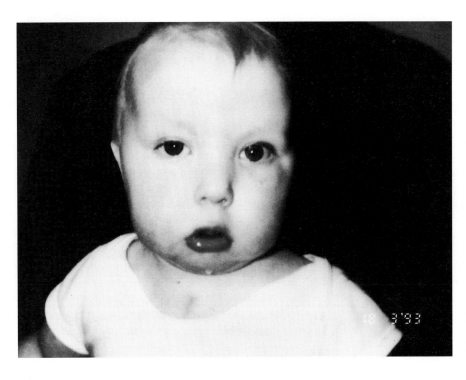

Fig. 17.8
Facial view of a child with the DiGeorge syndrome with a deletion of the chromosome 22 (courtesy of Dr. J. Goodship, University of Newcastle).

DiGeorge and Shprintzen syndromes

The DiGeorge syndrome is a rare disorder, usually occurring sporadically, characterised by a high incidence of cardiac malformations, particularly those involving the cardiac outflow tract, along with thymic and para-thyroid hypoplasia (p. 155). Molecular and FISH studies show that most if not all cases are due to a microdeletion involving the proximal long arm of chromosome 22 (22q11–2) (Fig.17.8).

Curiously, it has emerged that most children and adults with what was thought to be a separate syndrome known as Shprintzen's syndrome show a similar defect. This condition is characterised by similar cardiac malformations, cleft palate and a recognisable facial appearance. Several families showing apparent autosomal dominant inheritance have been described. It seems likely that in Shprintzen's syndrome there is a smaller deletion which does not convey such a high risk for a life-threatening malformation.

Perhaps even more curiously it has emerged that some families showing apparent clustering of isolated cardiac malformations, previously believed to be multifactorial in origin, are also segregating a 22q microdeletion. This is one of the first demonstrations of an important dominantly inherited susceptibility locus in an apparent multifactorial disorder, and if similar discoveries are forthcoming and confirmed in other so-called multifactorial conditions, this will necessitate a major reappraisal of contemporary understanding of the principles of multifactorial inheritance (p. 110).

TRIPLOIDY

Triploidy (69,XXX, 69,XXY, 69,XYY) is a relatively common finding in material cultured from spontaneous abortions, but is seen only rarely in a live-born infant. Such a child will almost always show severe intra-uterine growth retardation with relative preservation of head growth at the expense of a small thin trunk. Syndactyly involving the third and fourth fingers and/or the second and third toes is a common finding. Survival beyond the early neonatal period is extremely unusual.

Most diagnosed cases of triploidy are due to dispermy or to fertilisation by a diploid sperm. Such a double paternal contribution can lead to partial hydatidiform changes in the placenta (p. 70).

Hypomelanosis of Ito

Several children with mosaicism for diploidy/triploidy have been identified. These can demonstrate the clinical picture seen in full triploidy but in a milder form. An alternative presentation is as the condition known as hypomelanosis of Ito. In this curious disorder the skin shows alternating patterns of normally pigmented and depigmented streaks which correspond to the embryological developmental lines of the skin known as Blaschko's lines (Plate 14). Most children with hypomelanosis of Ito are moderately retarded and have convulsions which can be particularly difficult to treat. There is increasing evidence that this clinical picture represents a non-specific embryological response to cell or tissue mosaicism. A similar skin pattern of distribution of changes in the pigmentation of the skin is sometimes seen in women with one of the rare X-linked dominant disorders (p. 84) with skin involvement, such as incontinentia pigmenti. Such women can be considered as being mosaic, as some cells will be expressing the normal gene whereas others will be expressing only the mutant gene.

DISORDERS OF THE SEX CHROMOSOMES

KLINEFELTER'S SYNDROME (47,XXY)

First described in 1942, this relatively common condition with an incidence equal to 1 in 1000 male live births, was shown to be due to the presence of an additional X chromosome in 1959.

Clinical features

In childhood the diagnosis can be suspected in a male presenting with clumsiness or mild learning difficulties, particularly in relation to verbal skills. The overall verbal IQ is reduced by 10–20 points below that of unaffected siblings and controls. Adults with Klinefelter's syndrome tend to be slightly taller than average with long lower limbs. Approximately 30% of adult males with Klinefelter's syndrome show moderately severe gynaecomastia (enlargement of the breasts) and all are infertile with small soft testes. There is an increased incidence of leg ulcers, osteoporosis and carcinoma of the breast in adult life. Treatment with testosterone from puberty onwards is beneficial for the development of secondary sexual characteristics and the long-term prevention of osteoporosis.

Chromosome findings

Usually the karyotype shows an additional X chromosome. Molecular studies have shown that there is a roughly equal chance that this will have been inherited from the mother or from the father. The maternally derived cases are associated with advancing maternal age. A small proportion of cases show mosaicism, i.e. 46,XY/47,XXY. Rarely, a male with more than two X chromosomes can be encountered e.g. 48,XXXY or 49,XXXXY. These individuals are usually quite severely retarded.

TURNER'S SYNDROME (45,X)

This condition was first described in 1938. The absence of a Barr body, consistent with the presence of only one X chromosome, was noted in 1954 and cytogenetic confirmation of this was achieved in 1959. Whilst common at conception and in spontaneous abortions (Table 17.1), the incidence in live-born female infants is low, with estimates ranging from 1 in 5000 to 1 in 10 000.

Clinical features

Presentation can be at any time from pregnancy to adult life. Increasingly Turner's syndrome is being detected during the second trimester as a result of routine detailed ultrasound scanning which can reveal either generalised oedema (hydrops) or swelling localised to the neck (nuchal cyst or thickened nuchal pad) (Fig. 22.2). At birth some babies with Turner's syndrome look entirely normal. Others show the residue of intra-uterine oedema with puffy hands and feet, hyperconvex or concave nails and neck webbing (Fig. 17.9). Other findings can include a low posterior hair-line, increased carrying angles at the elbows, short fourth metacarpals, widely spaced nipples

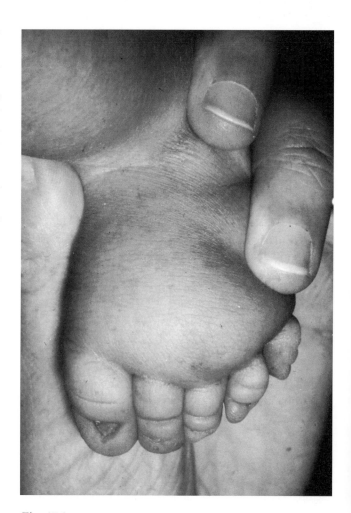

Fig. 17.9
The foot of an infant with Turner's syndrome showing oedema and small convex nails.

and, clinically important, coarctation of the aorta in 15% of females with Turner's syndrome.

Intelligence in Turner's syndrome is normal. The two main medical problems are short stature and ovarian failure. The short stature becomes apparent by mid-childhood, and without growth hormone treatment the average adult height is 145 cm. Ovarian failure commences during the second half of intra-uterine life and almost invariably leads to primary amenorrhoea and infertility. Oestrogen replacement therapy should be initiated at adolescence for development of secondary sexual characteristics and long-term prevention of osteoporosis. In vitro fertilisation using donor eggs offers the prospect of pregnancy for women with Turner's syndrome.

Chromosome findings

These are summarised in Table 17.8. The most common finding is 45,X, sometimes erroneously referred to as 45,XO. It has been found that Turner's syndrome arises in 75% of instances through a sex chromosome (X or Y) being lost in paternal meiosis.

XXX FEMALES

Birth surveys have shown that approximately 0.1% of all females have a 47,XXX karyotype. These women usually have no physical abnormalities but can show a mild reduction of between 10 and 20 points in intellectual skills. This is rarely sufficiently severe to require special education. Studies have shown that the additional X chromosome is of maternal origin in 90% of cases and usually arises from an error in meiosis I. Women with a 47,XXX karyotype usually show normal fertility and have children with normal karyotypes.

As with males who have more than two X chromosomes women with more than three X chromosomes show a high incidence of mental retardation, the severity of which is directly related to the number of X chromosomes present.

Table 17.8 Chromosome findings in Turner's syndrome

Karyotype	Frequency (%)
Monosomy X– 45,X	55
Mosaicism – e.g. 45,X/46,XX	10
Isochromosome – 46,X,i (Xq)	20
Ring – 46,X,r(X)	5
Deletion – 46,X,del (Xp)	5
Other	5

XYY MALES

This condition shows an incidence of 1 in 1000 in males in newborn surveys but is found in 2–3% of males who are in institutions because of mental retardation or antisocial criminal behaviour. However, it is important to stress that most 47,XYY men are neither mentally retarded nor in possession of a criminal record, although they can show emotional immaturity and impulsive behaviour.

Physical appearance is normal and stature is usually above average. Intelligence is mildly impaired with an overall IQ score of 10 to 20 points below a control sample. The additional Y chromosome must arise as a result of non-disjunction in paternal meiosis II or as a postzygotic event.

THE FRAGILE X SYNDROME

This condition, which could equally well be classified as a single gene disorder rather than a chromosome abnormality, has the unique distinction of being both the most common inherited cause of mental retardation and the first disorder in which a dynamic mutation was identified (p. 17). First described in 1969, the significance of the chromosome abnormality was not really fully realised until 1977 and it was only in 1991 that the underlying molecular defect was discovered.

Incidence

The Fragile X syndrome affects approximately 1 in 2000 males and accounts for 4–8% of all males with mental retardation.

Clinical features

Older boys and adult males usually have a recognisable facial appearance with high forehead, large ears, long face and prominent jaw (Fig. 17.10). After puberty most affected males have large testes (macro-orchidism). There can also be evidence of connective tissue weakness with hyperextensible joints, stretch marks on the skin (striae) and mitral valve prolapse. The mental retardation is moderate to severe and many affected boys show autistic features and/or hyperactive behaviour. Speech tends to be halting and repetitive. Female carriers can show some of the facial features and approximately 50% of women with the full mutation are mildly or moderately mentally retarded.

The Fragile X chromosome

The Fragile X syndrome takes its name from the appearance of the X chromosome which shows a *fragile site*

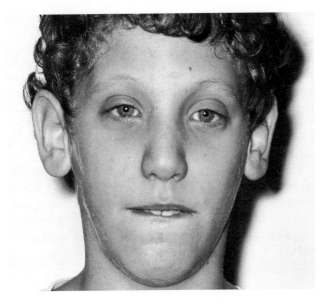

Fig. 17.10
Facial view of a boy with the Fragile X syndrome.

close to the telomere at the end of the long arm at Xq27.3 (Fig. 17.11). A fragile site is a non-staining gap usually involving both chromatids at a point at which the chromosome is liable to break. In this condition, detection of the fragile site involves the use of special culture techniques such as folate or thymidine depletion, which can result in the fragile site being detectable in up to 50% of cells from affected males. Demonstration of the fragile site in female carriers is much less commonly detected and cytogenetic studies alone are not a reliable means of carrier detection, in that although a positive result con-

firms carrier status, the absence of the fragile site does not exclude a woman being a carrier.

The molecular defect

It is now known that the Fragile X mutation consists of an increase in the size of a region in the 5'-untranslated region of the Fragile X mental retardation (FMR-1) gene. This region contains a long CGG trinucleotide repeat sequence. In the DNA of a normal person there are between 10 and 50 copies of this triplet repeat and these are inherited in a stable fashion. However, a small increase to between 50 and 200 renders this repeat sequence unstable, a condition in which it is referred to as a *premutation*.

A man who carries a premutation is known as a 'normal transmitting male'. All of his daughters will inherit the premutation and will be of normal intelligence, but when these daughters come to have sons there is a significant risk that the premutation will undergo a further increase in size during meiosis. If this reaches a critical size of greater than 200 CGG triplets it becomes a full mutation. This process is sometimes referred to as *expansion* of the triplet repeat sequence.

The full mutation is unstable not only during female meiosis but also in somatic mitotic divisions. Consequently in an affected male, gel electrophoresis shows a 'smear' of DNA consisting of many different sized alleles rather than a single band (Fig. 17.12). At the molecular level this appears to suppress transcription of the FMR-1 gene and possibly of adjacent genes also, and this in turn is thought to be responsible for the clinical features seen in males, and to a lesser extent in females who have a large expansion (Table 17.9).

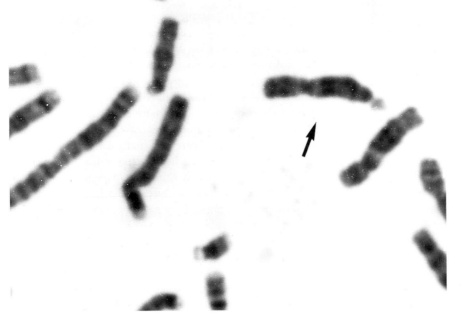

Fig. 17.11
Metaphase spread with arrow indicating an X chromosome with a fragile site at Xq27 (courtesy of Mr A. Monk, Cytogenetics Unit, City Hospital, Nottingham).

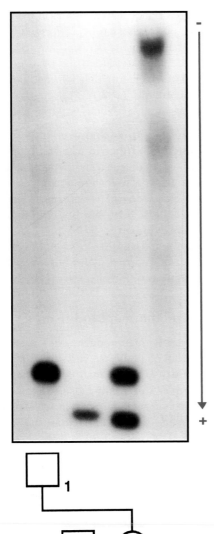

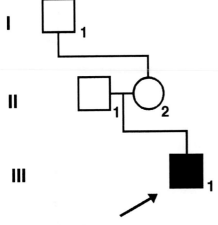

Table 17.9 The Fragile X syndrome–genotype–phenotype correlations

Number of triplet repeats (Normal range = 10–50)	Fragile site detectable	Intelligence
Males		
50–200 (premutation)	No	Normal (normal transmitting male)
200–2000 (full mutation)	Yes (in up to 50% of cells)	Moderate to severe mental retardation
Females		
50–200 (premutation)	No	Normal
200–2000 (full mutation)	Yes (usually < 10% of cells)	50% – normal, 50% mild mental retardation

Their male offspring are at risk of inheriting either the premutation or a full mutation. This risk is probably dependent on the size of the premutation in the mother, but unfortunately it is not possible at present to give such a woman an accurate indication of the risk that she will have either an affected son or a mildly affected 'carrier' daughter.

For women who carry a full mutation there is a risk of 1 in 2 that each of their sons will be affected with the full syndrome and that each of their daughters will inherit the full mutation. Since approximately 50% of females with the full mutation are mildly retarded, the risk that a female carrier of a full mutation will have a retarded daughter equals 1/2 x 1/2, i.e. 1/4. Prenatal diagnosis can be offered based on analysis of DNA from chorionic villi, but in the event of a female fetus with a full mutation accurate prediction of phenotype cannot be made.

The Fragile X syndrome is a condition for which screening could be offered, either amongst selected high risk groups such as mentally retarded males, or on a widespread general population basis. Such programmes will have to surmount major ethical, financial and logistical concerns if they are to achieve widespread acceptance (p. 269).

Fig. 17.12
Southern blot of DNA from a family showing expansion of the CTG triplet repeat being passed from a normal transmitting male through his obligate carrier daughter to her son with Fragile X mental retardation (courtesy Dr. G. Taylor, Regional DNA Laboratory, St. James's Hospital, Leeds).

Genetic counselling and the Fragile X syndrome

This common cause of mental retardation presents a major counselling problem. Inheritance can be regarded as modified or atypical X-linked. All the daughters of a normal transmitting male will carry the premutation.

DISORDERS OF SEXUAL DIFFERENTIATION

The process of sexual differentiation has been described in Chapter 5 (p. 71). Given the complexity of the sequential cascade of events which take place between 6 and 14 weeks of embryonic life it is not surprising that errors can occur. Many of these errors can lead to sexual ambiguity or to discordance between the chromosomal sex and the appearance of the external genitalia or what are also sometimes known as various forms of *intersex* (Table 17.10).

Table 17.10 Disorders of sexual differentiation and development

Seminiferous tubule dysgenesis (Klinefelter's syndrome)
47,XXY, 48,XXXY, 48,XXYY, 49,XXXXY

Ovarian dysgenesis (Turner's syndrome)
45,X, 46,X,i (Xq), 46,X, del (Xp), 46,X,r (X)

True hermaphroditism
46,XX with Y derived sequences
46,XX/46,XY chimaerism

Male pseudohermaphroditism
Androgen insensitivity
complete – testicular feminisation
incomplete – Reifenstein syndrome
Inborn errors of testosterone biosynthesis
e.g. 5α reductase deficiency
45,X/46,XY mosaicism

Female pseudohermaphroditism
Congenital adrenal hyperplasia
Maternal androgen ingestion or androgen secreting tumour

True hermaphroditism

In this extremely rare condition an individual has both testicular and ovarian tissue often in association with ambiguous genitalia. When an exploratory operation is carried out in these patients an ovary can be found on one side and a testis on the other. Alternatively, there can be a mixture of ovarian and testicular tissue in the gonad which is known as an ovotestis. Most patients with true hermaphroditism have a 46,XX karyotype and in many of these individuals the paternally derived X chromosome carries Y chromosome specific DNA sequences as a result of crossing-over between the X and Y chromosomes during meiosis I in spermatogenesis.

A small proportion of patients with true hermaphroditism are found to be chimaeras with both 46,XX and 46,XY cell lines, a situation analogous to freemartins in cattle (p. 43).

Male pseudohermaphroditism

In pseudohermaphroditism there is gonadal tissue of only one sex. The external genitalia can be ambiguous or of the sex opposite to that of the chromosomes. Thus in male pseudohermaphroditism there is a 46,XY karyotype with ambiguous or female genitalia.

The most widely recognised cause of male pseudohermaphroditism is androgen insensitivity (p. 134). In this condition, which is also known as the testicular feminisation syndrome, the karyotype is normal male and the external phenotype is essentially that of a normal female. Internally the vagina ends blindly and the uterus and fallopian tubes are absent. Testes are located in the abdomen or in the inguinal canal where they can be mistaken for inguinal herniae. This condition is caused by the absence of androgen receptors in the target organs, so that although testosterone is formed normally, its peripheral masculinising effects are blocked. These androgen receptors are coded for by a gene on the X chromosome in which both deletions and point mutations have been identified.

Other causes of male pseudohermaphroditism include:

1. An incomplete form of androgen insensitivity known as Reifenstein syndrome in which affected males have hypospadias, small testes and gynaecomastia
2. Enzyme defects in testosterone synthesis such as 5α-reductase deficiency in which the external genitalia are ambiguous at birth but undergo masculinisation (virilisation) at puberty
3. Chromosome mosaicism (45,X/46,XY) in which most individuals are normal males but a small proportion have ambiguous or female external genitalia.

Female pseudohermaphroditism

In female pseudohermaphroditism, the karyotype is female and the external genitalia are virilised so that they either resemble those of a normal male or are ambiguous.

By far the most important cause of female pseudohermaphroditism is congenital adrenal hyperplasia (p. 134). This can be caused by several different enzyme defects in the adrenal cortex, all of which show autosomal recessive inheritance. Reduced cortisol production leads to an increase in ACTH secretion which in turn causes hyperplasia of the adrenal glands. In the most common form of congenital adrenal hyperplasia due to 21-hydroxylase deficiency, hormone synthesis switches from the manufacture of cortisol and aldosterone to the androgen pathway (Fig. 10.4) leading to striking virilisation of a female fetus (Fig. 10.5). The lack of cortisol and aldosterone will usually lead to rapid collapse shortly after birth which can prove fatal unless appropriate hormone and electrolyte supplementation are initiated.

The gene for 21-hydroxylase deficiency is located on chromosome 6 where it is tightly linked to the histocompatability complex.

Rarer causes of female pseudohermaphroditism include an androgen secreting tumour and maternal androgen ingestion during pregnancy.

CHROMOSOME BREAKAGE SYNDROMES

Constitutional and acquired chromosome abnormalities which predispose to malignancy are considered in Chapter 13. In addition to these conditions, it is recognised that a small number of hereditary disorders are

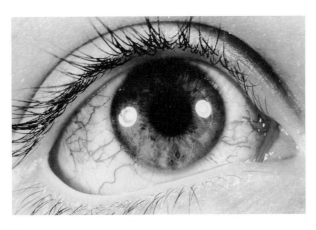

Fig. 17.13
Ocular telangiectasia in a child with ataxia telangiectasia.

characterised by an excess of chromosome breaks and gaps as well as an increased susceptibility to neoplasia.

ATAXIA TELANGIECTASIA

This is an autosomal recessive disorder which presents in early childhood with ataxia, oculocutaneous telangiectasia (Fig. 17.13) and susceptibility to sinus and pulmonary infection (p. 156). There is a 10–20% risk of developing leukaemia or lymphoma. Cells from patients show an increase in spontaneous chromosome abnormalities, such as chromatid gaps and breaks, which are enhanced by radiation.

BLOOM'S SYNDROME

Children with this autosomal recessive disorder are small with a light-sensitive facial rash and reduced immunoglobulin levels (IgA and IgM). The risk of lymphoreticular malignancy is approximately 20%. The basic defect lies in deficiency of DNA ligase 1 which repairs DNA damage caused by agents such as ultraviolet (UV) light. Cultured cells show an increased frequency of chromosome breaks particularly if they are exposed in vitro to UV light.

FANCONI'S ANAEMIA

This autosomal recessive disorder is associated with upper limb abnormalities involving the radius and thumb, increased pigmentation and a failure of the bone marrow leading to deficiency of all types of blood cells, i.e. pancytopenia. There is also an increased risk of neoplasia, particularly leukaemia, lymphoma and hepatic carcinoma. Multiple chromosomal breaks are observed

in cultured cells (Fig. 17.14) and the basic defect lies in the repair of DNA strand cross-links.

XERODERMA PIGMENTOSA

This exists in several different forms, all of which show autosomal recessive inheritance. Patients present with a light-sensitive pigmented rash and usually die of skin malignancy in sun-exposed areas before the age of 20 years. Cells cultured from these patients only show chromosome abnormalities after exposure to ultraviolet (UV) light. This disorder is due to defects in the excision and repair of UV-induced DNA damage.

CHROMOSOME BREAKAGE AND SISTER CHROMATID EXCHANGE

Strong evidence of increased *chromosome instability* is provided by the demonstration of an increased number of *sister chromatid exchanges* (SCEs) in cultured cells. An SCE is an exchange (crossing-over) of genetic material between the two chromatids of a chromosome in mitosis, in contrast to recombination in meiosis I which is between homologous chromatids. SCEs can be demonstrated by differences in the uptake of certain stains by the two chromatids of each metaphase chromosome after two rounds of cell division in the presence of the thymidine analogue 5-bromodeoxyuridine (BudR), which becomes incorporated in the newly synthesised DNA (Fig. 17.15). There are normally about ten SCEs per cell but the number is greatly increased in cells from patients with Bloom's syndrome and xeroderma pigmentosa. In the latter condition this is only apparent after the cells have been exposed to UV light.

At present it is not clear how SCEs relate to the increase in chromosome breakage observed in these two disorders, but it is thought that the explanation could involve one of the steps in DNA replication. It is also of interest that the number of SCEs in normal cells is increased on exposure to certain carcinogens and chemical mutagens. For this reason the frequency of SCEs in cells in culture has been suggested as a useful in vitro test of the carcinogenicity and mutagenicity of chemical compounds (p. 20).

INDICATIONS FOR CHROMOSOME ANALYSIS

It should be apparent from the contents of this chapter that chromosome abnormalities can present in many different ways. Consequently it is appropriate to consider the indications for chromosome analysis under a number of different headings (Table 17.11).

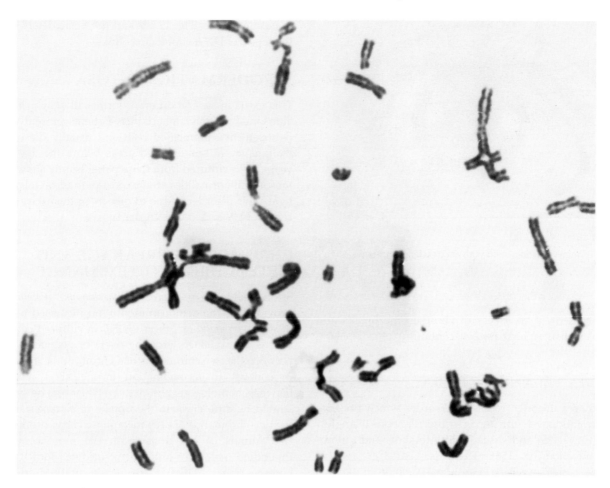

Fig. 17.14
Multiple chromosome breaks and gaps in a metaphase spread prepared from a child with Fanconi's anaemia.

MULTIPLE CONGENITAL ABNORMALITIES

Every child with multiple congenital abnormalities should have chromosome studies undertaken. This is important for several reasons:

1. Establishing a chromosomal diagnosis will prevent further potentially unpleasant investigations being undertaken.

Table 17.11 Indications for chromosome analysis

Multiple congenital abnormalities
Unexplained mental retardation
Sexual ambiguity or abnormality in sexual development
Infertility
Recurrent miscarriage
Unexplained stillbirth
Malignancy and chromosome breakage syndromes

2. Information about the prognosis can be provided along with details of the relevant lay society and an offer of contact with other families.
3. A chromosomal diagnosis should facilitate the provision of accurate information about the recurrence risk for future siblings.

Although it can be very distressing for parents to be told that their child has a chromosome abnormality, often, in fact, they will be relieved that an explanation for the problems in the child has been found.

UNEXPLAINED MENTAL RETARDATION

Chromosome abnormalities cause at least one third of the 50% of mental retardation which is attributable to genetic factors. Whilst most children with a chromosome abnormality will have other features such as growth retardation and physical anomalies, this is not always so. If the Fragile X syndrome is a possibility it is important that the cytogenetics laboratory is informed so that the

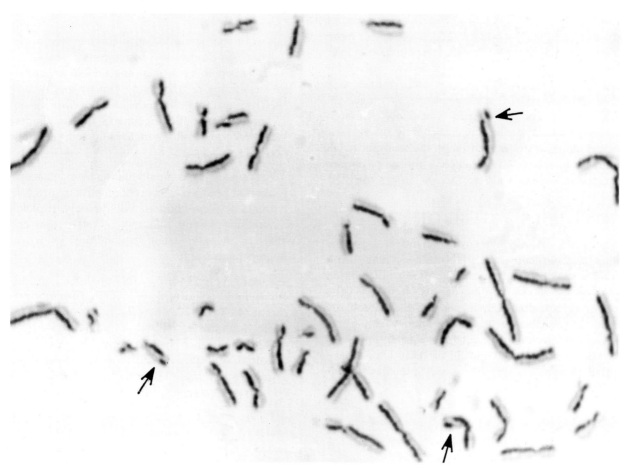

Fig. 17.15
Chromosome preparation showing sister chromatid exchanges (arrowed).

correct culture conditions are used (p. 224). It is also important that DNA analysis of a sample be carried out, especially if the diagnosis of the Fragile X syndrome is being considered in a female with unexplained mental retardation.

SEXUAL AMBIGUITY OR ABNORMALITY IN SEXUAL DEVELOPMENT

The birth of a child with ambiguous genitalia should be regarded as a medical emergency not only for the emotional consideration of easing the inevitable parental anxiety, but also because of the importance of ruling out the potentially life-threatening diagnosis of salt-losing congenital adrenal hyperplasia (p. 134). A chromosome analysis should be amongst the first investigations undertaken.

Disorders of sexual development presenting in later life with problems such as delayed puberty, primary amenorrhoea or male gynaecomastia are also strong indications for chromosome analysis as a first line inves-

tigation. This can provide a diagnosis such as Turner's syndrome (45,X) or Klinefelter's syndrome (47,XXY). Alternatively a normal karyotype will stimulate a search for other possible explanations such as an endocrine abnormality.

INFERTILITY

Unexplained involuntary infertility should prompt a request for chromosome studies, particularly if investigations reveal evidence of azoospermia in the male partner. At least 5% of such men are found to have Klinefelter's syndrome. More rarely a complex chromosome rearrangement such as a translocation can cause such severe mechanical disruption in meiosis that complete failure of gametogenesis ensues.

RECURRENT MISCARRIAGE

At least 15% of all recognised pregnancies end in spontaneous miscarriage and in 50% of cases this is because of a chromosome abnormality (pp. 193, 215).

Unfortunately, some couples experience recurrent pregnancy loss, which is usually defined as three or more spontaneous miscarriages. Often no explanation is ever found and many such couples go on to have successful pregnancies. However, in 3–6% of such couples, one partner is found to carry a chromosome rearrangement which predisposes to severe imbalance through malsegregation at meiosis. Consequently it is now standard practice to offer chromosome analysis to all couples who have experienced three or more spontaneous pregnancy losses.

UNEXPLAINED STILLBIRTH

The presence of growth retardation and at least one congenital abnormality in a stillbirth or neonatal death would be an indication for chromosome studies based on analysis of blood or skin collected from the baby before or as soon after death as possible. Skin fibroblasts continue to be viable for several days after death. Chromosome abnormalities account for 5% of all stillbirths and neonatal deaths and not all of these babies have multiple abnormalities which would immediately suggest a chromosomal cause.

MALIGNANCY AND CHROMOSOME BREAKAGE SYNDROMES

As already mentioned (p. 226), certain types of leukaemia (p. 167), lymphomas and solid tumours, such as retinoblastoma (p. 170) and Wilms' tumour (p. 220), are associated with specific chromosomal abnormalities which can be of both diagnostic and prognostic value. Clinical features suggestive of a chromosome breakage syndrome, such as a combination of photosensitivity and short stature, should also lead to appropriate chromosome fragility studies such as sister chromatid exchange.

ELEMENTS

1 Chromosome abnormalities account for 50% of all spontaneous miscarriages and are present in 0.5–1.0% of all newborn infants.

2 Down's syndrome is the most common autosomal syndrome and shows a strong association between increasing incidence and advancing maternal age. 95% of all cases are caused by trisomy 21. Chromosome studies are necessary in all cases so that the rare but important cases due to unbalanced familial Robertsonian translocations can be identified.

3 An increasing number of chromosome microdeletion syndromes are being recognised. These have helped in gene mapping and in enhancing understanding of underlying genetic mechanisms such as imprinting. Microdeletions of chromosome 15 are found in both Angelman's and the Prader–Willi syndrome and are maternally and paternally derived respectively.

4 Triploidy is a common finding in spontaneously aborted products of conception but rare in a liveborn infant. Some children with diploidy/triploidy mosaicism present with mental retardation and areas of depigmentation, a condition known as hypomelanosis of Ito.

5 Sex chromosome abnormalities include Klinefelter's syndrome (47,XXY), Turner's syndrome (45,X), the XYY syndrome (47,XYY) and the triple X syndrome (47,XXX). In all of these conditions intelligence is either normal or only mildly impaired. Infertility is the rule in Klinefelter's and Turner's syndromes. Fertility is normal in the XYY and the triple X syndrome.

6 The Fragile X syndrome is the most common inherited cause of mental retardation. It is associated with a fragile site on the long arm of the X chromosome and shows modified X-linked inheritance. Affected males are moderately to severely mentally retarded; carrier females can show mild mental retardation. At the molecular level there is expansion of a CGG triplet repeat which can exist as a premutation or a full mutation.

7 Disorders of sexual differentiation include true and pseudohermaphroditism. True hermaphroditism is extremely rare. Male pseudohermaphroditism is caused most commonly by androgen insensitivity, an X-linked disorder involving formation of androgen receptors. The most common cause of female pseudohermaphroditism is congenital adrenal hyperplasia, in which virilised infants can collapse with adrenal failure during the first week of life.

8 The chromosome breakage syndromes are rare autosomal recessive disorders characterised by increased chromosome breakage in cultured cells and an increased tendency to neoplasia such as leukaemia and lymphoma.

FURTHER READING

De Grouchy J, Turleau C 1984 Clinical atlas of human chromosomes, 2nd edn. John Wiley, Chichester
A lavishly illustrated atlas of known chromosomal syndromes.

Gardner R J M, Sutherland G R 1989 Chromosome abnormalities and genetic counselling. Oxford University Press, Oxford
A useful and practical guide for genetic counselling in families with a chromosome disorder.

Hagerman R J, Silverman A C (eds) 1991 Fragile X syndrome. Diagnosis, treatment and research. Johns Hopkins University Press, Baltimore
A detailed account of the clinical and genetic aspects of the Fragile X syndrome.

Jacobs P A, Browne C, Gregson N, Joyce C, White H 1992 Estimates of the frequency of chromosome abnormalities detectable in unselected newborns using moderate levels of banding. Journal of Medical Genetics 29: 103–108
A review of the results of over 14 000 prenatal diagnoses with estimates of the incidence of chromosome abnormalities in term infants.

CHAPTER 18 | Single gene disorders

Reference has been made to the dramatic explosion in knowledge which has led to the recognition of over 6000 single gene traits and disorders (p. 6). The majority of these are individually extremely rare. Some, however, are relatively common and their management in families has presented a major challenge for clinical genetics and closely allied specialties.

In this chapter, rather than produce a brief description of a long list of disorders, three of the most common disorders, each of which shows a different mode of single gene inheritance, will be considered in detail. Neurofibromatosis, cystic fibrosis and Duchenne muscular dystrophy are all serious conditions with implications for the extended family. In each of these disorders there has been rapid progress over the last decade. The cloning of the relevant genes, identification of their mutational basis and isolation of their protein products serve to illustrate important genetic principles and represent major scientific achievements.

NEUROFIBROMATOSIS

References to the clinical features of neurofibromatosis first appeared in the eighteenth century medical literature, but historically the disorder is most commonly associated with the name von Recklinghausen, a German pathologist, who coined the term 'neurofibroma' in 1882. He also noted that the condition could feature brown pigmented spots and be familial. Neurofibromatosis is now known to be one of the most common autosomal dominant disorders in humans and gained public notoriety when it was suggested that Joseph Merrick, the 'Elephant Man', was probably affected. Recent review of Merrick's photographs and skeleton indicates, however, that he probably had a different and much rarer condition known as the Proteus syndrome.

INCIDENCE

There are two main types of neurofibromatosis known as NF1 and NF2. NF1 is by far the more common with an incidence at birth of approximately 1 in 3000 in all ethnic communities. NF2 has an incidence of approximately 1 in 35 000 and a prevalence of 1 in 200 000.

CLINICAL FEATURES

The two major features of NF1 are small pigmented skin lesions, known as café-au-lait spots, and small soft fleshy lumps known as neurofibromata (Fig. 18.1). Café-au-lait spots first appear in early childhood and can be very numerous. A minimum of six café-au-lait spots at least 1 cm in diameter are required to support the diagnosis. Neurofibromata are benign tumours which arise most commonly in the skin. They usually appear in late childhood and adult life and increase in number with age.

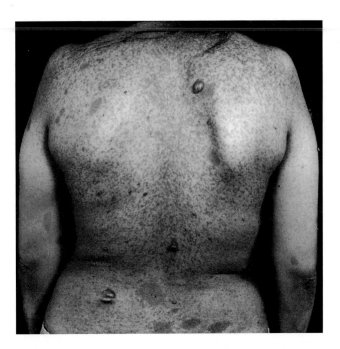

Fig. 18.1
A patient with neurofibromatosis 1 showing truncal freckling, café-au-lait spots and multiple neurofibromata.

Table 18.1 Clinical features of NF1 (Incidence figures derived from Huson and Hughes, 1994)

Feature	%
Minor	
Café-au-lait spots	100
Dermal neurofibromata	100
Axillary freckling	67
Lisch nodules	~90
Macrocephaly	45
Short stature	32
Major	
Large 'plexiform' neurofibromata	30
Mental retardation	~5
Epilepsy	4
CNS tumours	4
Other malignancy	3
Scoliosis	10

Other features and complications of NF1 can be considered under the headings of minor and major (Table 18.1). Minor features, which are useful diagnostically but are of no clinical importance, include axillary freckling and Lisch nodules, which are small harmless pigmented hamartomata of the iris (Plate 15). Many individuals with NF1 enjoy a normal healthy life and are not inconvenienced by their condition. Unfortunately the major complications, such as epilepsy, CNS tumours, and mental retardation, affect between 3% and 5% of patients, so that NF1 can cause serious morbidity and mortality.

In NF2 both café-au-lait spots and neurofibromata can occur, but these are much less common than in NF1. The most characteristic feature of NF2 is the development in early adult life of tumours involving the eighth cranial nerves. These used to be called acoustic neuromas and are now known as vestibular Schwannomas.

MODE OF INHERITANCE

NF1 shows autosomal dominant inheritance with almost complete penetrance by the age of 5 years, when almost all heterozygotes will have developed six or more café-au-lait spots. Expression is very variable and affected members of the same family can show striking differences in disease severity. The features in affected identical twins are usually very similar so that variable *expressivity* in family members, who must have the same mutation, is probably due to the effects of modifying genes at other loci.

Between 30% and 50% of cases of NF1 are due to new mutations, so that the mutation rate is approximately 1 per 10 000 gametes. This is one of the highest known mutation rates in humans.

Reports of multiple affected children born to un-

affected healthy parents probably represent examples of parental gonadal mosaicism (p. 87). Somatic mosaicism can manifest with features of NF1 limited to a particular part of the body. This is referred to as segmental NF (p. 87).

MAPPING OF THE NF1 LOCUS

The development of polymorphic DNA markers for each autosome, coupled with the willingness of large numbers of families to participate in research, led to an international collaborative effort to map the NF1 gene. Linkage to markers on chromosome 17 was established in 1987. Refined mapping using multipoint linkage analysis pinpointed the NF1 locus to the long arm of chromosome 17 closely adjacent to the centromere.

ISOLATING THE NF1 GENE

Shortly after the successful mapping of the NF1 locus to chromosome 17q, two patients with NF1 and balanced translocations involving breakpoints at 17q11.2 were identified. Somatic cell hybrids containing only the translocation chromosomes were constructed from both patients. A cosmid clone was identified which contained both translocation breakpoints and the region in which the NF1 gene could be located was narrowed down to a 600 kb genomic fragment.

A search for transcripts from this region yielded four genes, one of which was shown to be the NF1 gene. This occupies 300 kb of genomic DNA, contains approximately 50 exons and produces an RNA transcript of between 11 and 13 kb. Curiously, the other three genes identified in this region are located within a single intron of the NF1 gene and are transcribed in the opposite direction from the complementary strand (p. 14).

Several different types of mutations have been identified in the NF1 gene. These include deletions, point mutations and an insertion consisting of an Alu repetitive sequence (p. 11). No relationship between genotype and phenotype has been recognised, nor has any explanation emerged for the very high mutation rate.

NF1 GENE PRODUCT AND FUNCTION

Sequence analysis of the NF1 gene shows that it encodes a protein with structural homology to the GTPase-activating protein (GAP), which has an important role in regulating mitogenic signalling (p. 169). This is consistent with the NF1 gene being involved in cell turn-over. Loss of heterozygosity (p. 171) for chromosome 17 markers has been noted in several NF1 tumours. These observations suggest that the NF1 gene functions as a tumour suppressor gene (p. 170) with tumour development resulting from loss of both alleles. In tumours it is the normal 'wild-type' allele which is lost.

The gene product has been identified and is known as *neurofibromin*. It contains 2818 amino acids and has a molecular weight of 250 kDa. In cells it is located in the cytoplasmic microtubules which are believed to play a crucial role in mitosis and cell division. Neurofibromin consists of several apparently functional domains and the function of only the GAP domain is understood.

Other genes, including p53 on the short arm of chromosome 17 (p. 172), are involved in tumour development and progression in NF1. It is also known that the NF1 gene is implicated in the development of sporadic tumours not associated with neurofibromatosis, including carcinoma of the colon, neuroblastoma and malignant melanoma. These observations indicate that the NF1 gene plays an important role in cell growth and differentiation.

NF2

The NF2 locus has been mapped to chromosome 22q by linkage analysis. This chromosome was predicted to be the location of the NF2 locus because tumours from patients with NF2 had been found to show loss of chromosome 22 alleles. Similar allele loss has been demonstrated in sporadic Schwannomas and meningiomas. The NF2 gene was cloned in 1993 and is believed to encode a structural membrane associated protein which acts as a tumour suppressor gene in a manner, as yet, uncharacterised.

CLINICAL APPLICATIONS AND FUTURE PROSPECTS

Mapping of the NF1 gene has provided a means of offering presymptomatic and prenatal diagnosis to families which are informative for closely linked polymorphic markers. Intragenic markers have also been identified. Direct mutation analysis enables specific presymptomatic and prenatal diagnosis and potentially is very valuable in families containing only a single affected individual. However, each family appears to have a unique mutation so that detection of specific mutations within the NF1 gene is proving to be very laborious with currently available mutation detection systems. In practice direct mutation analysis is usually not available at present.

NF1 is a disorder for which effective gene therapy is not likely to be forthcoming in the near future. In the short term it is more probable that the major impact of the cloning of the NF1 and NF2 genes will be in the achievement of better understanding of the processes involved in the development of the nervous system and in tumour formation.

CYSTIC FIBROSIS

Cystic fibrosis (CF) was first recognised as a discrete entity in 1936 and is the most common autosomal recessive disorder in Caucasian populations. It used to be known as *mucoviscidosis* because of the thick mucus secretions which accumulate leading to blockage of the airways and secondary infection. Recurrent pulmonary infection is the most common cause of death. Antibiotics and physiotherapy have been very effective in increasing the average life expectancy of a child with CF from less than 5 years in 1955 to at least 25 years at present. Nevertheless, CF is still a significant cause of chronic ill-health and mortality in childhood and early adult life.

INCIDENCE

In Western European Caucasians the incidence of CF varies from 1 in 2000 to 1 in 3000, with slightly lower figures applying in Eastern and Southern Europe. CF is much rarer in other populations with incidences of 1 in 9000 in Hawaiian Orientals and 1 in 17 000 in North Americans of Afro-Caribbean origin.

CLINICAL FEATURES

The organs most commonly affected in persons affected with CF are the lungs and the pancreas. Chronic lung disease due to recurrent infection occurs in almost 100% of patients. This usually leads to irreversible lung damage which imposes a strain on the function of the right ventricle so that cardiac failure can also occur. This is known as *cor pulmonale*. In the event of this complication the only hope for long-term survival rests in a successful heart–lung transplant.

In 85% of persons with CF, pancreatic function is impaired with reduced enzyme secretion due to blockage of the pancreatic ducts by inspissated secretions. This causes malabsorption with an increase in the fat content of the stools. This complication of CF can be treated very successfully with oral supplements of pancreatic enzymes.

Other systems can also be involved (Table 18.2). 10% of children with CF present in the newborn period with obstruction of the small bowel due to thickened meconium, a condition known as *meconium ileus*. A similar proportion of patients with CF develop liver damage which can lead to cirrhosis. Almost all males with CF are sterile because of absence or atrophy of the vas deferens.

CONFIRMATION OF THE DIAGNOSIS

When the diagnosis of CF is suspected it can be confirmed by finding elevated levels of sodium and chloride in the sweat. A screening test for newborn infants has

Table 18.2 Possible clinical problems in cystic fibrosis

Chronic pulmonary infection
Cor pulmonale
Malabsorption
Meconium ileus
Rectal prolapse
Nasal polyps
Cirrhosis
Diabetes mellitus
Male subfertility

been developed based on measurement of the level of immunoreactive trypsin (IRT) in blood (p. 273). This is thought to be elevated because of blockage of the pancreatic ducts.

MAPPING OF THE CF LOCUS

In the absence of either clinical or cytogenetic clues about the position of the CF locus, the only option for mapping the gene was to use linkage analysis based on study of the segregation of the disease with polymorphic markers. In this way the locus was mapped to chromosome 7q31 in 1985. Shortly afterwards two polymorphic DNA marker loci known as MET and D7S8 were shown to be closely linked to and flanking the CF locus.

The region involved was scrutinised for the presence of HTF or CpG islands, which are known to be present close to the 5' end of most genes (p. 61). This resulted in the identification of several DNA markers, such as D7S23, which are very tightly linked to the CF locus with recombination frequencies of less than 1%. These loci were found to be in linkage disequilibrium with the CF locus (p. 101). The CF mutation was found to be associated with one particular haplotype in 84% of cases, in contrast to the 16% incidence of the same haploytpe in non-CF chromosomes. This discovery of linkage disequilibrium was consistent with the concept of a single original mutation being responsible for a large proportion of all CF alleles.

ISOLATION OF THE CF GENE

Using linkage analysis the position of the CF locus was narrowed down to a stretch of approximately 500 kilobases of DNA. A search was undertaken for genes in this 500 kb segment looking specifically for genes expressed in tissues involved in CF such as lung and pancreas and also for conserved genes present in other species, i.e. a zoo blot (p. 61).

By screening cDNA libraries from tissues affected in CF and looking for cross-species hybridisation, the CF gene was isolated in 1989 by two groups of scientists working in Canada and the USA. It was found to span a genomic region of approximately 250 000 base pairs and to contain 27 exons.

Mutations in the CF gene

The first mutation to be identified was a deletion of three adjacent base pairs at the 508th codon in the gene which results in the loss of a phenylalanine residue. This mutation is known as ΔF508 (Δ for deletion and F for phenylalanine) and it has been shown to account for approximately 70% of all mutations in the CF gene with the highest incidence of 88% being in Denmark (Table 18.3). The ΔF508 mutation can be demonstrated relatively easily by PCR (p. 48) using primers which flank the 508th codon (Fig. 18.2).

Over 300 other mutations in the CF gene have now been identified. These include missense and nonsense point mutations as well as deletions and insertions which result in an alteration of the reading frame. These mutations are all individually rare and usually account for less than 2–3% of all CF mutations in any one population. This striking heterogeneity at the molecular level has important implications for the planning of community screening programmes (p. 274).

Studies of the correlation between phenotype and genotype have shown that the ΔF508 mutation is strongly associated with pancreatic insufficiency, whereas several other mutations do not usually affect pancreatic function. The influence of genotype on the course of lung disease is less clear. While ΔF508 homozygotes tend to have more severe lung disease than compound heterozygotes with one ΔF508 mutation, studies have shown wide variation in lung involvement. In addition, affected

Table 18.3 Contribution of ΔF508 mutation to all CF mutations (data from European Working Group on CF Genetics (EWGCFG) Gradient of distribution in Europe of the major CF mutation and of its associated haplotype. Human Genetics 1990; 85: 436–441, and Worldwide survey of the ΔF508 mutation – report from the cystic fibrosis genetic analysis consortium. American Journal of Human Genetics 1990; 47: 354–359)

Country	%
Denmark	88
Netherlands	79
United Kingdom	78
Ireland	75
France	75
Germany	65
Poland	55
Italy	50
Turkey	30

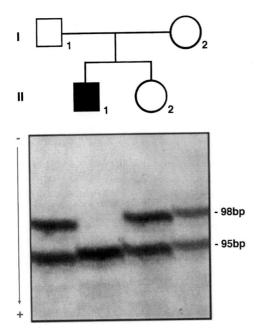

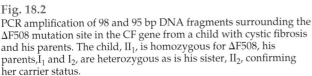

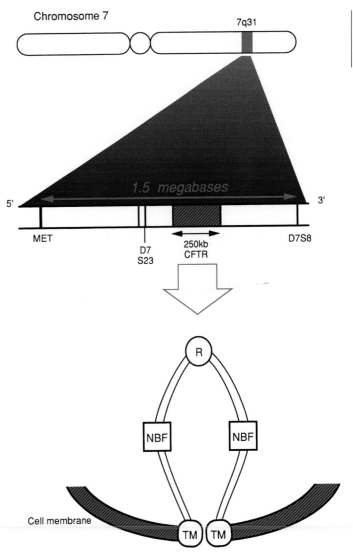

Fig. 18.2
PCR amplification of 98 and 95 bp DNA fragments surrounding the ΔF508 mutation site in the CF gene from a child with cystic fibrosis and his parents. The child, II₁, is homozygous for ΔF508, his parents, I₁ and I₂, are heterozygous as is his sister, II₂, confirming her carrier status.

siblings, who will have the same mutations, often show quite different degrees of lung disease.

A few patients with CF who are very mildly affected have been reported. These individuals usually have one or two of the rarer mutations in the CF gene and clinical involvement can be limited to absence of the vas deferens. This is now a recognised cause of males presenting with infertility due to azoospermia.

THE GENE PRODUCT – CYSTIC FIBROSIS TRANSMEMBRANE CONDUCTANCE REGULATOR (CFTR) PROTEIN

The product of the cystic fibrosis gene is known as the *cystic fibrosis transmembrane conductance regulator* or *CFTR* protein and by convention the gene is now known as the CFTR gene. The CFTR protein has a molecular weight of 168 kDa and is 1480 amino acids in length. It consists of two transmembrane (TM) domains which anchor it to the cell membrane, two nucleotide binding folds (NBF) which bind ATP, and a regulatory (R) domain, which has several phosphorylation sites (Fig. 18.3).

Initially it was thought that the CFTR protein acted as a chloride channel, but it is now believed to be responsible for both chloride transport and mucin secretion. The protein can be either open or closed. Opening is achieved by phosphorylation of the R domain followed by binding of ATP to the NBF domains, thereby

Fig. 18.3
Schematic representation of the cystic fibrosis locus, gene and protein product (R = regulatory domain, NBF = nucleotide binding fold, TM = transmembrane domain) (adapted from Estivill X 1993 Molecular genetics of cystic fibrosis. The New Genetics. In: Baillière's Clinical Paediatrics, Young I D (ed) Vol 1, no. 2. Baillière Tindall, London, pp 395–413).

allowing chloride to move through the cell membrane and mucin to be secreted.

The ΔF508 mutation prevents normal maturation of the CFTR protein and causes failure of its normal localisation to the cell membrane. This is probably because absence of the phenylalanine residue results in abnormal folding of the protein's extremely complex three-dimensional structure.

CLINICAL APPLICATIONS

These are limited, to some extent, by the extensive heterogeneity seen at the molecular level.

Prenatal diagnosis

Parents of an affected child can almost always be offered prenatal diagnosis, either by direct mutational analysis of DNA from chorionic villi, or by linkage analysis if one or both of the mutations in the affected child cannot be identified. Several highly polymorphic intragenic micro-satellites have been identified with which almost all nuclear families can be made informative.

Carrier detection in families – cascade screening

Knowledge of one or both of the mutations in an affected child permits the offer of carrier detection to close family relatives such as siblings, uncles, aunts and cousins. It is now standard practice to offer what is known as *cascade screening* to all families in which there is or has been an affected child.

Carrier detection in a community – population screening

In countries such as the United Kingdom, in which the ΔF508 mutation accounts for a high proportion of all CF mutations, screening programmes have been proposed for the general population (p. 274). Enthusiasm for these programmes amongst both the general population and health care professionals will almost certainly increase when it becomes possible to detect relatively easily all CF mutations. At present a relatively simple multiplex PCR technique allows approximately 85% of all mutations to be detected.

FUTURE PROSPECTS

The discovery of the CFTR gene and its protein product has opened up new opportunities for therapy. New pharmaceutical approaches are being tried using aerosols containing drugs such as ATP and amiloride, the latter of which blocks sodium uptake. Recognition that DNA released from bacteria contributes to the increased mucus viscosity has prompted the use of genetically engineered DNase with beneficial effect. Gene transfer studies have been carried out using transfected adenoviruses and CFTR cDNA liposome complexes administered to CF transgenic mice produced by homologous recombination. Initial results have been encouraging and similar pilot studies of gene therapy in humans (p. 278) are underway in small groups of CF patients. It is probable that, because of the relative ease of access to the crucial target organ, i.e. the lung, cystic fibrosis will be amongst the first disorders for which gene therapy will be successfully developed.

DUCHENNE MUSCULAR DYSTROPHY

Duchenne muscular dystrophy (DMD) shows X-linked recessive inheritance. It is characterised by progressive muscle weakness and a relentless downhill course. At present there is no effective treatment. The name for this disorder is derived from the French neurologist Guillaume Duchenne who described a case in 1861, although an English physician, Edward Meryon, had presented details of eight affected boys in three families 10 years previously. A similar but milder condition known as Becker muscular dystrophy (BMD) is now known to be due to mutations in the same gene.

INCIDENCE

DMD affects approximately 1 in 3500 males with no evidence of significant ethnic variation. BMD has a much lower incidence of around 1 in 20 000, so that the combined incidence of these two disorders is close to 1 in 3000 male births.

CLINICAL FEATURES

Most boys with DMD present between the ages of 3 and 5 years with muscle weakness manifesting as an awkward gait, inability to run and difficulty in climbing stairs. A particular problem is encountered in rising from the floor which the child can achieve only by pushing on or 'climbing up' his legs and thighs, or what is known as Gowers' sign. Over 50% of boys with DMD, however, are delayed in learning to walk, with an average age of walking of 18 months in contrast to 13 months in unaffected boys. Delay in walking in a male child should suggest the possibility of DMD.

As the disease progresses a lumbar lordosis becomes more pronounced and weakness of proximal pelvic muscles increases leading to increasing difficulty with walking. Most affected boys have to use a wheelchair by the age of 11 years. Subsequent deterioration leads to increasing disability and weakness with joint contractures, respiratory failure and occasionally cardiac failure with death occurring at a mean age of 18 years.

Examination of boys with DMD shows striking weakness and wasting of proximal muscles in all limbs. During the early stages, the calf muscles show an apparent increase in size, which is in fact due to replacement of muscle fibres by fat and connective tissue. This is referred to as *pseudohypertrophy* and DMD is sometimes also known as pseudohypertrophic muscular dystrophy.

Approximately one third of boys with DMD show mild to moderate intellectual impairment and the overall IQ distribution curve is shifted to the left with a mean value of 83. This suggests that intellectual impairment is a pleiotropic effect of mutations in the DMD gene.

In BMD the clinical features are similar but the disease process runs a much less aggressive course. The mean age of onset is 11 years and many patients remain ambulant until well into adult life. Overall life expectancy is only slightly reduced.

CONFIRMATION OF THE DIAGNOSIS

Until molecular methods were available, the diagnosis of DMD was confirmed by assay of creatine kinase activity in serum and histological examination of a muscle biopsy. Creatine kinase activity in serum is grossly elevated to levels of between 1000 and 20 000 i.u. as opposed to an upper limit of 200 in unaffected boys. This enzyme catalyses the formation of creatine and ATP in muscle, and is released by muscle which is damaged, either because of a dystrophic process as in DMD, or by physical agents such as anoxia or trauma. The muscle biopsy from boys with DMD shows an increased variation in fibre size in the early stages followed by necrosis with replacement of muscle fibres by fat and connective tissue.

MODE OF INHERITANCE

William Gowers, a London physician, whose name is associated with the Gowers' manoeuvre or sign, recognised over 100 years ago that DMD was limited almost exclusively to males and was inherited through the female line. X-linked recessive inheritance is now well established. Affected males rarely, if ever, have children of their own. Therefore, as genetic fitness equals zero, the mutation rate equals the incidence in affected males divided by three (p. 95), which approximates to 1 in 10 000.

CARRIER FEMALES

Clinically most carrier females are perfectly healthy. Approximately 5% have some degree of muscle weakness which can vary from mild to the full-blown clinical syndrome. In most of these women the muscle weakness is due to skewed X chromosome inactivation (p. 74). In a small proportion there is an alternative explanation such as Turner's syndrome or an X-autosome translocation (p. 84).

Many different approaches have been used to try to detect carriers. These have included careful clinical examination, muscle biopsy, electromyography and muscle ultrasonography. Until molecular techniques became available, the only test of proven value was assay of creatine kinase activity in serum. This is elevated in two-thirds of obligate carriers, and when plotted on a logarithmic scale, overlapping normal distribution curves for creatine kinase activity in obligate carriers and controls are obtained. Statistical analysis of such overlapping curves allows a conditional probability to be determined for carrier status for any particular value of creatine kinase activity (Fig. 19.1). This conditional probability or odds ratio can be included in a Bayesian calculation to determine the overall probability that a particular female relative is a carrier (p. 258).

MAPPING OF THE DMD LOCUS

The first clue to the site of the DMD locus was provided by reports of several affected females who had a balanced X-autosome translocation with the X chromosome breakpoint located at Xp21. In such women, cells in which the derivative translocation chromosome containing the X centromere with attached autosome segment is inactivated will have a biological disadvantage, as the inactivation process will extend to the autosomal segment of the chromosome with deleterious effects (Fig. 18.4). Consequently cells in which this chromosome is active are much more likely to survive so that X-inactivation appears to be skewed (p. 74). In reality the process of inactivation is not skewed; it is the pattern of cell survival thereafter which is altered.

The net result in such females of this process is that the derivative X-autosome is active in most if not all of their cells. If the breakpoint has damaged an important gene, then the woman will be affected by the disease resulting from damage to that gene.

This probable location of the DMD gene at Xp21 was soon confirmed by the identification of boys with visible microdeletions involving Xp21 (pp. 62, 219) and by linkage analysis using polymorphic DNA markers closely adjacent to Xp21. These provided the first molecular means of attempting carrier detection and offered reasonably accurate prenatal diagnosis. Previously, women thought to be at high risk of having an affected son had to choose between having no children, taking their chances, or aborting all male pregnancies.

INTRAGENIC DNA MARKERS AND CLONING THE GENE

In 1985 two series of intragenic probes within the DMD gene labelled XJ and pERT were identified. The XJ probes were isolated by cloning of the X-autosome breakpoint in an affected female (p. 84); hence 'J' stood for junction. The pERT probes were obtained by hybridising DNA from a DMD boy with a cyto-genetically visible microdeletion involving Xp21 with DNA from a male with a 49,XXXXY karyotype (p. 62). Portions of DNA from this male which did not hybridise with DNA from the DMD boy were likely to be derived from the region of the DMD locus.

Using subclones from the XJ and pERT probes, a

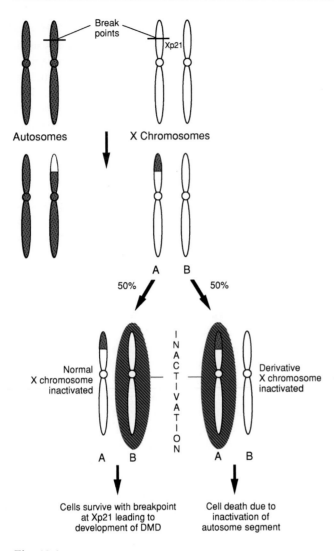

Fig. 18.4
Shows the generation of an X-autosome translocation with breakpoint at Xp21 in a female and how this results in the development of DMD.

search was made for sequences which were conserved across the animal kingdom, i.e. a zoo blot (p. 61). Such sequences were soon identified in muscle cDNA libraries and were found to consist of exons from the actual DMD gene. The full transcribed sequence was isolated in 1987 in a series of overlapping cDNA clones.

THE DMD GENE

The DMD gene is the largest yet identified in man and consists of 2300 kilobases (kb) of genomic DNA, of which only 14 kb are transcribed into mRNA. The gene contains at least 79 exons and is expressed in muscle and, perhaps not surprisingly given the reports of learning difficulties in a small but significant proportion of boys with DMD, in neurones of the cerebral cortex. The large size of this gene probably accounts for the high

mutation rate and explains why several women with X-autosome translocations were identified.

Mutations in the DMD gene

Using Southern blot analysis with cDNA probes it has been shown that approximately two-thirds of DMD boys have a deletion of part of the DMD gene. These deletions differ in their size and in their position, and probably arise due to either unequal crossing over or to breakage and fusion within a small inversion loop during maternal meiosis (Fig. 18.5). A small number of boys with the other outcome of this event, i.e. duplications, have also been described.

Two deletion 'hot spots' in the DMD gene have been identified. One involves the first 20 exons of the gene and the other is located in the centre of the gene around exons 45–53. The size of the deletion in the DMD gene does not correlate with disease severity or with the presence of mental retardation in an affected boy. However, deletions causing DMD usually disturb the translational reading frame (pp. 15, 17). In contrast, deletions seen in males with BMD in general do not alter the reading frame so that the amino acid sequence downstream of the deletion is usually normal. Interestingly, one of the deletion breakpoint 'hotspots' in intron 7 has been found to contain a cluster of transposon-like repetitive DNA sequences which could lead to misalignment in meiosis and a subsequent cross-over could lead to deletion or duplication products. This could also provide an explanation for the frequent occurrence of mutations in this region of the dystrophin gene.

Mutations in the remaining one-third of boys who do not have a deletion can sometimes be identified by systematic analysis of PCR amplified genomic or cDNA. This can be laborious to carry out because of the large size of the gene. Mutations identified in the DMD gene to date include stop codons, frameshift mutations, altered splicing signals and promoter mutations. Provisional data suggest that these mutations in the DMD gene are more likely to arise during spermatogenesis than oogenesis, presumably because of the greater number of opportunities for a copy error to occur in mitosis in the male than in the female (p. 32).

The gene product – dystrophin

The DMD gene produces a 427 kDa protein known as *dystrophin*. This contains at least three distinct functional domains consisting of a C terminal domain, a central repeat spectrin-like rod domain and an N terminal domain with sequence homology to the actin-binding domain of actinin.

Dystrophin is located at or close to the muscle

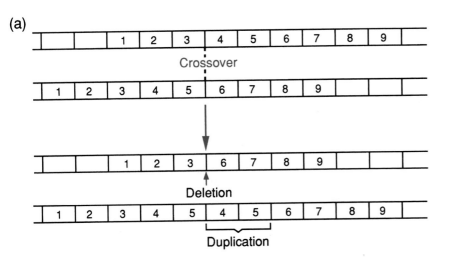

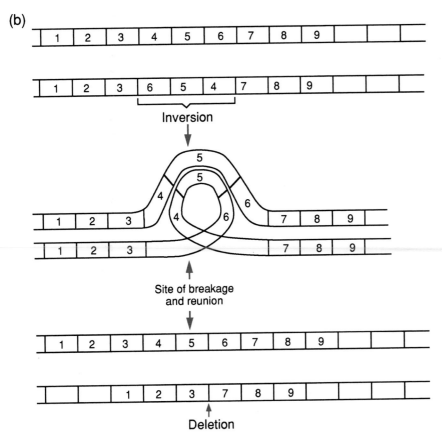

Fig. 18.5
Shows the generation of a deletion in the DMD gene by (a) unequal crossing over or (b) by breakage and fusion within a small inversion loop during maternal meiosis.

membrane where it is thought to act as a link between extracellular laminin and intra-cellular actin (Fig. 18.6). The sequence of events leading to muscle damage in DMD is unknown. Plausible theories include a metabolic role for dystrophin in maintaining muscle membrane calcium permeability and a physical role as a sort of shock absorber to prevent shearing damage when the muscle fibre contracts. The function of dystrophin in cerebral neurones is unknown.

Muscle studies in boys with DMD have shown that the quantity of dystrophin present is much reduced and that carboxy terminal domains are absent. This is consistent with a frameshift mutation causing formation of a truncated molecule. In BMD, dystrophin is also reduced in quantity but to a lesser extent than in DMD, and usually the amino and carboxy domains are both present. This is consistent with BMD deletions leading to loss of part of the central repeat rod domain.

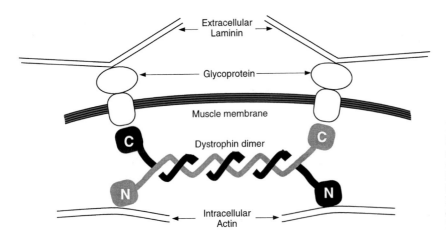

Fig. 18.6
Schematic representation of the probable structure of the dystrophin protein molecule which is depicted as a dimer linking intracellular actin with extracellular laminin (adapted from Ervasti J M, Campbell K P 1991 Membrane organization of the dystrophin–glycoprotein complex. Cell 66: 1121–1131).

A protein with sequence homology to dystrophin has been identified known as *utrophin* which is on chromosome 6. The role of this protein is unknown although it has been suggested that it could represent an early fetal or embryonic form of dystrophin, just as there are embryonic precursor forms of globin (p. 115).

CLINICAL APPLICATIONS

The discovery of the DMD/BMD gene and its protein product, dystrophin, has several useful clinical applications.

Diagnosis in affected boys

The identification of a DMD gene deletion provides confirmation of a suspected clinical diagnosis without the need for a muscle biopsy. Characterisation of the deletion in an isolated case and establishing whether or not it disturbs the reading frame can allow prediction of likely disease severity.

Carrier detection in females

Accurate carrier detection can now be achieved for most female relatives of DMD/BMD males by using polymorphic intragenic DNA markers. Microsatellites have been identified both in and closely adjacent to the dystrophin gene. If a microsatellite maps to the site of a deletion, then study of the segregation of that microsatellite marker in a family will provide conclusive evidence of carrier status in relevant female relatives (Fig. 19.2).

Prenatal diagnosis

The demonstration of a deletion in an affected boy allows reliable prenatal diagnosis to be offered to all female relatives who are at risk of being carriers, based on analysis of DNA obtained from chorionic villi (pp. 247, 262). Alternatively linked DNA markers can be used, although this is less satisfactory than direct mutation analysis because of the possibility of a predictive error occurring due to the small but significant chance of recombination between the site of the mutation and the linked DNA marker.

FUTURE PROSPECTS

Vigorous efforts are being made to utilise these new discoveries in gene therapy using transgenic and naturally occurring mutant mice with dystrophin negative muscular dystrophy. Several approaches have been used. These include direct injection of recombinant DNA, myoblast implantation, and transfection with retroviral or adenoviral vectors containing a dystrophin *minigene*. Results to date are not very encouraging. However, the fact that mice with dystrophin negative muscular dystrophy show spontaneous muscle repair suggests that there could be a way of switching on an alternative or compensatory protein such as the aforementioned dystrophin-like protein known as utrophin. Future strategies are likely to focus on attempts to 'upregulate' utrophin and dystrophin production.

CONCLUSION

These three conditions illustrate the diversity of clinical problems which can occur in single gene disorders in humans and show how combined clinical and molecular research has led to elucidation of their basic defects. Neurofibromatosis is characterised by variable expression, pleiotropy and heterogeneity which is both allelic and non-allelic. The discovery of the NF1 gene has shed light on tumour formation both in NF1 and in general. Cystic fibrosis is characterised by striking molecular heterogeneity, with the most common ΔF508 mutation showing linkage disequilibrium, an observation consistent with a single original mutation and heterozygote advantage. Duchenne and Becker muscular dystrophy emphasise the importance and difficulties of carrier detection and demonstrate how disturbance or maintenance of the reading frame provides an explanation for the relationship between genotype and phenotype.

A factor common to all of these disorders has been the recent isolation of the causal gene using the approach known as positional cloning (p. 61). Initially this involves mapping of the disease locus to a particular chromosome either by linkage analysis or by the serendipitous finding of an associated chromosome abnormality in an individual with a single gene disorder. Refined linkage studies help to pinpoint the locus more precisely. This is followed by physical mapping of the region concerned and a search for transcripts which are conserved in different species and expressed in disease affected organs. The finding of mutations in the putative disease gene in affected individuals provides absolute confirmation of its identity.

By employing these techniques the genes and their protein products have been identified for all three of these disorders, thereby opening up new opportunities and strategies for treatment including the possibility of effective gene therapy (p. 278).

ELEMENTS

1 Neurofibromatosis type 1 (NF1) shows autosomal dominant inheritance with complete penetrance and variable expression. The NF1 gene has been mapped to chromosome 17q11.2 by linkage analysis aided by two affected individuals with translocations in that region of chromosome 17. The gene product, neurofibromin, is involved in the regulation of cell division and probably acts as a tumour suppressor.

2 Cystic fibrosis (CF) shows autosomal recessive inheritance and causes recurrent chest infection and malabsorption. The CF locus has been mapped to chromosome 7q31 by linkage analysis. The gene is known as the CFTR gene and its protein product, CFTR, is involved in chloride transport and mucin secretion through the cell membrane. The most common mutation in the CFTR gene is caused by a deletion of the 508th codon and is known as ΔF508.

3 Duchenne muscular dystrophy (DMD) shows X-linked recessive inheritance, with most carriers being entirely healthy. The locus has been mapped to Xp21 by the discovery of several affected females with X-autosome translocations and subsequent linkage analysis. Two-thirds of males with DMD have an identifiable gene deletion. The protein product is known as dystrophin.

4 Positional cloning techniques have been successful in mapping and cloning the NF1, CFTR and DMD genes as well as the genes for many other important single gene disorders. The isolation of these genes has enhanced the prospect of successful gene therapy.

FURTHER READING

Dodge J A, Brock D J H, Widdicombe J H (eds) 1993 Cystic fibrosis. Current topics. John Wiley, Chichester
A comprehensive contemporary review of the clinical, genetic and molecular aspects of cystic fibrosis.
Emery A E H 1993 Duchenne muscular dystrophy, 2nd edn. Oxford University Press, Oxford
A detailed monograph reviewing the history, clinical features and genetics of Duchenne and Becker muscular dystrophy.
Huson S M, Hughes R A C (eds) 1994 The neurofibromatoses. Chapman and Hall, London
A very thorough description of the different types of neurofibromatosis. Includes a chapter on the Elephant Man.
McKusick V A 1994 Mendelian inheritance in man, 11th edn. Johns Hopkins University Press, Baltimore
The regularly updated definitive catalogue of all known single gene disorders and traits.

CHAPTER 19

Carrier detection and presymptomatic diagnosis

If it was easy to recognise carriers of autosomal and X-linked recessive disorders and persons who are heterozygous for autosomal dominant disorders which show reduced penetrance or a late age of onset, much doubt and uncertainty would be removed from genetic counselling. A number of tests of different types are available to detect carriers for autosomal and X-linked recessive disorders and for presymptomatic diagnosis of heterozygotes for autosomal disorders.

CARRIER TESTING

In a number of autosomal recessive disorders, such as some of the inborn errors of metabolism, e.g. Tay–Sachs disease (p. 137), and the haemoglobinopathies, e.g. sickle-cell disease (p. 119), carriers can be recognised with a high degree of certainty using biochemical techniques. In other single gene disorders, it is possible to detect or confirm carrier status by biochemical means in a proportion of carriers, e.g. the presence of abnormal coagulation studies in a woman at risk of being a carrier for haemophilia. However, a significant proportion of obligate carriers of haemophilia will have normal results, so that a normal result in a woman at risk does not exclude her from being a carrier.

There are several possible ways in which carriers of genetic diseases can be recognised.

CLINICAL MANIFESTATIONS IN CARRIERS

Occasionally, carriers for certain disorders can have mild clinical manifestations of the disease (Table 19.1). This is particularly true of some X-linked disorders.

These manifestations are usually so slight that they will only be obvious on careful clinical examination. Such manifestations, even though minimal, are unmistakably pathological, as in the mosaic pattern of retinal pigmentation seen in manifesting female carriers of X-linked ocular albinism (Plate 7). Unfortunately, in many conditions there are either no manifestations at all in the carrier or they are so slight as to be consistent with

Table 19.1 Clinical and biochemical abnormalities used in carrier detection of X-linked disorders

Disorder	Abnormality
Clinical	
Ocular albinism	mosaic retinal pigmentary pattern
Retinitis pigmentosa	mosaic retinal pigmentation, abnormal electroretinogram
Anhidrotic ectodermal dysplasia	sweat pore counts reduced, dental anomalies
Lowe's syndrome	lens opacities
Alport's syndrome	haematuria
Biochemical	
Haemophilia A	reduced factor VIII activity: antigen ratio
Haemophilia B	reduced levels of factor IX
G6PD deficiency	erythrocyte G6PD activity reduced
Lesch–Nyhan syndrome	reduced hypoxanthine-guanine phosphoribosyl transferase activity in skin fibroblasts
Hunter's syndrome	reduced sulphoiduronate sulphatase activity in skin fibroblasts
Vitamin D resistant rickets	serum phosphate level reduced
Duchenne muscular dystrophy	elevated serum creatine kinase level
Becker muscular dystrophy	elevated serum creatine kinase level
Fabry's disease	reduced α-galactosidase activity in hair root follicles

normal variation. This is so in some carriers of haemophilia, who have a tendency to bruise easily. Thus clinical manifestations are only of importance in detecting carriers when they are unmistakably pathological, and this is the exception rather than the rule with most single-gene disorders.

BIOCHEMICAL ABNORMALITIES IN CARRIERS

By far the most important approach to this problem has been the demonstration of detectable biochemical abnormalities in carriers of certain diseases (Table 19.1). In some diseases the biochemical abnormality is a direct result of the action of the gene and the carrier state can be tested for with confidence. This is so in carriers of Tay–Sachs disease, in whom the range of enzyme activity is intermediate between levels found in normal and affected persons. In many disorders the activity levels overlap with the normal range so that it is not possible to reliably distinguish between carriers and normal individuals.

In many single-gene disorders, however, the biochemical abnormality in the affected individual is not a direct result of gene action but the consequence of some secondary process. Such abnormalities are probably farther from the primary action of the gene and are even less likely to be useful in distinguishing carriers from the general population. For example, in Duchenne muscular dystrophy there appears to be an increased permeability of the muscle membrane as a result of the dystrophic process which results in an escape of muscle enzymes into the blood. An elevated serum creatine kinase is used as one of the confirmatory clinical investigations of the diagnosis in a boy presenting with features of the disorder (p. 239). Obligate carriers of DMD have, on average, serum creatine kinase levels which are elevated when compared to the general female population (Fig. 19.1) but there is overlap between normals and obligate carriers. This information can be used to help predict the likelihood of a woman being a carrier for this disorder, in conjunction with pedigree risk information (p. 258) and the results of linked DNA markers (p. 259).

There is a further reason for possible difficulty in the case of X-linked recessive disorders. Random inactivation of the X chromosome in females (p. 72) means that a proportion of carriers of X-linked disorders are unlikely to be detectable by biochemical methods, except one which involves analysis of cloned cells to identify two populations, as has been done in some of the X-linked immunodeficiency syndromes (p. 156).

LINKAGE BETWEEN A DISEASE LOCUS AND A POLYMORPHIC MARKER

Demonstration of linkage between a hereditary disorder and a polymorphic marker can be used in determining the carrier status of persons at risk in a family.

Biochemical and blood group polymorphic markers

The close linkage between the loci for G6PD (p. 145) and haemophilia A (p. 82) could provide a possible means of determining carrier status for females at risk of being carriers for haemophilia A. Unfortunately, polymorphisms at the G6PD locus are not found in most populations so that this linkage is usually uninformative for determining carrier status of females at risk.

DNA polymorphic markers

Developments in recombinant DNA technology have revolutionised the approach to carrier detection. The large number of different types of DNA sequence variants (p. 52) in the human genome means that if sufficient families are available, it should be possible to demonstrate linkage of a DNA marker with any disease locus. The demonstration of linkage between a DNA sequence variant and a disease locus overcomes the need for an identifiable biochemical defect or marker and the necessity for the enzyme or marker to be expressed in accessible

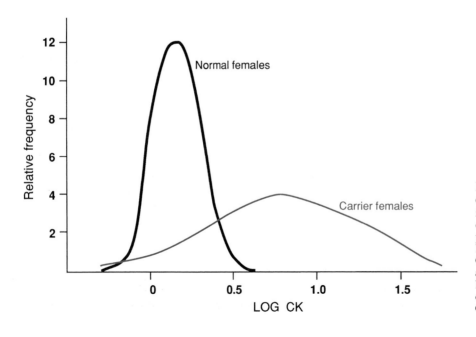

Fig. 19.1
Creatine kinase levels in obligate carrier females of Duchenne muscular dystrophy and women from the general population (adapted from Tippett P A, Dennis N R, Machin D, Price C P, Clayton B E 1982 Creatine kinase activity in the detection of carriers of Duchenne muscular dystrophy: comparison of two methods. Clinica Chemica Acta 121: 345–359).

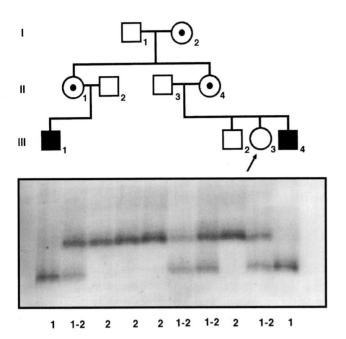

Fig. 19.2
Family with Duchenne muscular dystrophy showing segregation of the CA repeat 5′ to the dystrophin gene known as Dys 5′II (courtesy of J Noble, Regional DNA Laboratory, St James's Hospital, Leeds).

tissues. This also overcomes the difficulties of carrier detection in X-linked disorders due to X-inactivation in females.

Linked DNA markers are frequently used in determining the carrier status of females in families at risk for Duchenne muscular dystrophy. In Figure 19.2 individual III$_3$ presents for genetic counselling wanting to know whether she is a carrier and at risk for having sons affected with DMD. Analysis of the pedigree reveals that her mother, II$_4$, along with her sister, II$_1$, and their mother I$_2$, are all obligate carriers. The family is informative for a polymorphic CA dinucleotide repeat (p. 56) in the closely flanking region 5′ to the dystrophin gene known as Dys 5′ II which can be demonstrated by PCR (p. 48). The mutation in the dystrophin gene in the family is segregating with allele 1 and since individual III$_3$ has inherited this allele from her mother, she is likely to be a carrier. In the absence of identifying a specific mutation in the dystrophin gene in the affected males in the family, linked markers can be used for prenatal diagnosis to predict whether a male fetus is likely to be affected with DMD (p. 247).

Problems with DNA markers

There are a number of important factors to keep in mind with the use of linked markers. The first is the chance of recombination between the DNA marker and disease locus. This risk can be minimised, in most instances, by the identification of intragenic or closely flanking

markers. However, the dystrophin gene appears to be a 'hot-spot' for recombination (p. 240). Even with closely flanking and intragenic markers there appears to be a minimal chance of approximately 5% that recombination will occur in any meiosis in a female. This needs to be taken into account when combining the results of linked markers with pedigree risks and the results of CPK testing for women at risk of being carriers of DMD (p. 258).

The use of linked markers means that samples from the appropriate members of the family are required and this necessitates their cooperation. This can prove difficult depending on relationships within the family and the need for confidentiality of individual family members. In addition, families and physicians with individuals affected with lethal inherited disorders such as DMD and the autosomal recessive disorder spinal muscular atrophy, need to have the foresight to arrange for DNA to be banked from the affected person(s). For example, it is not unusual that by the time a younger sister of a male with DMD seeks advice about her carrier status, the affected male will no longer be alive. If the family structure is suitable, e.g. there is an unaffected male(s) in the pedigree, it is often possible to 'reconstruct' the likely markers in the affected male. This will, however, affect the risk estimation in the pedigree as the phase of the marker in the affected male will not be known with certainty (p. 99).

Another problem which can be encountered in the use of linked DNA markers is whether the family possesses the necessary variation in a linked marker to be what is known as *informative*. This occurs much less frequently now with the availability of a large number of different types of DNA sequence variants in the human genome. In addition, this also will become less of a problem with specific mutational analysis becoming available for an increasingly greater number of single gene disorders.

PRESYMPTOMATIC DIAGNOSIS OF AUTOSOMAL DOMINANT DISORDERS

There are a number of single gene disorders inherited in an autosomal dominant manner which either have a delayed age of onset or exhibit reduced penetrance. The results of clinical examination, specialist investigations, biochemical studies and family DNA studies can allow prediction of whether a person has inherited the gene before the onset of symptoms or signs. This is known as *presymptomatic diagnosis* (Table 19.2).

CLINICAL EXAMINATION

In a number of dominantly inherited disorders simple clinical means can be used for presymptomatic diagnosis, taking into account possible pleiotropic effects of a gene

Table 19.2 Autosomal dominant disorders which show a delayed age of onset or exhibit reduced penetrance in which linked DNA markers or specific mutational analysis can be used to offer presymptomatic diagnosis

Adult polycystic kidney disease

Familial adenomatous polyposis

Familial hypercholesterolaemia

Hereditary motor and sensory neuropathy type I

Huntington's disease

Marfan's syndrome

Myotonic dystrophy

Neurofibromatosis type 1

Neurofibromatosis type 2

Retinitis pigmentosa

Tuberous sclerosis

von Hippel Lindau disease

(p. 78). For example, persons with the dominantly inherited disorder known as neurofibromatosis type 1 (NF1) can have a number of different clinical features (p. 233). It is not unusual to examine an apparently unaffected relative of someone with NF1 who has had no medical problems, only to discover that they have sufficient numbers of a major diagnostic feature such as café-au-lait spots or cutaneous neurofibroma(ta), to indicate that they are affected.

SPECIALIST INVESTIGATION

The involvement of multiple different systems of the body in a number of autosomal dominantly inherited disorders can be utilised as a means of presymptomatic diagnosis. For example, in persons at risk for inheriting NF1, the presence of characteristic areas of pigmentation of the iris, known as Lisch nodules (Plate 15) would suggest that they have inherited the gene. It is important to realise, however, that 15% of the general population

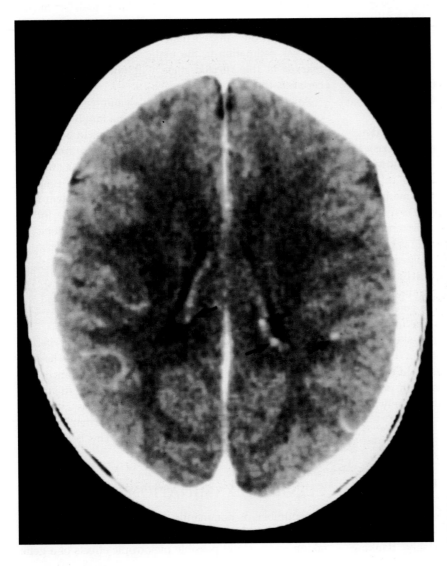

Fig. 19.3
Intracranial calcification (arrowed) in an asymptomatic person with tuberous sclerosis.

can have a few Lisch nodules, so that their presence in a person at risk for NF1 does not prove that they have inherited the NF1 gene. The presence of other features of NF1, such as café-au-lait spots or cutaneous neurofibroma(ta), would need to be present to confirm the diagnosis (p. 234).

Persons affected with the dominantly inherited disorder known as tuberous sclerosis (TSC) usually have evidence of involvement in a number of systems of the body. This can include intracranial calcification in the central nervous system (Fig. 19.3) and cysts or a disordered growth in the kidneys known as an angiomyolipoma(ta) (Fig. 19.4). In relatives of persons with TSC use of relatively non-invasive tests such as computerised axial tomography of the central nervous system or renal ultrasound can detect evidence of the TSC gene in asymptomatic persons.

In myotonic dystrophy, a dominantly inherited muscle disorder, in which affected persons have an inability to relax muscles normally, an electromyogram (EMG) can be used to confirm the diagnosis by detecting the presence of an abnormal spontaneous discharge of electrical activity which occurs with the insertion of the electrode into the muscle. This discharge does not occur in muscle from unaffected persons (Fig. 19.5). In persons at risk for inheriting myotonic dystrophy, an EMG can be used as a presymptomatic test, although this is rapidly being replaced by specific DNA mutational analysis looking for expansion of the CTG triplet repeat in the 3' end of the gene (pp. 17, 86).

Persons with myotonic dystrophy are also at an increased risk of developing early cataracts. The type of cataract seen in myotonic dystrophy is different from the common, so-called, senile cataract and can be detected by slit-lamp examination of the lens which shows refractile opacities (Plate 16). The presence of this type of cataract in an asymptomatic person at risk for myotonic dystrophy would confirm that they had inherited the gene.

It is important to point out, however, that the absence of these findings on clinical or specialist investigation does not exclude the diagnosis of the disorder being tested for but does reduce the likelihood of the person concerned having inherited the gene. If the relative

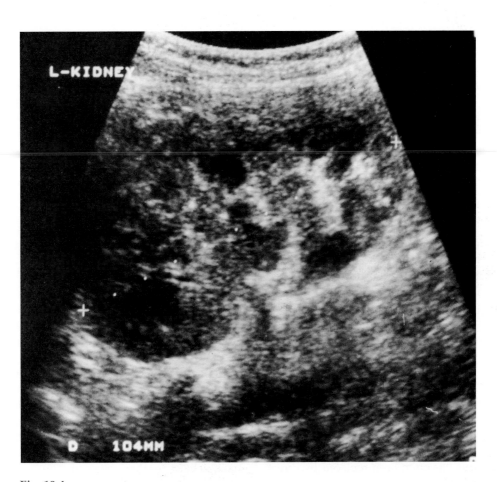

Fig. 19.4
Renal ultrasound of an asymptomatic person with tuberous sclerosis showing abnormal echogenicity due to presumed angiomyoplipomata.

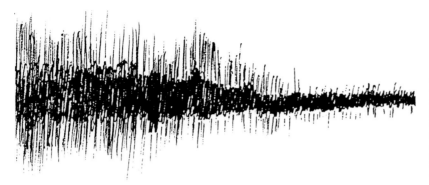

Fig. 19.5
An electromyogram from a person with myotonic dystrophy showing the characteristic abnormal spontaneous electrical discharge seen with insertion of the electrode into the muscle which decreases with time (courtesy of Dr A. DaCosta, Dept of Neurophysiology, St James's Hospital, Leeds).

frequencies of such findings in persons with the disorder and in persons from the general population are known, it is possible to give the person at risk a relative likelihood of having inherited the gene. This information can be used in conjunction with other information, such as the pedigree risk, in genetic counselling (pp. 208, 253).

BIOCHEMICAL TESTS

In a number of autosomal dominant disorders biochemical tests can determine whether or not a person at risk has inherited a gene. Examples include the use of serum cholesterol levels in persons at risk for familial hypercholesterolaemia (p. 134) and assay of the appropriate urinary porphyrins or enzyme in the various dominant porphyrias (p. 138).

LINKED MARKERS

Linked biochemical or DNA polymorphic markers can be used in presymptomatic diagnosis of dominantly inherited disorders.

Biochemical and blood group markers

The linkage of secretor status for the ABO blood group to myotonic dystrophy was one of the first examples of the use of this approach (p. 158). Unfortunately most families are uninformative for this polymorphism. In addition, there is a significant chance of a cross-over occurring in meiosis between the two loci resulting in this approach being of little use.

DNA markers

The availability of linked DNA markers has found widespread use in presymptomatic and predictive testing for a number of single gene disorders inherited in an autosomal dominant manner. With the cloning of the gene responsible, this has often been replaced by direct mutational analysis as has occurred in presymptomatic, or *predictive testing* for persons at risk for Huntington's disease.

ETHICAL CONSIDERATIONS

There are often clear advantages in being able to determine the carrier status for a person at risk of being a carrier for an autosomal or X-linked recessive disorder. These primarily centre around a couple being able to make an informed choice when having children (p. 209).

In those at risk for the late onset autosomal dominant disorders, there can also be a clear advantage in presymptomatic diagnosis. For example, in persons at risk for familial adenomatous polyposis (p. 173), colonoscopy looking for the presence of colonic polyps can be offered as a regular screening procedure to those shown to be at high risk by molecular studies.

In contrast, in persons at risk for Huntington's disease, in which there is, as yet, no effective treatment to delay the onset or progression of the disorder, the benefit of predictive testing is not immediately obvious. While choice is often considered to be of paramount importance in genetic counselling for persons at risk for inherited disorders, it is important to remember that those considering presymptomatic testing should only proceed if they can give truly informed consent and are free from coercion from any outside influence. It is increasingly likely that employers, life insurance companies and society in general will put indirect and, on occasion, direct pressure on persons at risk for inherited disorders (p. 290).

Another problem raised by this technology is that presymptomatic testing can be carried out on children. The issue of predictive testing in childhood is very contentious with many persons arguing, particularly when no obvious advantage accrues to the child in carrying out such testing, that it is best left until they can make a choice for themselves (p. 289).

ELEMENTS

1 Determination of carrier status for autosomal recessive and X-linked disorders can involve detailed clinical examination looking for specific minor features, specialist clinical investigations, biochemical tests and family studies using linked biochemical, blood group or DNA polymorphic markers.

2 Presymptomatic or predictive testing for persons at risk for autosomal dominant disorders with reduced penetrance or a delayed age of onset can also be carried out by detailed clinical examination for specific features, specialist investigations, biochemical testing and the use of linked biochemical or DNA polymorphisms.

3 Consideration should be given to the advantages and disadvantages of presymptomatic or predictive testing both from a practical and an ethical point of view.

FURTHER READING

Bakker E, Hofker M H, Goor N et al 1985 Prenatal diagnosis and carrier detection of Duchenne muscular dystrophy with closely linked RFLPs. Lancet i: 655–658
A paper which illustrates in more detail the principle of the use of linked DNA polymorphisms in carrier detection.
Pauli R, Motulsky A G 1981 Risk counselling in autosomal dominant disorders with undetermined penetrance. J Med Genet 18: 340–343
A paper which considers the problem of counselling for autosomal dominant disorders with reduced penetrance.
Pembrey M E, Davies K E, Winter R M, Elles R G, Williamson R, Fazzone T E, Walker C 1984 Clinical use of DNA markers linked to the gene for Duchenne muscular dystrophy. Arch Dis Child 59: 208–216
A useful discussion of how DNA markers can be used for carrier detection in Duchenne muscular dystrophy.
Harper P S 1993 Practical genetic counselling, 4th edn. Butterworth Heinemann, Oxford
As the title suggests, a practical book which serves as a good starting point in almost every aspect of genetic counselling including carrier testing.

CHAPTER 20 | Risk calculation

INTRODUCTION

One of the most important aspects of genetic counselling is the provision of a risk figure. This is often referred to as a recurrence risk. Usually estimation of the recurrence risk will require careful consideration taking into account:

1. The diagnosis and its mode of inheritance
2. Analysis of the family pedigree
3. The results of tests which can include linkage studies using DNA markers.

Sometimes the provision of a risk figure can be quite easy, but in a surprisingly large number of situations complicating factors arise which can make the calculation very difficult. For example, the mother of a boy who is an isolated case of a sex-linked recessive disorder could very reasonably wish to know the recurrence risk for her next child. This is a very simple question, but the solution is far from straightforward, as will become clear later in this chapter.

Before proceeding any further, it is necessary to clarify what we mean by probability and review the different ways in which it can be expressed. The *probability* of an outcome can be defined as the number or, more correctly, the proportion of times it occurs in a large series of events. Conventionally, probability is indicated as a proportion of one, so that a probability of zero implies that an outcome will never be observed, whereas a probability of one implies that it will always be observed. Therefore a probability of 0.25 indicates that, on average, a particular outcome or event will be observed on 1 in 4 or 25% of occasions. The probability that the outcome will not occur is 0.75, which can also be expressed as 3 chances out of 4, or 75%. Alternatively, this probability could be expressed as odds of 3 to 1 against or 1 to 3 in favour of this particular outcome being observed. In this chapter fractions will be used where possible as these tend to be more easily understood than proportions of 1 expressed as decimals.

PROBABILITY THEORY

In order to calculate genetic risks it is necessary to have a basic understanding of probability theory. This will be discussed in so far as it is relevant to the skills required for genetic counselling.

LAWS OF ADDITION AND MULTIPLICATION

When considering the probability of two different events or outcomes, it is essential to clarify whether they are mutually exclusive or independent. If the events are mutually exclusive then the probability that *either* one *or* the other will occur equals the *sum* of their individual probabilities. This is known as the *law of addition*.

If, however, two or more events or outcomes are independent, then the probability that *both* the first *and* the second will occur equals the product of their individual probabilities. This is known as the *law of multiplication*.

As a simple illustration of these laws consider parents who have embarked upon their first pregnancy. The probability that the baby will be *either* a boy *or* a girl equals 1, i.e. 1/2 + 1/2. An ultrasound scan reveals that the mother is carrying non-identical twins. The probability that both the first and the second twin will be boys equals 1/4, i.e. 1/2 x 1/2.

BAYES' THEOREM

Bayes' theorem, which was first formulated in 1763, is widely used in genetic counselling. Essentially it provides a very valuable method for determining the overall probability of an event or outcome, such as carrier status, by considering all initial possibilities, e.g. carrier or non-carrier, and then modifying or 'conditioning' these by incorporating information, such as test results, which indicates which is the more likely.

The initial probability of each event is known as its *prior probability*, which is based on ancestral or *anterior information*. The observations which modify these prior

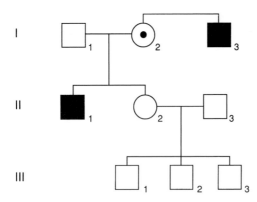

Fig. 20.1
A pedigree showing sex-linked recessive inheritance. When calculating the probability that II_2 is a carrier it is necessary to take into account her three unaffected sons.

Table 20.1	Bayesian calculation from Figure 20.1

Probability	II_2 is a carrier	II_2 is not a carrier
Prior	1/2	1/2
Conditional 3 healthy sons	1/8	1
Joint	1/16	1/2

Perhaps by now the use of Bayes' theorem will be a little more clear. Some of the following applications of Bayes' theorem could help shed further light!

AUTOSOMAL DOMINANT INHERITANCE

For someone with an autosomal dominant disorder, the risk that each of his or her children will inherit the mutant gene equals 1 in 2. This will apply whether the affected individual inherited the disorder from a parent or developed the condition as a result of a new mutation. Therefore the provision of risks for disorders showing autosomal dominant inheritance is usually straightforward as long as there is a clear family history, the condition is characterised by being fully penetrant and there is a reliable means of diagnosing heterozygotes. However, if penetrance is incomplete or if there is a delay in the age of onset so that heterozygotes cannot always be diagnosed, then risk calculation becomes more complicated. Two examples will be discussed to illustrate the sort of problems which can arise.

REDUCED PENETRANCE

A disorder is said to show reduced penetrance when it has clearly been demonstrated that individuals who must possess the abnormal gene, who by pedigree analysis must be obligate heterozygotes, show absolutely no manifestations of the condition. For example, if someone who was completely unaffected had both a parent and a child with the same autosomal dominant disorder, then this would be an example of non-penetrance. Penetrance is usually quoted as a percentage, e.g. 80%, or as a proportion of 1, e.g. 0.8. This would imply that 80% of all heterozygotes express the condition in some way.

For a condition showing reduced penetrance, the risk that the child of an affected individual will be affected equals 1/2, i.e. the probability that the child will inherit the mutant allele, x P, the proportion of heterozygotes who are affected. Therefore for a disorder such as hereditary retinoblastoma, an embryonic eye tumour (p. 170) which shows dominant inheritance in some families with a penetrance of P = 0.8, the risk that the child of an

probabilities allow *conditional probabilities* to be determined. In genetic counselling these are usually based on numbers of offspring and the results of tests. This is *posterior information*. The resulting probability for each event or outcome is known as its *joint probability*. The final probability for each event is known as its *posterior* or *relative probability* and is obtained by dividing the joint probability for that event by the sum of all the joint probabilities.

This is not an easy concept to grasp! To try to make it a little more comprehensible consider a pedigree with two males, I_3 and II_1, who have a sex-linked recessive disorder (Fig. 20.1). The sister, II_2, of one of these men wishes to know the probability that she is a carrier. Her mother, I_2, must be a carrier as she has both an affected brother and an affected son, i.e. she is an obligate carrier. Therefore the prior probability that II_2 is a carrier equals 1/2. Similarly the prior probability that II_2 is not a carrier equals 1/2.

The fact that II_2 already has three healthy sons must be taken into consideration, as intuitively this makes it rather unlikely that she is a carrier. Bayes' theorem provides a way to quantify this intuition. These three healthy sons provide posterior information. The conditional probability that II_2 would have three healthy sons if she is a carrier equals 1/2 x 1/2 x 1/2, which equals 1/8. These values of 1/2 are multiplied as they are independent events in that the health of one son is not influenced by the health of his brother(s). The conditional probability that II_2 would have three healthy sons if she is not a carrier equals 1.

This information is now incorporated into a Bayesian calculation (Table 20.1). From this table the posterior probability that II_2 is a carrier equals 1/16 / (1/16 + 1/2) which reduces to 1/9. Similarly the posterior probability that II_2 is not a carrier equals 1/2 / (1/16 + 1/2) which reduces to 8/9. Thus by taking into account the fact that II_2 has three healthy sons, we have been able to reduce her risk of being a carrier from 1 in 2 to 1 in 9.

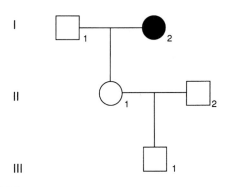

Fig. 20.2
I_2 has an autosomal dominant disorder which shows reduced penetrance. The probability that III_1 will be affected has to take into account the possibility that his mother (II_1) is a non-penetrant heterozygote.

affected parent will develop a tumour equals $1/2 \times 0.8$ or 0.4.

A more difficult calculation arises when a risk is sought for the future child of someone who is healthy but whose parent has or had an autosomal dominant disorder showing reduced penetrance (Fig. 20.2).

Let us assume that the penetrance, P, equals 0.8. Calculation of the risk that III_1 will be affected can be approached in two ways. The first simply involves a little logic. The second utilises Bayes' theorem.

1. Imagine that I_2 has 10 children. On average five children will inherit the gene but as $P = 0.8$ only four will be affected (Fig. 20.3). Therefore six out of the ten children will be unaffected. II_1 is unaffected so that there is therefore a probability of 1 in 6 that she is, in fact, a heterozygote. Consequently the probability that III_1 will both inherit the mutant gene and be affected equals $1/6 \times 1/2 \times P$ which equals 1/15 if P is 0.8.

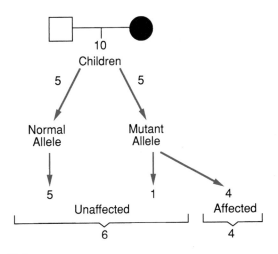

Fig. 20.3
The expected genotypes and phenotypes in 10 children born to an individual with an autosomal dominant disorder with penetrance equal to 0.8.

Table 20.2 Bayesian calculation from Figure 20.2

Probability	II_1 is heterozygous	II_1 is not heterozygous
Prior	1/2	1/2
Conditional not affected	1–P	1
Joint	1/2 (1–P)	1/2

2. Now consider II_1 in Figure 20.2. The prior probability that she is a heterozygote equals 1/2. Similarly the prior probability that she is not a heterozygote equals 1/2. Now a Bayesian table can be constructed to determine how these prior probabilities are modified by the fact that II_1 is not affected (Table 20.2).

The posterior probability that II_1 is a heterozygote equals $1/2(1 - P) / [1/2(1 - P) + 1/2]$ which reduces to $1 - P/2 - P$. Therefore, the risk that III_1 will both inherit the mutant allele and be affected equals $[(1 - P/2 - P)] \times 1/2 \times P$ which reduces to $(P - P^2)/(4 - 2P)$. If P equals 0.8, this expression equals 1/15 or 0.067.

By substituting different values of P in the above expression, it can be shown that the maximum risk for III_1 being affected equals 0.086, approximately 1/12, which is obtained when P equals 0.6. This maximal risk figure is often used in counselling persons at risk for late onset autosomal disorders with reduced penetrance in which their parent is unaffected but they have an affected grandparent.

DELAYED AGE OF ONSET

Many autosomal dominant disorders do not present until well into adult life (p. 247). Healthy members of families in which these disorders are segregating often wish to know whether they themselves will develop the

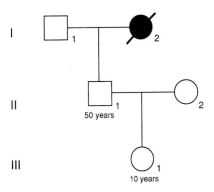

Fig. 20.4
I_2 had an autosomal dominant disorder showing delayed age of onset. When calculating the probability that III_1 will develop the disorder it is necessary to determine the probability that II_1 is a heterozygote who is not yet clinically affected.

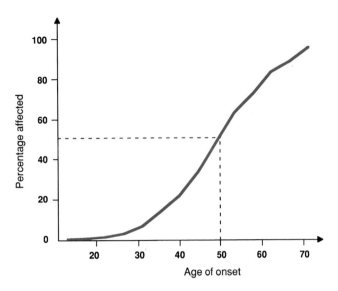

Fig. 20.5
Graph showing age of onset in years of clinical expression in Huntington's disease heterozygotes. Approximately 50% show clinical signs or symptoms by age 50 years (data from R G Newcombe 1981 A life table for onset of Huntington's chorea. Ann Hum Genet 45: 375–385).

condition and/or pass it on to their children. Risks for these individuals can be calculated in the following way.

Consider someone who has died with a confirmed diagnosis of Huntington's disease (Fig. 20.4). This is a late onset autosomal dominant disorder. The son of I_2 is entirely healthy at age 50 years and wishes to know the probability that his 10 year old daughter, III_1, will develop Huntington's disease in later life. In this condition the first signs usually appear between the ages of 30 and 60 years, and approximately 50% of all heterozygotes have shown signs by the age of 50 years (Fig. 20.5).

The probability that II_1 has inherited the gene, given that he shows no signs of the condition, can be determined by a simple Bayesian calculation (Table 20.3).

The posterior probability that II_1 is heterozygous equals $1/4 / (1/4 + 1/2)$ which equals $1/3$. Therefore the prior probability that his daughter III_1 will have inherited the disorder equals $1/3 \times 1/2$ or $1/6$.

There is a temptation when doing calculations such as this to conclude that the overall risk for II_1 being a hete-

rozygote simply equals $1/2 \times 1/2$, the prior probability that he will have inherited the mutant gene times the probability that a heterozygote will be unaffected at age 50 years, giving a risk of $1/4$. This is correct in as much as it gives the joint probability for these two events, but it does not take into account all the possibilities. Consider the possibility that I_2 has four children. On average two will inherit the mutant allele, one of whom will be affected by the age of 50 years. The remaining two children will not inherit the mutant allele. By the time these children have grown up and reached the age of 50 years, on average one will be affected and three will not. Therefore, on average one third of the *healthy* 50 year old offspring of I_2 will be heterozygotes. Hence the correct risk for II_1 is $1/3$ and not $1/4$.

AUTOSOMAL RECESSIVE INHERITANCE

With an autosomal recessive condition, the parents of an affected child are both heterozygotes. There are two possible exceptions, both of which are very rare. These arise when only one parent is a heterozygote, in which case a child can be affected if either a new mutation occurs on the gamete inherited from the other parent, or uniparental disomy occurs resulting in the child inheriting two copies of the heterozygous parent's mutant allele (p. 88).

When both parents are heterozygotes, the risk that each of their children will be affected equals 1 in 4. On average three of their four children will be unaffected, of whom, on average, two will be carriers (Fig. 20.6).

Therefore the probability that the healthy sibling of someone with an autosomal recessive disorder will be a

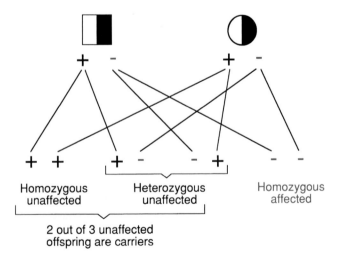

Fig. 20.6
The possible genotypes and phenotypes in the offspring of parents who are both carriers of an autosomal recessive disorder. On average 2 out of 3 healthy offspring are carriers.

Table 20.3	Bayesian calculation from Figure 20.4	
Probability	**II_1 is heterozygous**	**II_1 is not heterozygous**
Prior	1/2	1/2
Conditional unaffected at age 50 years	1/2	1
Joint	1/4	1/2

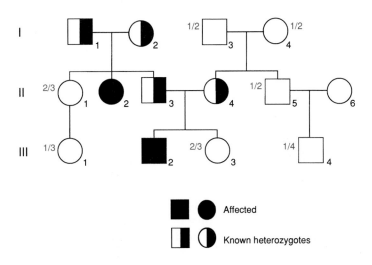

Affected

Known heterozygotes

Fig. 20.7
The probabilities of various relatives being carriers of an autosomal recessive disorder.

carrier equals 2/3. Carrier risks can be derived for other family members (Fig. 20.7).

When calculating risks in autosomal recessive inheritance the underlying principle is to establish the probability that each prospective parent is a carrier, and then multiply the product of these probabilities by 1/4, this being the risk that any child born to two carriers will be affected. Therefore, in Figure 20.7, if the sister, III_3, of the affected boy was to marry her first cousin, III_4, then the probability that their first baby would be affected would equal $2/3 \times 1/4 \times 1/4$, i.e. the probability that III_3 is a carrier times the probability that III_4 is a carrier times the probability that a child of two carriers will be affected. This gives a total risk of 1/24.

If this same sister, III_3, was to marry a healthy unrelated individual, the probability that their first child would be affected would equal $2/3 \times 2pq \times 1/4$, i.e. the probability that III_3 is a carrier times the carrier frequency in the general population (p. 95) times the probability that a child of two carriers will be affected. For a condition such as cystic fibrosis, with a disease incidence of approximately 1 in 2000, $q2 = 1/2000$ and therefore

$q = 1/44$ and thus $2pq = 1/22$. Therefore, the final risk would be $2/3 \times 1/22 \times 1/4$ or 1 in 132.

SEX-LINKED RECESSIVE INHERITANCE

This pattern of inheritance tends to generate the most complicated risk calculations when counselling for Mendelian disorders. In severe sex-linked conditions, affected males often do not survive long enough to have their own children. Consequently these conditions are usually transmitted only by healthy female carriers. The carrier of a sex-linked recessive disorder transmits the gene on average to half of her daughters who are therefore carriers, and to half of her sons who will thus be affected. If an affected male does have children, then he will transmit his Y chromosome to all of his sons who will be unaffected, and his X chromosome to all of his daughters who will be carriers (Fig. 20.8).

An example of how the birth of unaffected sons to a possible carrier of a sex-linked disorder results in a

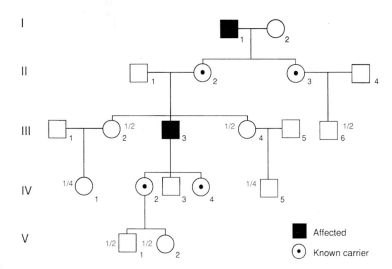

Affected

Known carrier

Fig. 20.8
The probabilities of male relatives being affected and female relatives being carriers of an X-linked recessive disorder. All the daughters of an affected male are obligate carriers.

reduction of her carrier risk has already been discussed in the introductory section on Bayes' theorem (p. 254). In this section we shall consider two further factors which can complicate risk calculation in sex-linked recessive disorders.

THE ISOLATED CASE

If a woman has only one affected son, then in the absence of a positive family history there are three possible ways in which this can occur:

1. The woman is a carrier of the mutant allele, in which case there is a risk of 1/2 that any future son will be affected.
2. The disorder in the son arose as a new mutation which occurred during meiosis in the gamete which led to his conception. The recurrence risk in this situation is negligible.
3. The woman is a gonadal mosaic for the mutation which occurred in an early mitotic division during her own embryonic development. The recurrence risk will be equal to the proportion of ova which carry the mutant allele, i.e. between 0% and 50%.

In practice it is usually very difficult to distinguish between these three possibilities unless reliable tests are available for carrier detection. If a woman is found to be a carrier then risk calculation is straightforward. If the tests indicate that she is not a carrier, then the recurrence risk is probably low, but not negligible because of the possibility of gonadal mosaicism.

For example, in Duchenne muscular dystrophy, it has been estimated that amongst the mothers of isolated cases approximately two-thirds are carriers, 5–10% are gonadal mosaics and in the remaining 25–30% the disease has arisen as a new mutation in meiosis.

INCORPORATING CARRIER TEST RESULTS

Several biochemical tests are available for detecting carriers of sex-linked recessive disorders (p. 246). Unfortunately there is often overlap in the values obtained for controls and women known to be carriers, i.e. obligate carriers. Although an abnormal result in a potential carrier would suggest that she is very likely to be a carrier, a normal test result does not exclude a woman being a carrier. Whilst for many sex-linked recessive disorders this problem can be overcome by using linked DNA markers (p. 247), the difficulties presented by overlapping biochemical test results arise sufficiently often to justify further consideration.

For example, in Duchenne muscular dystrophy, serum creatine kinase is elevated in approximately two out of three obligate carriers (Fig.19.1). Therefore, if a possible

Table 20.4 Bayesian calculation from Figure 20.1

Probability	II$_2$ is a carrier	II$_2$ is not a carrier
Prior	1/2	1/2
Conditional		
3 healthy sons	1/8	1
normal creatine kinase	1/3	1
Joint	1/48	1/2

carrier such as II$_2$ in Figure 20.1 is found to have a normal level of creatine kinase, this would provide further support for her not being a carrier. The test result therefore provides a conditional probability, which is included in a new Bayesian calculation (Table 20.4).

The posterior probability that II$_2$ is a carrier equals 1/48 / (1/48 + 1/2) or 1/25. Consequently by taking into account firstly this woman's three healthy sons and secondly her normal creatine kinase test result we have been able to reduce her carrier risk from 1 in 2 to 1 in 9 and then to 1 in 25.

THE USE OF LINKED MARKERS

As a result of the developments which have taken place in molecular biology over the last 15 years, many of the more common single gene disorders have been mapped to the human genome (p. 63). For many conditions the gene has been isolated and characterised so that specific mutation analysis is available. This now applies to disorders such as Huntington's disease and sickle-cell disease, and is also the case for many families in which

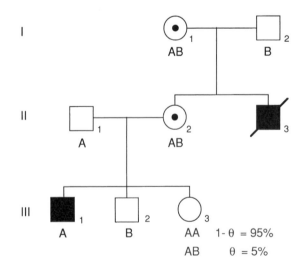

Fig. 20.9
A pedigree showing sex-linked recessive inheritance. A and B represent alleles at a locus closely linked to the disease locus.

Duchenne muscular dystrophy is present. However, in conditions such as Duchenne muscular dystrophy in which each family usually has its own unique mutation, direct mutation analysis is not always possible if, for example, there are no surviving affected males. In these families DNA markers at a locus closely linked to the disease locus can be used to assist in carrier detection.

As an illustration of the potential value of this approach, consider the sister of a boy affected with Duchenne muscular dystrophy (DMD), whose mother is an obligate carrier as she herself had an affected brother (Fig. 20.9).

A DNA marker with alleles A and B is available and is known to be closely linked to the DMD disease locus with a recombination fraction (θ) equal to 0.05 (pp. 99, 247). The disease allele must be in coupling with the A marker allele in II_2 as this woman has inherited both the A allele and the DMD allele on the X chromosome from her mother. Therefore, if III_3 inherits this A allele from her mother, the probability that she will also inherit the disease allele and be a carrier equals $1-\theta$, i.e. the probability that a crossover will not occur between the disease and marker loci in the meiosis of the ova which resulted in her conception. For a value of θ equal to 0.05 this gives a carrier risk of 0.95 or 95%. Similarly the probability that III_3 will be a carrier if she inherits the B allele from her mother equals 0.05 or 5%.

Closely linked DNA markers are now available for most single gene disorders and these are widely used in genetic counselling for carrier detection and prenatal diagnosis. The smaller the value of θ, then the smaller the likelihood of a predictive error. If DNA markers are available which 'bridge' or 'flank' the disease locus, this greatly reduces the risk of a predictive error as only a double crossover will go undetected.

EMPIRIC RISKS

Up to this point risks have been calculated for single gene disorders using knowledge of basic Mendelian genetics and applied probability theory. In many counselling situations it is not possible to arrive at an accurate risk figure in this way, either because the disorder in question does not show single gene inheritance or because the clinical diagnosis with which the family has been referred shows causal heterogeneity (pp. 81, 260). In these situations it is usually necessary to resort to the use of observed or *empiric risks*. These are based on observations derived from family studies rather than theoretical calculations.

MULTIFACTORIAL DISORDERS

One of the basic principles of multifactorial inheritance

Table 20.5 Empiric recurrence risks for common multifactorial disorders

Disorder	Incidence (per 1000)	Sex ratio	Unaffected parents having a second affected child (%)	Affected parents having an affected child (%)
Cleft lip +/− cleft palate	1–2	3:2	4	4
Club foot (talipes)	1–2	2:1	3	3
Congenital heart defects	8	1:1	1–4	2 (father affected) 6 (mother affected)
Congenital dislocation of the hip	1	1:6	6	12
Hypospadias (in males)	2	–	10	10
Manic-depressive psychosis	4	2:3	10–15	10–15
Neural tube defects				
anencephaly	1.5	1:2	4–5	–
spina bifida	2.5	2:3	4–5	4
Pyloric stenosis				
male index	2.5	–	2	4
female index	0.5	–	10	17
Schizophrenia	10	1:1	14	16

is that the risk of recurrence in first degree relatives, siblings and offspring, equals the square root of the incidence of the disease in the general population (p. 108), i.e. $P^{1/2}$ where P equals the general population incidence. The theoretical risks for second and third degree relatives can be shown to approximate to $P^{3/4}$ and $P^{7/8}$ respectively. Therefore, if there is strong support for multifactorial inheritance, it is reasonable to use these theoretical risks when counselling close family relatives.

However when using this approach it is important to remember that the confirmation of multifactorial inheritance will often have been based on the study of observed recurrence risks. As a consequence it is generally more appropriate to refer back to the original family studies and counsel on the basis of the risks derived in these (Table 20.5).

Ideally reference should be made to local studies as recurrence risks can differ quite substantially in different communities, ethnic groups, and geographical locations. For example, the recurrence risk for neural tube defects in siblings is quoted as 4–5%. This is essentially an average risk. The actual risk varies from 2–3% in South-East England up to 8% in Northern Ireland, and also

Table 20.6 Empiric recurrence risks for conditions showing causal heterogeneity

Disorder	Incidence (per 1000)	Sex ratio	Unaffected parents having a second affected child (%)	Affected parents having an affected child (%)
Autism	0:2	3:1	2	–
Epilepsy (idiopathic)	5	1:1	5	5
Hydrocephalus	0.5	1:1	3	–
Mental retardation (idiopathic)	3	1:1	3–5	10
Profound childhood sensorineural deafness	1	1:1	10–15	5–10

shows an inverse relationship with the family's socio-economic status, being greatest in mothers of poorest circumstances.

Unfortunately empiric risks are rarely available for families in which there are several affected family members or for disorders with variable severity or different sex incidences. A computer program has been devised which allows theoretical estimates to be made in many of these more complex situations.

CONDITIONS SHOWING CAUSAL HETEROGENEITY

Many referrals to genetic clinics relate to a clinical phenotype rather than to a precise underlying diagnosis (Table 20.6). In these situations great care must be taken to ensure that all appropriate diagnostic investigations have been undertaken before resorting to the use of empiric risk data (p. 207).

It is worth emphasising that the use of empiric risks for conditions such as sensorineural deafness in childhood is at best a compromise as the figure quoted to an individual family will rarely be the correct one for their particular diagnosis. Nerve deafness in a young child is usually caused by either a single gene disorder, most commonly autosomal recessive but occasionally autosomal dominant or sex-linked recessive, or by an environmental condition such as rubella embryopathy. Therefore, for most families the correct risk of recurrence will be either 25% or 0%. In practice it is often not possible to establish the precise cause so that the only option available is to offer the family an empiric or 'average' risk.

ELEMENTS

1 Risk calculation in genetic counselling requires a knowledge and understanding of basic probability theory. Bayes' theorem enables initial background 'prior' risks to be modified by 'conditional' information to give an overall probability or risk for a particular event such as carrier status.

2 For disorders showing autosomal dominant inheritance it is often necessary to consider factors such as reduced penetrance and delayed age of onset.

3 For disorders showing autosomal recessive inheritance, risks to offspring are determined by calculating the probability that each parent is a carrier and then multiplying the product of these probabilities by 1/4.

4 In sex-linked recessive inheritance a particular problem arises if only one male in a family is affected. The results of carrier tests which show overlap between carriers and non-carriers can be incorporated in a Bayesian calculation.

5 Polymorphic DNA markers linked to the disease locus can be used in many single gene disorders for carrier detection, preclinical diagnosis and prenatal diagnosis.

6 Empiric (observed) risks are available for multifactorial disorders and for aetiologically heterogeneous conditions such as non-syndromal sensorineural deafness.

FURTHER READING

Bayes T 1958 An essay towards solving a problem in the doctrine of chances. Biometrika 45: 296–315
A reproduction of the Reverend Bayes' original essay on probability theory which was first published, posthumously, in 1763.
Emery A E H 1986 Methodology in medical genetics, 2nd edn. Churchill Livingstone, Edinburgh
An introduction to statistical methods of analysis in human and medical genetics.
Murphy E A, Chase G A 1975 Principles of genetic counselling. Year Book Medical Publication, Chicago
A very thorough explanation of the use of Bayes' theorem in genetic counselling.
Young I D 1991 Introduction to risk calculation in genetic counselling. Oxford University Press, Oxford
A short introductory guide to all aspects of risk calculation in genetic counselling. Highly recommended!

CHAPTER 21

Prenatal diagnosis of genetic disease

In the past, couples at high risk of having a child with a genetic disorder had to choose between taking the risk or considering other reproductive options such as long term contraception, sterilisation and termination of all pregnancies. Other alternatives included adoption, long term fostering and *artificial insemination by donor sperm* (AID).

Over the last three decades *prenatal diagnosis*, the ability to detect abnormalities in an unborn child, has been widely used. While it is never easy for a couple to decide to pursue prenatal diagnosis, because of the possibility of subsequently having to consider termination of pregnancy, this is an option which is chosen by many couples at high risk of having a child with a serious hereditary disorder.

The ethical issues surrounding prenatal diagnosis and selective termination of pregnancy are both complex and emotive, and are considered more fully in Chapter 24 (p. 287). In this chapter we shall focus on the practical aspects of prenatal diagnosis, which can be considered under the headings of the techniques which are used and the indications for offering each of these various procedures.

TECHNIQUES USED IN PRENATAL DIAGNOSIS

There are several techniques which can be utilised for the prenatal diagnosis of hereditary disorders and structural abnormalities (Table 21.1).

AMNIOCENTESIS

Amniocentesis involves the aspiration of 10–20 ml of amniotic fluid through the abdominal wall under ultrasound guidance (Fig. 21.1). This is usually performed around the sixteenth week of gestation. The sample is spun down to yield a pellet of cells and supernatant fluid. The fluid can be used in the prenatal diagnosis of neural tube defects by assay of alpha-fetoprotein. The cell pellet is resuspended in culture medium with fetal

Table 21.1 Standard techniques used in prenatal diagnosis

Technique	Optimal time (in weeks)	Disorders diagnosed
Non-invasive		
Maternal serum screening		
alpha fetoprotein	16	neural tube defects
triple test	16	Down's syndrome
Ultrasound	18	structural abnormalities, e.g. CNS, heart, kidneys and limbs
Invasive		
Amniocentesis	16	
fluid		neural tube defects
cells		chromosome abnormalities, metabolic disorders, molecular defects
Chorionic villus sampling	10–12	chromosome abnormalities, metabolic disorders, molecular defects
Fetoscopy		
blood		chromosome abnormalities, haematological disorders, congenital infection
liver		metabolic disorders, e.g. ornithine transcarbamylase deficiency
skin		hereditary skin disorders, e.g. epidermolysis bullosa

calf serum which stimulates cell growth. Whilst most of these cells, which have been shed from the amnion, fetal skin and urinary tract epithelium, will be non-viable, a small proportion will grow. After approximately 14 days there are usually sufficient cells for chromosome analysis, although a longer period is usually needed before enough cells are obtained for biochemical or DNA studies.

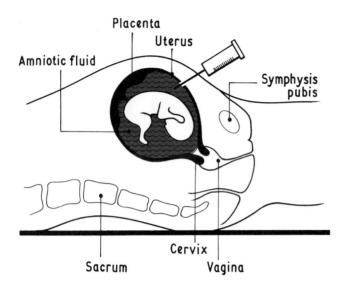

Fig. 21.1
The technique of amniocentesis.

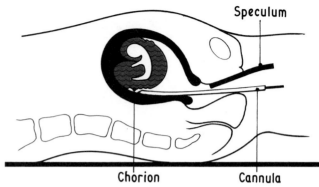

Fig. 21.2
The technique of transvaginal chorionic villus sampling.

When a couple are considering amniocentesis as an option they should be informed of the 0.5% to 1% risk of miscarriage associated with the procedure and that if the result is abnormal they will be facing the possibility of a late mid-trimester termination of pregnancy.

Recent trials carrying out amniocentesis earlier in pregnancy, at 12 to 14 weeks gestation, have yielded comparable rates of success in obtaining results and in the associated risk of miscarriage. However, this approach does not allow the option of a first trimester termination of pregnancy.

CHORIONIC VILLUS SAMPLING

In contrast to amniocentesis, *chorionic villus sampling*, which was first developed in China, enables prenatal diagnosis to be undertaken during the first trimester. This procedure is usually carried out at 10 to 11 weeks gestation under ultrasound guidance by either transcervical or transabdominal aspiration of chorionic villi (Fig. 21.2). These are fetal in origin being derived from the outer cell layer of the blastocyst, i.e. the trophoblast. Maternal decidua, normally present in the biopsy sample, must be removed before the sample is analysed.

Chromosome analysis can be undertaken either directly, looking at metaphase spreads from actively dividing cells, or following culture. Direct analysis usually gives a result within 24 hours. For single gene disorders, sufficient tissue is usually obtained to allow prenatal diagnosis by biochemical assay or DNA analysis using uncultured villi.

The major advantages of chorionic villus sampling are that it offers first trimester prenatal diagnosis and that chorionic villi provide a rich source of DNA. A disadvantage is that even in experienced hands this pro-

cedure conveys a risk of 2–3% for causing miscarriage. There is also evidence that this technique can cause limb abnormalities in the embryo if it is carried out before 9 weeks gestation.

ULTRASOUND

Ultrasound offers a valuable means of prenatal diagnosis. It can be used not only for obstetric indications, such as placental localisation and the diagnosis of multiple pregnancies, but also for the prenatal diagnosis of structural abnormalities which are not associated with known chromosomal, biochemical or molecular defects. Ultrasound is particularly valuable because it is non-invasive and conveys no known risk to the fetus or to the mother. It does, however, require specialised expensive equipment and an experienced operator.

Until recently, detailed ultrasound scanning for structural abnormalities was offered only to couples who had a child with a genetic disorder or syndrome for which there was no chromosomal, biochemical or molecular marker. For example, a search could be made for polydactyly as a diagnostic feature of a multiple abnormality syndrome, such as one of the autosomal recessive short limb polydactyly syndromes which are associated with severe pulmonary hypoplasia and are invariably lethal (Fig. 21.3). Similarly, a scan can reveal that the fetus has a small jaw which can be associated with a posterior cleft palate and other more serious abnormalities in several single gene syndromes (Fig. 21.4).

Increasingly, detailed 'fetal anomaly' scanning is now being offered routinely to all pregnant women around 18 weeks gestation as a screening procedure for structural abnormalities such as neural tube defects and cardiac anomalies. This technique can also identify features which suggest the presence of an underlying chromosomal abnormality (p. 273). Such a finding would lead to an offer of amniocentesis for definitive chromosome analysis.

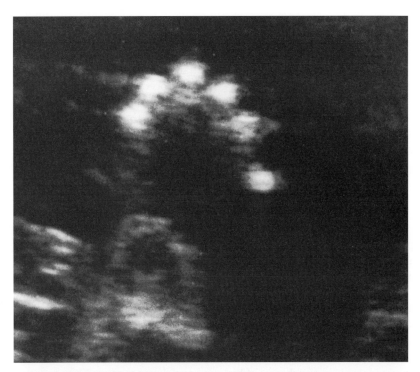

Fig. 21.3
Ultrasound image of a transverse section of the hand of a fetus showing polydactyly (courtesy of Dr D. Martinez, The General Infirmary at Leeds).

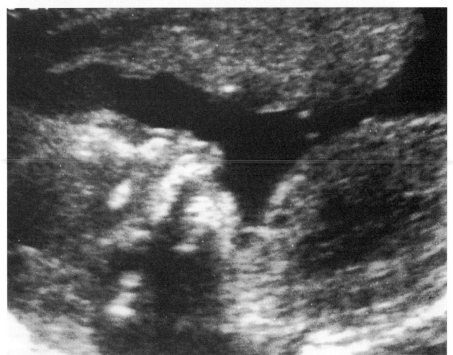

Fig. 21.4
Longitudinal sagittal ultrasound image of the head and upper chest of a fetus showing micrognathia (small jaw) (courtesy of Dr D. Martinez, The General Infirmary at Leeds).

FETOSCOPY

Fetoscopy involves visualisation of the fetus by means of an endoscope. Increasingly this technique is being superseded by detailed ultrasound scanning although occasionally fetoscopy is still undertaken during the second trimester to try to detect the presence of subtle structural abnormalities which would point to a serious underlying diagnosis.

Fetoscopy can also be used to obtain samples of tissue from the fetus which can be analysed as a means of achieving the prenatal diagnosis of several rare disorders. These include inherited skin disorders such as epidermolysis bullosa and metabolic disorders in which the enzyme is expressed only in certain tissues or organs such as liver, e.g. ornithine transcarbamylase deficiency (p. 132). Fetoscopy also allows a small sample of fetal blood to be obtained from one of the umbilical cord vessels in the procedure known as *cordocentesis*. This can be used for chromosome analysis to resolve problems associated with possible mosaicism.

Fetoscopy is associated with a 3–5% risk of miscarriage. This relatively high risk, coupled with the increasing sensitivity of ultrasound scanning and the rapid discovery of DNA markers for single gene disorders, explains why this technique is used only infrequently and in highly specialised prenatal diagnostic centres.

RADIOGRAPHY

The fetal skeleton can be visualised by radiography from 10 weeks onwards and this technique was used in the past to diagnose inherited skeletal dysplasias. This is now rarely if ever employed because of the dangers of radiography to the fetus (p. 18) and the widespread availability of the much safer approach of detailed ultrasound scanning.

MATERNAL SERUM SCREENING

In many centres it is now standard practice to offer screening for neural tube defects and Down's syndrome using a blood sample obtained from the mother at 16 weeks gestation. In this way up to 75% of all cases of open neural tube defect and 60% of all cases of Down's syndrome can be detected. This approach is considered further in the next chapter on screening (p. 270).

PREIMPLANTATION DIAGNOSIS

A technique which is still being developed and which will almost certainly find increasing use as a reproductive option for some couples is *preimplantation diagnosis*. In this procedure, an egg is removed from the female partner and fertilised in vitro using techniques developed for couples undergoing in vitro fertilisation (IVF) for infertility. The fertilised oocyte is cultured in the laboratory up to the 8 cell stage. A single cell, which is known as a *blastomere*, is removed and analysed by PCR (p. 48) to see if the zygote is affected by the disorder for which it is at risk. If not, it is implanted into the mother's uterus. This approach avoids the couple having to consider the possibility of termination of pregnancy. Preimplantation diagnosis has been used diagnostically in a limited number of instances to determine the sex of the zygote in the case of a couple at risk for Duchenne muscular dystrophy and for the prenatal diagnosis of cystic fibrosis.

The use of this technique requires caution. Despite the potential value of PCR, it is not surprising that, even in the best hands a procedure using only a single cell has a 10–20% failure rate. In addition, there is a significant risk that a false result will be obtained because of contamination. For example, desquamated skin from the laboratory worker carrying out the procedure could contaminate the reaction and would overwhelm the signal from the single cell of the zygote. For these reasons, centres developing this technique usually recommend that the mother subsequently undergoes an invasive form of prenatal diagnosis such as chorionic villus sampling in order to confirm the predicted result.

In the small number of cases in which preimplantation diagnosis has been carried out, the manipulation and removal of a cell from the zygote has not appeared to affect the subsequent development of the remaining cells. A variation of this technique, which it is believed could reduce the risk of any potential harm to the developing embryo, involves the removal of the first polar body from the unfertilised oocyte, which remains adjacent to the secondary oocyte under the zona pelludica. The oocyte and first polar body divide from each other during meiosis I and therefore contain different members of each pair of homologous chromosomes. Therefore it is unlikely that a genetic defect identified in the polar body will be present in the oocyte, which can then be fertilised and implanted in the uterus.

It is important to emphasise that in most centres carrying out IVF the likelihood that a couple will have a successful pregnancy, even without the manipulation involved in preimplantation diagnosis, is still relatively low. Therefore, preimplantation diagnosis should be regarded as a highly specialised and largely experimental technique.

DETECTION OF FETAL CELLS IN THE MATERNAL CIRCULATION

Finally, it is possible that an entirely non-invasive means of prenatal diagnosis for chromosome and DNA abnormalities will soon be developed. Using antibodies raised to cells of the fetal trophoblast, there is evidence that fetal cells are present in the maternal circulation in the first trimester. The validity of these claims has been substantiated by the use of PCR to detect the presence of paternally derived DNA markers in blood taken from women during early pregnancy. Although immunological techniques using antibodies to fetal trophoblast can be used to enrich fetal cells in the maternal circulation, problems can be encountered in obtaining a reliable signal of fetal origin and in excluding the possibility of significant maternal cell contamination in the sample being analysed. In addition, the use of this approach still requires a couple to have to consider termination of pregnancy as a possible outcome.

INDICATIONS FOR PRENATAL DIAGNOSIS

There are many indications for offering prenatal diagnosis. Ideally couples at high prior risk of having a baby with an abnormality should be identified and assessed before embarking upon a pregnancy so that they can be counselled at leisure. A less satisfactory but acceptable alternative is that such couples be identified early in pregnancy so that they still have an opportunity to consider all available prenatal diagnostic options. Unfortunately many couples with an increased risk, because of their family history or previous reproductive history, are not recognised or referred until mid-pregnancy, when it can be too late to offer the most appropriate prenatal diagnostic investigations.

ADVANCED MATERNAL AGE

This is the commonest indication for offering prenatal diagnosis. There is a well recognised association of advancing maternal age with increased risk of Down's syndrome (Table 17.4) and other trisomy syndromes. No standard criterion exists for determining at what age a mother should be offered the option of an invasive technique for fetal chromosome analysis. Most centres routinely offer amniocentesis or chorionic villus sampling to women aged 37 years or over, and the option is often discussed with women from the age of 35 years onwards. These ages relate to the maternal age at the expected date of delivery. The risk figures for Down's syndrome at the time of chorionic villus sampling, amniocentesis and delivery differ (Fig. 17.1) because a proportion of Down's syndrome pregnancies are lost spontaneously during the first and second trimesters.

PREVIOUS CHILD WITH A CHROMOSOME ABNORMALITY

For couples who have had a child with Down's syndrome due to non-disjunction, i.e. trisomy 21, or to a de novo unbalanced Robertsonian translocation, the risk in a subsequent pregnancy is the mother's age related risk plus approximately 0.5%. If one of the parents has been found to carry a balanced chromosome rearrangement which has caused a previous child to have a serious chromosome abnormality, then the recurrence risk is likely to be between 5% and 10% although the precise risk will depend on the nature of the parental rearrangement (p. 218).

FAMILY HISTORY OF A CHROMOSOME ABNORMALITY

Couples are often referred for possible prenatal diagnosis because of a family history of a chromosome abnormality, most commonly Down's syndrome. Usually there will be no increase in risk to the pregnancy as most cases of Down's syndrome and other chromosomal syndromes will have arisen as a result of non-disjunction rather than a familial rearrangement. However, each situation should be carefully evaluated, either by confirming the nature of the chromosome abnormality in the affected individual or, if this is not possible, by urgent chromosome analysis of blood from the relevant parent. A result can usually be obtained within 3–4 days and this will often mean that an invasive prenatal diagnostic procedure is not necessary.

FAMILY HISTORY OF A SINGLE GENE DISORDER

If prospective parents have already had a child with a serious single gene disorder, or if one of the parents has a positive family history which conveys a significant risk to offspring, then an offer of prenatal diagnosis is indicated. This can now be achieved for over 300 single gene disorders by either biochemical or molecular analysis.

FAMILY HISTORY OF A NEURAL TUBE DEFECT

Careful evaluation of the pedigree is necessary to determine the risk which applies to each pregnancy. Risks can be determined based on empiric data (p. 259). In high risk situations amniocentesis with assay of alpha-fetoprotein has been used for prenatal diagnosis in the past. Ultrasound examination of the fetus in conjunction with assay of maternal serum alpha-fetoprotein has proved equally reliable. Even with the best possible equipment small closed neural tube defects can be missed. Fortunately these do not usually cause the serious problems associated with open neural tube defects.

FAMILY HISTORY OF OTHER CONGENITAL STRUCTURAL ABNORMALITIES

As with neural tube defects, evaluation of the family pedigree should enable the provision of a risk derived from the results of empiric studies. If the risk to a pregnancy is increased, detailed ultrasound examination can be offered at around 16–18 weeks gestation. This technique will detect most serious cranial, cardiac, renal and limb malformations. Some couples request detailed ultrasound scanning not because they wish to pursue the option of termination of pregnancy but because they wish to prepare themselves for the stressful events surrounding delivery if the baby is found to be affected.

ABNORMALITIES IDENTIFIED IN PREGNANCY

The widespread introduction of prenatal diagnostic screening procedures, such as triple testing and fetal anomaly scanning, has meant that many couples are presented with diagnostic uncertainty which can only be resolved by an invasive procedure such as amniocentesis. Other factors such as poor fetal growth can also be an indication for prenatal chromosome analysis, as confirmation of a serious and non-viable chromosome abnormality such as triploidy can influence subsequent management of the pregnancy and mode of delivery.

OTHER HIGH RISK FACTORS

These include parental consanguinity, poor obstetric history and maternal illness. Parental consanguinity conveys an increased risk that a child will have a hereditary disorder or congenital abnormality (p. 210). Consequently, if the parents are concerned, it is appropriate to offer detailed ultrasonography to try to exclude a serious structural abnormality. A poor obstetric history such as recurrent miscarriage or previous unexplained stillbirth could indicate an increased risk of problems in a future pregnancy and would be an indication for detailed ultrasound monitoring. A history of three or more unexplained miscarriages should be investigated by parental chromosome studies (p. 229). A maternal illness such as poorly controlled insulin dependent diabetes mellitus or a history of ingestion of drugs such as sodium valproate (p. 203) would also be indications for detailed ultrasonography as both of these factors convey an increased risk of structural abnormality in a fetus.

PROBLEMS IN PRENATAL DIAGNOSIS

While the significance of the result of a prenatal diagnostic investigation is usually clear, situations can arise which pose major problems of interpretation. Problems also occur if the diagnostic investigation is unsuccessful or if an unexpected result is obtained.

AMNIOCENTESIS AND CHORIONIC VILLUS SAMPLING

Failure to obtain a sample or culture failure

It is important that every woman undergoing one of these techniques is alerted to the possibility that it can prove impossible to obtain a suitable sample or that subsequently the cells obtained fail to grow. Fortunately both of these risks are less than 1%.

An ambiguous chromosome result

In approximately 1% of cases, chorionic villus sampling shows evidence of apparent chromosome mosaicism, i.e. the presence of 2 or more cell lines with different chromosome constitutions. This can occur for several reasons:

1. The sample is contaminated by maternal cells. This is more likely to be seen using cultured cells than with direct preparations.
2. The mosaicism is a culture artefact. Usually several cell cultures are established. If mosaicism is present in only one culture then it is probably not a true reflection of the fetal karyotype.
3. The mosaicism is limited to a portion of the placenta, i.e. *confined placental mosaicism*. This arises due to an error in mitosis during the formation and development of the trophoblast.
4. There is true fetal mosaicism.

In order to resolve the uncertainty generated by the finding of mosaicism using chorionic villi it is often necessary to proceed to amniocentesis. If this yields a normal result then it is concluded that the result obtained from chorionic villi was not a true indication of the fetal karyotype.

In the case of amniocentesis it is routine in most laboratories for the sample to be split and for two or three separate cultures to be established. If a single abnormal cell is identified in only one culture this is assumed to be a culture artefact, what is termed level 1 mosaicism or *pseudomosaicism*. If the mosaicism extends to two or more cells in two or more cultures this is taken as evidence of true mosaicism or what is known as level 3 mosaicism. The most difficult situation to interpret is when mosaicism is present in two or more cells in only one culture, what is termed level 2 mosaicism. This is most likely to represent a culture artefact but there is a risk of up to 20% that the mosaicism will be present in the fetus.

Counselling couples who find themselves in this situation is always extremely difficult. Even if true mosaicism is confirmed it can be impossible to predict the probable phenotypic outcome. An attempt can be made to resolve ambiguous findings by proceeding to fetal blood sampling for urgent karyotype analysis. Whatever the parents decide, it is important that tissue such as placenta or blood is obtained for chromosome analysis after delivery for confirmation of the findings.

An unexpected chromosome result

Three different situations can arise. Firstly, a diagnosis other than Down's syndrome can be obtained, such as one of the sex chromosome aneuploidy syndromes, e.g. 45,X, 47,XXX, 47,XXY, 47,XYY. Ideally all women undergoing amniocentesis should be alerted to this possibility before the test is carried out although in practice this is not always done. When a diagnosis such as Turner's syndrome (45,X) or Klinefelter's syndrome (47,XXY) is obtained it is essential that the parents be given full details of the nature and consequences of the diagnosis. Recent studies have shown that when objective and informed counselling is available, less than 50% of the parents of a fetus with an 'incidental' diagnosis of a sex chromosome abnormality opt for termination of pregnancy.

The second situation involves the discovery of an apparently balanced chromosome rearrangement, such as an inversion or translocation. If parental chromosome studies show that this is familial, then the parents can be reassured that it is very unlikely that this will cause any problems in the fetus. The opportunity should also be taken to investigate the extended family. If, however, the apparently balanced rearrangement has occurred as a de novo event, then there is a risk of between 5% and 10% that the fetus will have physical abnormalities or show subsequent mental handicap. Presumably this reflects subtle imbalance, which is not perceptible, or damage to a critical gene at one or both of the rearrangement break-

points. It is not surprising that couples who find themselves in this situation can have great difficulty in deciding what to do. Detailed ultrasonography, if normal, can provide some, but not complete, reassurance.

The third situation which presents a difficult counselling problem is the discovery of a small additional chromosome known as a *marker chromosome*. If this is present in one of the parents, then it is unlikely that it will be of significance to the fetus. If, on the other hand, it is a de novo finding, there is a risk of up to 15% that the fetus will be phenotypically abnormal. The risk is lower if the marker chromosome has satellites (p. 23) and contains heterochromatin (p. 24), than if it does not have satellites and contains euchromatin (p. 24).

ULTRASOUND

The increasing sophistication of mid-trimester ultrasonography has resulted in the identification of subtle anomalies, the significance of which is not always clear. For example, choroid plexus cysts are sometimes seen in the cerebral ventricles (Fig. 21.5). Initially it was thought that these were invariably associated with the fetus having trisomy 18. It is now known that choroid plexus

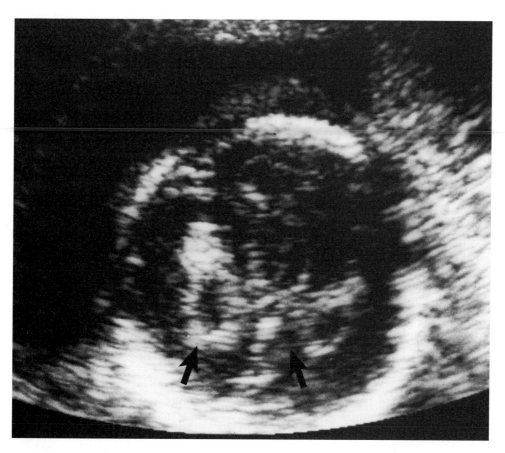

Fig. 21.5
Ultrasound scan of a fetal brain showing bilateral choroid plexus cysts (arrowed) (courtesy of Dr D. Martinez, The General Infirmary at Leeds).

cysts occur frequently in normal fetuses, although if they are very large and do not disappear spontaneously they can be indicative of a chromosome abnormality.

This example of difficulty in distinguishing normal from abnormal variation coupled with lack of knowledge of the natural history of other commonly observed findings, such as mild enlargement of the cerebral ventricles, emphasises the importance of viewing new reports of apparent ultrasound abnormalities and their association(s) with caution.

TERMINATION OF PREGNANCY

The presence of a serious abnormality in a fetus is an acceptable legal indication for termination of pregnancy. This does not mean that this is an easy decision for a couple to make. It is essential that all couples undergoing any form of prenatal diagnostic investigation, whether invasive or non-invasive, be provided with information about the practical aspects of termination of pregnancy. This should include an explanation that while termination in the first trimester is carried out by surgical means under general anaesthetic, a woman undergoing a mid-trimester termination will have to experience labour and delivery.

PRENATAL DIAGNOSIS AND TREATMENT

So far in this chapter attention has focused on the prenatal diagnosis of abnormalities with the subsequent option of termination of pregnancy. While this applies in most situations, there is cautious optimism that with the advent of gene therapy (p. 278) prenatal diagnosis will, in time, lead not to termination but to effective intra-uterine treatment.

A model for successful prenatal treatment is provided by the autosomal recessive disorder congenital adrenal hyperplasia (pp. 134, 226). Affected female infants are born with virilisation of the external genitalia. There is evidence that in a proportion of cases this can be prevented if the mother takes a powerful steroid known as dexamethasone in a very small dose from 4–5 weeks gestation onwards. Specific prenatal diagnosis can be achieved by DNA analysis of chorionic villi. If this procedure confirms that the fetus is both female and affected, then the mother continues to take low doses of dexamethasone throughout pregnancy. This suppresses the fetal pituitary–adrenal axis and prevents virilisation of the female fetus. If the fetus is not female and affected, the mother ceases to take dexamethasone and the pregnancy proceeds uneventfully.

When gene therapy has been proved to be both safe and effective, the fact that the fetus is immunologically tolerant should make it easier to commence such therapy

before birth rather than afterwards. This will have the added advantage of reducing the period in which irreversible damage can occur in organs such as the central nervous system, which is affected by progressive neurodegenerative disorders such as Tay–Sachs disease.

ELEMENTS

1 Prenatal diagnosis can be carried out by non-invasive procedures such as maternal serum alpha-fetoprotein screening for neural tube defects, the triple test for Down's syndrome and ultrasonography for structural abnormalities.

2 Specific prenatal diagnosis of chromosome and single gene disorders usually requires an invasive technique such as amniocentesis or chorionic villus sampling by which material of fetal origin can be obtained.

3 Invasive prenatal diagnostic procedures convey small risks for causing miscarriage, i.e. amniocentesis 0.5–1%, chorionic villus sampling 2–3%, fetoscopy 3–5%.

4 The commonest indication for prenatal diagnosis is advanced maternal age. Other conditions include a family history of a chromosome, single gene or structural abnormality and an increased risk predicted on the result of a screening test.

5 While the significance of most prenatal diagnostic findings is clear, situations can arise in which the implications for the fetus are very difficult to predict. When this occurs the parents should be given as much information as possible.

FURTHER READING

Brock D J H, Rodeck C H, Ferguson Smith M A (eds) 1992 Prenatal diagnosis and screening. Churchill Livingstone, Edinburgh
A very comprehensive multiauthor text-book covering all aspects of prenatal diagnosis.
Drife J O, Donnai D (eds) 1991 Antenatal diagnosis of fetal abnormalities. Springer-Verlag, London
The proceedings of a workshop on the practical aspects of prenatal diagnosis.
Lilford R J (ed) 1990 Prenatal diagnosis and prognosis. Butterworths, London
Provides useful information on recurrence risks for Down's syndrome, the prognosis for abnormalities detected by ultrasound, and decision analysis.
Whittle M J, Connor J M (eds) 1989 Prenatal diagnosis in obstetric practice. Blackwell Scientific Publications, Oxford
Describes prenatal diagnostic techniques and the types of abnormalities identified.

CHAPTER

CHAPTER 22 | Population screening and community genetics

Increasing awareness of the role of genetics in the aetiology of disease and its overall impact on the burden imposed on individuals, families and society has led to the introduction of several population genetic screening programmes. The branch of medical genetics which is concerned with screening and the prevention of genetic disease on a population basis is known as *community genetics*.

Population screening involves the offer of genetic testing on an equitable basis to all individuals in a defined population. Its primary objective is to enhance autonomy by enabling individuals to be better informed about genetic risks and reproductive options. A secondary goal is the prevention of morbidity due to genetic disease and alleviation of the suffering that this would impose.

CRITERIA FOR A SCREENING PROGRAMME

These can be considered under the headings of the disease, the test and the practical aspects of the programme (Table 22.1).

THE DISEASE

The disease should be relatively common and have potentially serious effects which are amenable to prevention or amelioration. This can involve the early introduction of treatment, as in the case of neonatally diagnosed

Table 22.1 Criteria for a screening programme

Disease	— high incidence in target population — serious effect on health — treatable or preventable
Test	— non-invasive and easily carried out — accurate and reliable — inexpensive
Programme	— widespread with equitable availability — voluntary participation — acceptable to the target population — full information and counselling provided

phenylketonuria (p. 129), or termination of pregnancy for disorders which cannot be treated effectively and which convey a high likelihood of serious ill-health.

THE TEST

The test should be accurate and reliable with high sensitivity and specificity. *Sensitivity* refers to the proportion of cases which are detected. A measure of sensitivity can be made by determining the proportion of *false-negative* results, i.e. how many cases are missed. *Specificity* refers to the extent to which the test detects only affected individuals. If unaffected persons are detected, these are referred to as *false-positives*.

THE PROGRAMME

The programme should be offered in a fair and equitable manner and should be widely available. It must also be morally acceptable to a substantial proportion of the population to which it is offered. Participation must be entirely voluntary. Easily understood information and well informed counselling should both be readily available.

It is often stated that the cost of a screening programme should be reasonable and affordable. This does not mean that the potential savings gained through a reduction in the number of affected cases requiring treatment has to exceed or even balance the cost of screening, although this is an argument which is popular with health administrators and planners who have to fund the programme. It is reasonable to point out that cost-benefit analyses also have to take into account non-tangible factors such as the emotional costs of human suffering borne by both the affected individuals and those who care for them.

PRENATAL SCREENING PROGRAMMES

NEURAL TUBE DEFECTS

In 1972 it was recognised that many pregnancies in which the baby had an open neural tube defect (NTD)

(p. 200) could be detected at 16 weeks gestation by assay of a protein in maternal serum known as alpha-fetoprotein (αFP). αFP is the fetal equivalent of albumin and is the major protein in fetal blood. If the fetus has an open NTD, the level of αFP is elevated in both the amniotic fluid and maternal serum as a result of leakage from the open defect.

Unfortunately maternal serum αFP screening for NTDs is neither 100% sensitive nor 100% specific. The curves for the levels of maternal serum αFP in normal and affected pregnancies overlap (Fig. 22.1), so that in practice an arbitrary cut-off level has to be introduced below which no further action is taken. This is usually either the 95th centile or 2.5 multiples of the median, and as a result around 75% of screened open spina bifida cases are detected. Those pregnant women with results which lie above this arbitrary cut-off level are offered further investigations such as detailed ultrasonography and possibly also amniocentesis, which gives a clearer distinction between the levels of αFP in normal and affected pregnancies.

Lack of specificity is due to the elevation in maternal serum αFP which can occur for other reasons (Table 22.2) such as a threatened miscarriage, twin pregnancy, or other fetal abnormality such as an exomphalos, in which there is a protrusion of abdominal contents through the umbilicus.

DOWN'S SYNDROME AND OTHER CHROMOSOME ABNORMALITIES

The triple test

Confirmation of a chromosome abnormality in an unborn baby requires cytogenetic studies using material obtained by an invasive procedure such as chorion villus sampling or amniocentesis (p. 261). However, chromosome abnormalities, and in particular Down's syndrome,

Table 22.2   Causes of elevated maternal serum αFP

Anencephaly
Open spina bifida
Incorrect gestational age
Intra-uterine fetal bleed
Threatened miscarriage
Multiple pregnancy
Congenital nephrotic syndrome
Abdominal wall defect

can be screened for in pregnancy by taking into account risk factors such as maternal age and the levels of three biochemical markers in maternal serum (Table 22.3).

This latter approach is based on the discovery that, at 16 weeks gestation, maternal serum αFP and unconjugated oestriol levels tend to be reduced in Down's syndrome pregnancies as compared with normal pregnancies, whereas the level of maternal serum human chorionic gonadotrophin is usually elevated. None of these parameters gives absolute discrimination, but taken together they provide a means of modifying a woman's prior age-related risk to give an overall probability that the unborn baby is affected. When this probability exceeds 1 in 250 amniocentesis is offered.

Table 22.3   Maternal risk factors for Down's syndrome

	MOM*
Advanced age (35 years or over)	
Maternal serum	
α-fetoprotein (αFP)	(0.75)
unconjugated oestriol (μE$_3$)	(0.73)
human chorionic gonadotrophin (hCG)	(2.05)

*Numbers in brackets refer to the mean values in affected pregnancies expressed as multiples of the median (MOM's) in normal pregnancies.

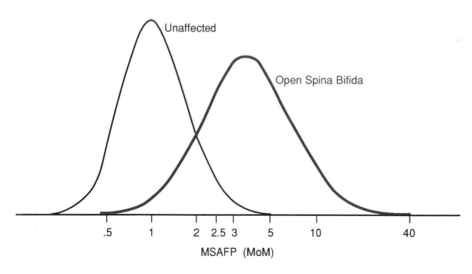

Fig. 22.1
Maternal serum αFP levels at 16 weeks gestation plotted on a logarithmic scale as multiples of the median (MOM's). Women with a value on or above 2.5 multiples of the median are offered further investigations.
(Adapted from Brock D J H, Rodeck C H, Ferguson-Smith M A (eds) 1992 Prenatal diagnosis and screening. Churchill Livingstone, Edinburgh.)

Table 22.4 Detection rates using different Down's syndrome screening strategies

Screening procedure	% of all pregnancies tested	% of Down's syndrome cases detected
Age alone		
40 years and over	1.5	15
35 years and over	7	35
Age + αFP	5	34
Age + αFP, μE₃ + hCG	5	61

Using age alone as a screening parameter, if all pregnant women aged 35 years and over opt for fetal chromosome analysis approximately 35% of all Down's syndrome pregnancies will be detected (Table 22.4). If the aforementioned three biochemical markers are also included, this being the so called *triple test*, 60% of all Down's syndrome pregnancies will be detected using a risk of 1 in 250 or greater as the criterion for offering amniocentesis. This approach will also result in the detection of approximately 50% of all cases of trisomy 18 (p. 218).

Ultrasonography

In many centres it is now standard practice to offer a detailed 'fetal anomaly' scan to all pregnant women at 18 weeks gestation. Although chromosome abnormalities cannot be diagnosed directly, their presence can be suspected by the detection of an abnormality such as nuchal oedema with generalised fetal hydrops (Fig. 22.2) or a rocker-bottom foot (Fig. 22.3) (Table 22.5). A chromosome abnormality is found in 50–60% of fetuses with a cystic hygroma identified at 18 weeks, and a rocker-bottom foot is a characteristic finding in babies with trisomy 18 (p. 218).

NEONATAL SCREENING PROGRAMMES

Routine biochemical screening of newborn infants for phenylketonuria was recommended by the Ministry of

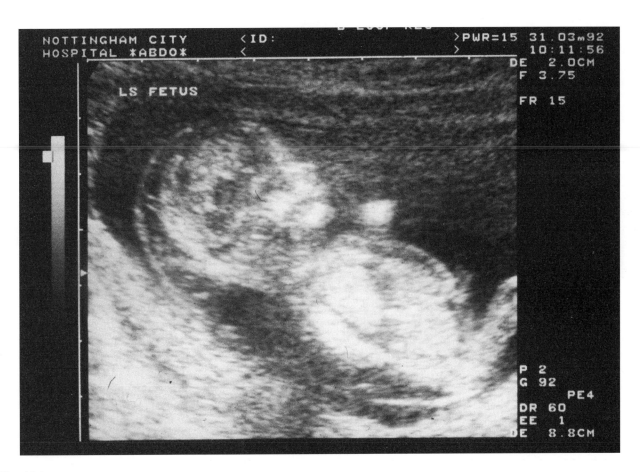

Fig. 22.2
Ultrasound scan at 18 weeks showing generalised oedema around the fetus, i.e. fetal hydrops (courtesy of Dr D. Rose, City Hospital, Nottingham).

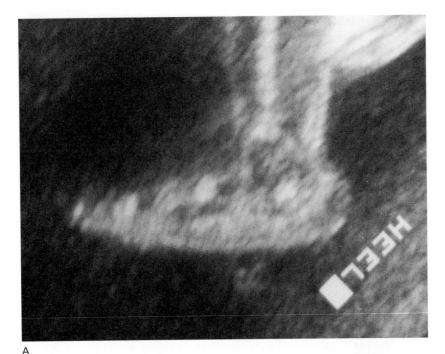

A

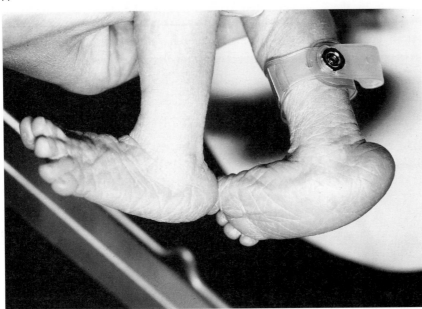

B

Fig. 22.3
(A) Ultrasound scan at 18 weeks showing a rocker-bottom foot in a fetus subsequently found to have trisomy 18, together with (B) a photograph of the feet of a newborn with trisomy 18 (courtesy of Dr D. Rose, City Hospital, Nottingham).

Health in the United Kingdom in 1968 after it had been shown that a low phenylalanine diet could prevent the severe mental retardation which previously had been a hallmark of this condition (p. 127). The screening test, which is sometimes known as the Guthrie test, is carried out on a small sample of blood obtained by heel-prick at age 7 days. An abnormal test result is further investigated by repeat analysis of phenylalanine in a venous blood sample. A low phenylalanine diet is extremely effective in preventing mental retardation, and, although it is not particularly palatable, most affected children can be persuaded to adhere to it until early adult life when it

can be relaxed. Any woman with phenylketonuria who is contemplating pregnancy should adhere, however, to a strict low phenylalanine diet to minimise the risk of brain damage to her unborn child (pp. 129, 203).

Neonatal biochemical screening programmes have been devised for several other disorders (Table 22.6), although not all of these conditions are included in every programme. The other condition for which neonatal screening is almost universal is congenital hypothyroidism. Strictly speaking, this condition should not be included in a discussion on screening for genetic disorders as it is usually not genetic in origin being due to absence of

Table 22.5 Prenatal ultrasound findings suggestive of a chromosome abnormality

Feature	Chromosome abnormality
Cardiac defect (especially common atrio-ventricular canal)	Trisomy 13, 18, 21
Choroid plexus cysts	Trisomy 18, 21
Clenched overlapping fingers	Trisomy 18
Cystic hygroma or fetal hydrops	Trisomy 13, 18, 21, Turner's syndrome
Duodenal atresia	Trisomy 21
Exomphalos	Trisomy 13, 18
Rocker bottom foot	Trisomy 18

Table 22.6 Conditions suitable for neonatal screening

Disorder	Test
Widely applied	
Phenylketonuria	Phenylalanine
Congenital hypothyroidism	Thyroid stimulating hormone
Specific populations only	
Congenital adrenal hyperplasia	17-hydroxyprogesterone
Cystic fibrosis	Immunoreactive trypsin
Duchenne muscular dystrophy	Creatine kinase
Sickle-cell disease	Haemoglobin electrophoresis

development of the thyroid gland. Life-long treatment with thyroxine is effective and the clinical picture of severe mental retardation formerly associated with 'cretinism' is now rarely encountered.

POPULATION CARRIER SCREENING

Widespread screening for carriers of autosomal recessive disorders in high incidence populations was first introduced for the haemoglobinopathies (p. 118) and has been extended to several other disorders (Table 22.7). The rationale behind these programmes is that carrier detection can be supported by genetic counselling so that carrier couples will have been forewarned of the 1 in 4 risk that each of their children could be affected.

Experience with the two common haemoglobinopathies, thalassaemia and sickle-cell disease, illustrates the extremes of success and failure which can result from well planned or poorly devised screening programmes.

THALASSAEMIA

α- and β-thalassaemia are caused by abnormal globin chain synthesis due to mutations involving the α- and β-

Table 22.7 Autosomal recessive disorders suitable for population carrier screening

Disorder	Ethnic group or community	Test
α-thalassaemia	China and eastern Asia	Mean corpuscular haemoglobin and haemoglobin electrophoresis
β-thalassaemia	Indian sub-continent and Mediterranean countries	Mean corpuscular haemoglobin and haemoglobin electrophoresis
Sickle-cell disease	Afro-Caribbeans	Sickle test and haemoglobin electrophoresis
Cystic fibrosis	Western European Caucasians	ΔF508 mutation analysis
Tay–Sachs disease	Ashkenazi Jews	Hexosaminidase A

globin genes respectively (p. 121). Both disorders show autosomal recessive inheritance, and both are extremely common in certain parts of the world, notably China (α-thalassaemia) and Cyprus, Italy and the Indian sub-continent (β-thalassaemia).

In Cyprus in 1974 the birth incidence of β-thalassaemia was 1 in 250. Following the introduction of a comprehensive screening programme to determine the carrier status of young adults, the incidence of affected babies declined by over 95% within 10 years. Similar programmes in Greece and Italy have seen a drop in the incidence of affected homozygotes of over 50%.

If it is acceptable to judge the success of these screening programmes on the basis of a reduction in the births of affected babies, then these programmes have certainly been successful, due largely to the efforts of highly motivated staff interacting with a well informed target population which has usually opted not to have affected children.

SICKLE-CELL DISEASE

In contrast to the Cypriot response to β-thalassaemia screening, early attempts to introduce sickle-cell carrier detection in the black population of North America were disastrous. Information pamphlets tended to confuse the sickle-cell carrier state, or trait, which is usually harmless, with the homozygous disease which conveys significant morbidity (p. 119). Several US states passed legislation making sickle-cell screening in blacks mandatory, and sickle-cell carriers began to be discriminated against by employers and insurance companies. It is not surprising that public criticism was aroused leading to abandonment of the screening programmes and amendment of the ill-conceived legislation.

This experience with sickle-cell carrier screening emphasises the importance of ensuring voluntary participation and providing adequate and appropriate information and counselling. More recent pilot studies in the United States and in Cuba have shown that individuals of Afro-Caribbean origin are perfectly receptive to well planned non-directive sickle-cell screening programmes.

CYSTIC FIBROSIS

The discovery in 1989 that the ΔF508 deletion/mutation accounts for a high proportion of all cystic fibrosis heterozygotes soon led to the suggestion that screening programmes could be implemented for carrier detection on a population basis. In the white population of the United Kingdom, the cystic fibrosis carrier frequency is approximately 1 in 22 and the ΔF508 mutation accounts for 75–80% of all heterozygotes. A further 10% of carriers can be detected relatively easily and cheaply using a multiplex PCR analytical procedure.

Initial studies of attitudes to cystic fibrosis carrier detection have yielded quite divergent results. A casual written invitation generates a poor take-up response of around 10%, whereas personal contact during early pregnancy, whether mediated through general practice or the ante-natal clinic, results in uptake rates of over 80%. Pilot studies are underway to explore attitudes to cystic fibrosis screening amongst specific groups such as school leavers and women in early pregnancy.

POSITIVE AND NEGATIVE ASPECTS OF POPULATION SCREENING

Well planned population screening enhances informed choice and offers the prospect of a significant reduction in the incidence of disabling genetic disorders. These potential advantages have to be weighed against the potential disadvantages which can arise from the over-enthusiastic pursuit of a poorly planned or ill-judged screening programme (Table 22.8). Experience to date indicates that in relatively small well informed groups, such as the Greek Cypriots and American Ashkenazi

Jews, community screening is welcomed. When screening is offered to larger populations the outcome is less certain.

GENETIC REGISTERS

Most clinical genetic units maintain what is known as a *genetics register* of families and individuals who are either affected by or at risk of developing a serious hereditary disorder. The primary purpose of a genetics register is to maintain two-way contact between a genetics unit and relevant family members (Table 22.9). This permits investigations to be offered as appropriate and ensures that families do not feel abandoned or excluded from a source of information and support.

Table 22.9 Roles of a genetics register

To maintain an informal two-way communication process between the family and the genetics unit

To offer carrier detection to relevant family members as they reach adult life

To coordinate presymptomatic and prenatal diagnosis when requested

To coordinate multidisciplinary management of patients with complex hereditary conditions such as the familial cancer syndromes

To ensure effective implementation of new technology and treatment

To provide a long-term source of information and support

Table 22.8 Potential advantages and disadvantages of genetic screening

Advantages
Informed choice
Improved understanding
Early treatment when available
Reduction in births of affected homozygotes

Disadvantages and hazards
Pressure to participate causing mistrust and suspicion
Stigmatisation of carriers (social, insurance and employment)
Inappropriate anxiety in carriers

Table 22.10 Disorders suitable for a genetics register

Disorder	Chromosome location
Autosomal dominant	
Adult polycystic kidney disease	16
Familial hypercholesterolaemia	19
Huntington's disease	4
Multiple endocrine neoplasia types 1 and 2	11/10
Myotonic dystrophy	19
Neurofibromatosis types 1 and 2	17/22
Polyposis coli	5
Retinoblastoma	13
Von Hippel Lindau syndrome	3
Autosomal recessive	
Cystic fibrosis	7
Sickle-cell disease	11
Thalassaemia	11/16
X-linked	
Duchenne/Becker muscular dystrophy	
Fragile X syndrome	
Haemophilia	
Retinitis pigmentosa	
Chromosomal	
Inversions	
Translocations	

Entry on to a genetics register is entirely voluntary and it is essential that confidentiality is not breached. Information is never revealed to outside agencies without the consent of the relevant individual.

Genetic registers are most appropriate for conditions which are relatively common, have potentially serious effects, convey high risks to other family members and in which complications can be treated or prevented (Table 22.10). They are particularly valuable for conditions which show a delayed age of onset or in which unaffected carriers could be at high risk of having seriously affected children.

Well-organised genetics registers can also play a key role in coordinating a multidisciplinary approach to the management of patients with conditions such as the familial cancer predisposing syndromes (p. 175). The management of such patients often involves the interpretation of molecular investigations and the organisation of regular visits to other hospital departments where screening for early signs of malignancy can be undertaken (p. 177). Programmes of this nature are much appreciated by family members and can make a major contribution to improving the quality of life for individuals and families at risk of developing serious genetic disease.

ELEMENTS

1 Population screening involves the offer of genetic testing to all members of a particular population, with the primary objective being the enhancement of informed personal choice.

2 Participation should be voluntary and each programme should be widely available, equitably distributed, acceptable to the target population and supported by full information and counselling.

3 Prenatal screening is now offered routinely for neural tube defects, by assay of maternal serum alpha-fetoprotein, and for chromosome abnormalities by assay of up to three biochemical markers using a technique known as the 'triple' test.

4 Neonatal screening is widely available for phenylketonuria and congenital hypothyroidism. Other conditions are screened for in specific populations.

5 Population screening programmes for carriers of β-thalassaemia have resulted in a major fall in the births of affected homozygotes. Similar programmes could be equally effective for sickle-cell disease and cystic fibrosis if care is taken to ensure that these are acceptable to their target populations.

6 Well organised genetic registers provide an effective means of maintaining two-way contact between genetics centres and families with hereditary disease.

FURTHER READING

Brock D J H, Rodeck C H, Ferguson Smith M A (eds) 1992 Prenatal diagnosis and screening. Churchill Livingstone, Edinburgh
A huge multiauthor text-book with excellent chapters on all aspects of genetic screening.
Modell B, Modell M 1992 Towards a healthy baby. Oxford University Press, Oxford
A clearly written and easily understood guide to genetic counselling and community genetics.

CHAPTER 23

New developments: gene therapy and the human genome project

Many genetic disorders are characterised by progressive disability or chronic ill-health for which there is no effective treatment. Consequently one of the most exciting aspects of the explosive developments in biotechnology is the prospect of successful gene therapy.

CONVENTIONAL APPROACHES TO TREATMENT

Most genetic disorders cannot be cured or even ameliorated using conventional methods. Often this is because the underlying gene and its product have not been identified so that there is little if any understanding of the basic metabolic or molecular defect. If, however, this is understood, then dietary restriction, as in phenylketonuria (p. 127) or hormone replacement, as in congenital adrenal hyperplasia (p. 134), can be used very successfully. In a few disorders, such as homocystinuria (p. 131) and some of the organic acidurias (p. 138), supplementation with a vitamin or coenzyme can increase the activity of the defective enzyme and have a beneficial effect (Table 23.1).

If a genetic disorder is found to be due to a deficiency of or an abnormality in an enzyme or protein then, in theory, the defective enzyme or protein can be replaced. An obviously successful example is the use of factor VIII concentrate in haemophilia A.

In most of the inborn errors of metabolism in which an enzyme deficiency has been identified, simple enzyme replacement has not been possible because, until recently, sufficient quantities of the enzyme or protein have not been available. In addition, even if available, it could be predicted that injection of the enzyme or protein would be unsuccessful as the metabolic processes involved are carried out within cells. Delivery systems, such as *liposomes*, allow proteins to cross the cell membrane. Liposomes are artificially prepared cell-like structures in which one or more bimolecular layers of phospholipid enclose one or more aqueous compartments, which can include proteins. Unfortunately, liposomes have met with little success in the treatment of disorders such as the mucopolysaccharidoses, in which it was hoped that such a therapy could be effective. Biochemical modification of the protein or enzyme, as has been carried out with β-glucosidase in the case of Gaucher's disease, allows normal cellular transport mechanisms to target the enzyme to the lysosomes and has met with some success as an effective form of treatment (p. 137).

In other genetic disorders drug therapy is possible, e.g. certain drugs can help lower cholesterol levels in familial hypercholesterolaemia (p. 134). In others, avoidance of drugs or certain foods, can prevent the manifestation of the disorder, e.g. sulphonamides in G6PD deficiency (p. 145).

Replacement of defective tissue is another option which became available with the advent of tissue typing (p. 159), e.g. renal transplantation in adult polycystic kidney disease. Removal of diseased tissue to prevent complications is a prophylactic or therapeutic option in many of the familial cancer predisposing syndromes (p. 179).

For a number of serious genetic disorders it is necessary to consider less frequently used and, on occasion, drastic and/or unproven therapeutic options. These include bone marrow transplantation for some of the neurodegenerative disorders. This approach has met with some success in the treatment of some of the mucopolysaccharidoses.

THERAPEUTIC APPLICATIONS OF RECOMBINANT DNA TECHNOLOGY

The advent of recombinant DNA technology, in the first instance, led to diagnostic tests and the beginning of an

Table 23.1 Examples of various methods for treating genetic disease

Treatment	Disorder
Enzyme induction by drugs	
phenobarbitone	congenital non-haemolytic jaundice
Replacement of deficient enzyme/protein	
tissue transplantation	
blood transfusion	SCID due to adenosine deaminase deficiency
bone marrow transplantation	mucopolysaccharidoses
enzyme/protein preparations	
trypsin	trypsinogen deficiency
α_1-antitrypsin	α_1-antitrypsin deficiency
cryoprecipitate/Factor VIII	haemophilia A
α-glucosidase	Gaucher's disease
Replacement of deficient vitamin or coenzyme	
B6	homocystinuria
B12	methylmalonicacidaemia
biotin	proprionicacidaemia
D	vitamin D resistant rickets
Replacement of deficient product	
cortisone	congenital adrenal hyperplasia
thyroxine	congenital hypothyroidism
Substrate restriction in diet	
amino acids	
phenylalanine	phenylketonuria
leucine, isoleucine, valine	maple syrup urine disease
carbohydrate	
galactose	galactosaemia
lipid	
cholesterol	familial hypercholesterolaemia
protein	urea cycle disorders
Drug therapy	
aminocaproic acid	angioneurotic oedema
dantrolene	malignant hyperthermia
cholestyramine	familial hypercholesterolaemia
pancreatic enzymes	cystic fibrosis
penicillamine	Wilson's disease, cystinuria
Drug/dietary avoidance	
sulphonamides	G6PD deficiency
barbiturates	porphyria
Replacement of diseased tissue	
kidney transplantation	adult polycystic kidney disease, Fabry's disease
bone marrow transplantation	X-linked SCID, Wiskott–Aldrich syndrome
Removal of diseased tissue	
colectomy	polyposis coli
splenectomy	hereditary spherocytosis

understanding of the molecular pathology of genetic diseases. Further developments have led rapidly to progress in the availability of *biosynthetic* gene products and the planning of strategies for successful gene therapy.

BIOSYNTHESIS OF GENE PRODUCTS

Until recently insulin used in the treatment of diabetes mellitus has been obtained from pig pancreas. This has to be very carefully purified for use and even then it

occasionally produces sensitivity reactions in patients. However, with recombinant DNA technology, microorganisms can be used to synthesise insulin from the human insulin gene. This is inserted, along with appropriate sequences to ensure efficient transcription and translation, into a plasmid and cloned in *E. coli*. In this way large quantities of insulin can be made. An artificial gene needs to be constructed for this purpose which is not identical with the natural gene. This is because synthetically produced genes must not contain the noncoding intervening sequences, or introns (p. 12), found in the majority of structural genes in eukaryotic organisms, as *E. coli* does not possess a means for splicing of the mRNA during transcription.

Recombinant DNA technology is being employed in the synthesis of a number of other substances (Table 23.2). The biosynthesis of medically important peptides in this way is usually more expensive than obtaining the product from conventional sources. However, this approach has the dual advantages of providing a pure product which is unlikely to induce a sensitivity reaction and which is free of the risk of contaminating viruses. In the past, the use of growth hormone from human cadaver pituitaries has been associated with the transmission of Jacob–Creutzfeldt disease, and the human immunodeficiency virus (HIV) has been a contaminant in cryoprecipitate used in the treatment of haemophilia A.

GENE THERAPY

Gene therapy can be defined as the replacement of a deficient gene product or correction of an abnormal gene. Conventional approaches to gene therapy by, for example, hormone supplementation have already been reviewed. New approaches to gene therapy have as their goal the introduction of a normal functional gene into somatic

Table 23.2 Proteins produced biosynthetically using recombinant DNA technology (? = effectiveness not yet proven)

Protein	Disease
Insulin	Insulin dependent diabetes mellitus
Growth hormone	Short stature due to growth hormone deficiency
Factor VIII	Haemophilia A
Factor IX	Haemophilia B
Interferon	Infections, cancer (?)
α_1-antitrypsin	Emphysema due to α_1-antitrypsin deficiency (?)
Somatostatin	Excess growth
Vaccines	Hepatitis B, malaria and other tropical diseases (?)

cells in patients who are deficient for the normal gene product.

Until recently the possibility of successful gene therapy belonged in the realms of science fiction. However, recent advances in molecular biology leading to the identification of many important human disease genes and their protein products have opened up new opportunities for research and raised the prospect of successful gene therapy for many genetic and non-genetic disorders. It is important to emphasise that although gene therapy is often presented as the new panacea in medicine, its impact, at least in the short term, will be limited and its application will be fraught with many practical difficulties.

REGULATORY REQUIREMENTS

Regulatory bodies have been established in several countries to oversee the technical, therapeutic and safety aspects of gene therapy programmes (p. 290). In the United States the Human Gene Therapy Subcommittee of the National Institutes of Health has produced guidelines for protocols of trials of gene therapy which must be submitted for approval to both the Food and Drug Administration and the Recombinant DNA Advisory Committee. A similar body in the United Kingdom, known as the Committee on the Ethics of Gene Therapy, has recommended that all gene therapy programmes must be approved by hospital research ethical committees.

There is universal agreement that *germ line gene therapy*, in which genetic changes could be distributed to both somatic and germ cells, and therefore be transmitted to future generations, is unacceptable. Therefore all programmes must focus only on *somatic cell gene therapy*, in which the alteration in genetic information is targeted to cells of specific organs.

TECHNICAL ASPECTS

Gene characterisation

One of the basic prerequisites of gene therapy is that the gene involved should have been cloned. This should include not only the structural gene which needs to be expressed but also the DNA sequences involved in the control and regulation of expression. While this prerequisite would seem obvious, some of the early attempts at gene therapy were carried out when little was known about the regulatory or control regions of structural genes needed for normal gene expression. In retrospect, it is clear that these early attempts at gene therapy were both premature and naive in their expectation of achieving success.

Target cells

The cells which are to be treated must be identifiable. Again this seems obvious. Some of the early attempts at treating the inherited disorders of haemoglobin, such as β-thalassaemia, involved removing bone marrow from affected individuals, treating it in vitro, and then returning it to the patient by transfusion. While in principle this could have worked, in order to have any likelihood of success, the particular cells which needed to be targeted were the stem cells from which the reticulocytes develop.

Vector system

The means by which a foreign gene is introduced needs to be both efficient and safe. If gene therapy is to be considered as a realistic alternative to conventional treatments, there should be unequivocal evidence from animal experiments that the inserted gene functions adequately with regulatory, promoter and enhancer sequences. In addition, it needs to be shown that the treated cell population has a reasonable life span, that the gene product continues to be expressed and that the body does not react adversely to the gene product, e.g. by producing antibodies to the protein product. Lastly, it is essential to demonstrate that introduction of the foreign gene has no deleterious effects, such as malignancy or a mutagenic effect on either the somatic or the germ cell lines, e.g. insertional mutagenesis (p. 166). This latter possibility needs to be considered even if the treatment is directed to somatic tissues.

METHODS OF GENE THERAPY

These can be divided into two main types, viral and physical.

Viral agents

A number of different viruses can be used to transport foreign genetic material into cells. Each of these has advantages and disadvantages.

Retroviruses

These are derived from a family of viruses which include the human immunodeficiency virus and viruses which can cause cancer in certain species (p. 164). They are the most extensively developed viral vector systems used so far. Retroviruses integrate into the host DNA by making a copy of their RNA molecule using the enzyme reverse transcriptase (p. 165). The provirus so formed is the template for the production of the mRNAs for the various viral gene products and the new genomic RNA of the virus. If the provirus is stably integrated into dividing stem cells, all subsequent progeny cells will inherit a copy of the viral genome.

Retroviruses used in gene therapy are rendered incapable of replication so as not to produce the side effects associated with infectivity. For this to be achieved, retroviruses used in gene therapy require 2 elements, a packaging cell line and a vector or helper virus.

Packaging cell line

The *packaging cell line* is a cell line which has been infected with a retrovirus in which the provirus is genetically engineered to lack the region of the proviral DNA called the *packaging sequence*. This means that the cells will produce all of the normal viral proteins but the provirus cannot be packaged into infectious virus particles.

Vector or helper virus

Another retroviral provirus is engineered with more than 90% of the viral genetic material removed, leaving only the minimal sequences necessary to produce copies of the viral RNA sequences along with the sequences necessary for packaging of the viral genomic RNA. This is the vector backbone into which the foreign DNA or gene can be inserted. If this vector, or *helper* virus, is introduced into the packaging cell line which contains the provirus which is missing the packaging sequences, the RNA produced by the vector provirus can be packaged into viruses. These *virions* can be used to infect, or what is more correctly called *transduce*, the particular target cells. Transduce is the more appropriate term as the virions do not replicate and produce further infective virions since the retrovirus vector cannot replicate because it lacks the sequences necessary for this to occur (Fig. 23.1).

Disadvantages

One of the disadvantages associated with the use of retroviruses as a vector system in gene therapy is that only a small amount of genetic information can be introduced into the target cells, usually less than 7 kb. For example, even if all of the introns were removed from the dystrophin gene (p. 240) for use in gene therapy of Duchenne muscular dystrophy, the gene would still be too large to be incorporated into a retroviral vector. In this instance, attempts have been made to insert a dystrophin gene in which a large amount of the gene has been deleted but which still has relatively normal function or what is known as a *minidystrophin* gene.

A second disadvantage of using retroviruses as vectors in gene therapy is that they can only infect dividing cells. This means that disorders affecting, for example, the central nervous system would not be amenable to this approach. In addition, at present, retroviruses can only be used in vitro. In theory, with identification of the receptors on cells for retroviruses, they could also be used to target specific cell types in vivo.

A further disadvantage of retroviruses is that they are unstable and cannot be purified for use in gene therapy without reducing their ability to transduce their target cells. As a consequence, retrovirus preparations from cultured cells cannot be fully characterised so that it is not possible to exclude contamination with replication competent retroviruses or packaging of cellular RNAs which could act as an oncogene. This is not simply a theoretical risk as there has been a report of lymphoma

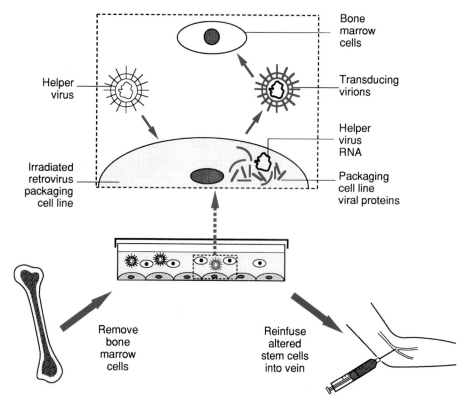

Bone marrow cells

Helper virus

Transducing virions

Irradiated retrovirus packaging cell line

Helper virus RNA

Packaging cell line viral proteins

Remove bone marrow cells

Reinfuse altered stem cells into vein

Fig. 23.1
Representation of retrovirus gene therapy using bone marrow cells.

occurring in Rhesus monkeys subjected to trials of retro-viral gene therapy.

Difficulties in controlling the level of expression of the introduced gene have been encountered in animal trials of retrovirus mediated gene therapy. Improvements in retrovirus mediated gene therapy are likely with targeting of specific cells, e.g. stem cells in bone marrow, and with inclusion of the appropriate control or regulatory sequences.

Adenoviruses

Adenoviruses can be used as vectors in gene therapy. They have advantages over retroviruses in that they are stable and can be easily purified to produce high titres for infection. In addition, they are suitable for targeted treatment of specific tissues such as the respiratory tract. Unlike retroviruses, they can infect non-dividing cells and they also carry larger segments of foreign DNA, up to 36 kb in length.

One disadvantage of adenoviruses is that they do not integrate into the host genome and as a consequence expression of the introduced gene is usually unstable and often transient. In addition, by virtue of their infectivity, they produce adverse effects secondary to infection and by stimulating the host immune response. Lastly, adenoviruses contain genes known to be involved in malignant transformation so that there is a potential risk that they could induce malignancy.

Herpes virus

Herpes viruses are neurotropic and, if suitably modified, could be used to target gene therapy to the central nervous system. An immediate disadvantage of using herpes viruses as a vector system is their direct toxic effects on nerve cells as well as the consequent immune response.

Herpes viruses do not integrate into the host genome and therefore it is likely that the expression of introduced genes would be unstable.

Other viruses

Other viruses, including the polio, vaccinia and a number of other RNA viruses could be used as vectors in gene therapy as they produce large quantities of gene product. However, many are likely to have problems similar to those seen with other vector systems.

Physical agents

Liposome mediated DNA transfer

This involves complexing plasmid DNA with liposomes which fuse with the cell membrane allowing the introduction of foreign DNA into the target cell (Fig. 23.2). A disadvantage of this technique is that expression of the foreign gene is transient, so that treatment has to be repeated. An advantage of using this technique is that a much larger amount of DNA can be introduced than with viral vector systems. This can be as large as an artificially constructed *minichromosome* which, in addition to a particular structural gene, can include elements for regulation of gene expression in a physiologically controlled fashion along with centromeric and telomeric elements which allow replication of the foreign DNA as a separate entity.

Receptor mediated endocytosis

A variation of liposome mediated gene transfer is to target the DNA to specific receptors on cells. A complex is made between plasmid DNA containing the foreign gene and specific polypeptide ligands for which the cell

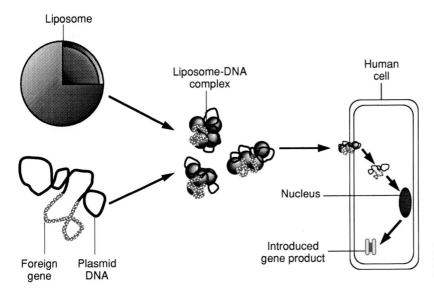

Fig. 23.2
Representation of liposome mediated gene therapy.

has a receptor. For example, DNA complexed to a glyco-protein containing galactose will be recognised by receptors on liver cells which are specific to glycoproteins with a terminal galactose. This results in internalisation of the complex into endocytic vesicles, which are then transported to the lysosomes where the complex is degraded. In order for the foreign gene to be expressed, it has to escape from the lysosome. The rate at which it escapes from the lysosomes can be increased by inclusion of adenovirus or fusogenic influenza gene products.

Oligonucleotides

It is possible to synthesise what are known as *antisense oligonucleotides* which bind to specific mRNA sequences. This can result in blocking of mRNA processing and protein synthesis of that particular mRNA species. Difficulties arise, however, in ensuring that the oligonucleotide enters the relevant target cells. Alternatively, an oligonucleotide can be synthesised to a sequence in a gene which will form a triple helical structure with double stranded genomic DNA. If the stretch of triple helix is then alkylated, then that gene can be disabled permanently. This latter approach is also of limited value as the oligonucleotide must be up to 15 to 18 bp in length and composed primarily of the purine nucleotides adenine and guanine, a combination which occurs only rarely in the coding sequences of most genes.

Future methods

It is likely that the development of vector systems for gene therapy in the future will involve a convergence of viral and non-viral technologies, such as virus targeted integration into a specific region of DNA in particular cell types through specific receptor mediated endocytosis.

Animal models

One of the basic prerequisites for assessing the suitability of gene therapy trials in humans is the existence of an animal model. While there are naturally occurring animal models for some inherited human diseases, for most there is no animal counterpart. Site directed DNA mutagenesis allows the targeted introduction of mutations into a gene (p. 53). If carried out in the embryonic cells of an inbred species, the subsequent offspring will be mosaics for the normal and mutated gene. These animals can then be interbred to produce animal models which will be homozygous for the introduced mutation. Several groups, using homologous recombination (p. 53), have been able to *knock out* the CFTR gene (p. 238) in mouse embryonic cells to produce a mouse model for cystic fibrosis. These mice have been confirmed as transgenic animal models

for cystic fibrosis by having symptoms and findings similar to those seen in humans with the disease. These mice also have an abnormal chloride channel. This animal model has been used to evaluate several types of gene therapy before trials in humans.

Target organs

In most instances gene therapy will need to and should be directed to a particular organ, tissue or body system.

Liver
Viral vectors for gene therapy of inherited hepatic disorders have been of limited use due to the lack of vectors which specifically target hepatocytes. Although liver cells are refractory to retroviruses in vivo, they are, somewhat surprisingly, susceptible to transduction by retroviruses in vitro. Cells removed from the liver by partial hepatectomy can be treated in vitro and then reinjected via the portal venous system from where they seed in the liver. The effectiveness of this approach has been demonstrated by the lowering of cholesterol levels in a rabbit animal model with a defect in the low density lipoprotein receptor. The injection of the hepatocytes into the portal venous system is, however, associated with a significant risk of thrombosis of the portal venous system which can lead to the complication of portal hypertension. Nevertheless, because of the serious outlook for homozygotes with mutations in the LDL receptor (p. 135), gene therapy by this means has been attempted in a woman homozygous for an LDL receptor defect. This has led, in the short term, to a reduction of LDL levels, although the long term benefit is, as yet, undetermined. Other disorders affecting or involving the liver in which a similar approach could be considered are phenylketonuria, α_1-antitrypsin deficiency and haemophilia A.

CNS
CNS directed vector systems are being developed in which replication defective neurotropic adenoviruses lacking the so-called E1 region can be produced and then be made infective by growing them in cells engineered to express the E1 genes.

Another approach which has been suggested in genetic disorders affecting the CNS is to transplant cells which have been genetically modified in vitro into specific regions of the brain, such as the caudate nucleus in Huntington's disease.

Muscle
Unlike other tissues, direct injection of foreign DNA into muscle has met with some success in terms of retention and expression of the foreign gene in the treated muscle. Alternatively, injection of myoblasts into muscle results in their incorporation into recipient muscle bundles. This

approach can be used to express the protein products of genes, transferred in vitro into myoblasts which are unrelated to muscle function, e.g. human growth hormone and factor VIII. Other primary cell types, such as fibroblasts treated in vitro, could also be transplanted back as skin grafts to deliver circulating gene products.

Bone marrow

In the treatment of disorders affecting the bone marrow problems arise due to the low frequency of stem cells, these being the cells which need to be transduced if there is be more than a transient response. Stem cells often constitute less than 1% of the total cells present. Pretreatment of the bone marrow to expand the number of stem cells has been tried for certain inherited immunological disorders by the use of growth factors such as the granulocyte-colony stimulating factor (G-CSF) and the cytotoxic agent 5-fluorouracil. Reliable identification of specific stem cell types would enable them to be enriched for thereby increasing the likelihood of success.

DISEASES AMENABLE TO GENE THERAPY

The disorders which are possible candidates for gene therapy include both genetic and non-genetic diseases (Table 23.3).

Genetic disorders

There are a number of single gene diseases which are obvious candidates for gene therapy. One of the first diseases for which gene therapy has been attempted in humans is the inherited immunodeficiency disorder due to adenosine deaminase (ADA) deficiency (p. 155). Somewhat surprisingly, it has been found that persons with this disorder respond to simple blood transfusions. The adenosine deaminase activity present in the transfused blood transiently corrects the immunodeficiency in the lymphocytes of the affected patients. Treatment with polyethylene conjugated adenosine deaminase increases the half-life of the enzyme in the circulation. Trials of treatment with ADA deficient lymphocytes transduced with a retroviral vector with the ADA gene are underway at present.

Attempts at treating thalassaemia and sickle-cell disease by gene therapy have not been effective as yet, primarily because of difficulties in the identification of sequences involved in the normal control of the expression of the globin genes (p. 115).

Double blind trials are being carried out in the United Kingdom and the United States treating cystic fibrosis patients using either a liposome–gene complex or an adenovirus vector sprayed into the nasal passages. Studies of their efficacy and safety involve looking for the

Table 23.3 Genetic and non-genetic diseases which can potentially be treated by gene therapy

Genetic disorder	Defect
Immune deficiency	Adenosine deaminase deficiency Purine nucleoside phosphorylase deficiency
	Chronic granulomatous disease
Hypercholesterolaemia	Low density lipoprotein receptor abnormalities
Haemophilia	Factor VIII deficiency (A) Factor IX deficiency (B)
Gaucher's disease	glucocerebrosidase deficiency
Mucopolysaccharidosis VII	β-glucuronidase deficiency
Emphysema	α_1-antitrypsin deficiency
Cystic fibrosis	CFTR mutations
Phenylketonuria	phenylalanine hydroxylase deficiency
Urea cycle abnormalities Hyperammonaemia	Ornithine transcarbamylase deficiency
Citrullinaemia	argininosuccinate synthetase deficiency
Muscular dystrophy	Dystrophin mutations
Thalassaemia/Sickle-cell disease	α and β globin mutations
Cancer Malignant melanoma Ovarian cancer Brain tumours Neuroblastoma Renal cancer Lung cancer	
Acquired immunodeficiency syndrome (AIDS)	
Cardiovascular diseases	
Rheumatoid arthritis	

presence of the introduced CFTR gene in biopsies of the nasal epithelium and measurement of ion transport in nasal epithelial cells.

Common multifactorial diseases

In the majority of human diseases, in which there is a genetic aetiology, both genes and environmental factors are involved (pp. 106, 181). Gene therapy will have a much more widespread impact in medicine if it can be used in this group of disorders. It is important, however, to remember that for most of the common non-genetic diseases in humans, the identification, and subsequent avoidance, of causative environmental factors is likely to be much more effective than gene therapy in its present form.

Cancer

Gene therapy for cancer involves the introduction of toxic genetic elements into tumour cells. This can be achieved in several different ways.

Supply tumour suppressor genes

It has been proposed that the targeted introduction of recognised tumour suppressor genes (p. 170), such as p53, to cancer cells could result in control of their growth. More detailed knowledge of the biology of cancer will be needed before this approach will be reliable.

Target immunological mitogen genes into tumour cells

Mitogens, such as interleukin-2, introduced in vivo into melanosomes which have been removed from patients with malignant melanoma and then reintroduced into the patient, could be used to activate the patient's immune response. The use of liposome bound plasmid DNA, containing foreign histocompatibility genes to transduce tumour cells to enhance the immune response has also been proposed as a possible form of gene therapy in cancer. Again, a better understanding of the malignant process and the body's immune response to malignancy will be necessary for this form of gene therapy to be effective.

Introduce genes which selectively damage cancer cells

The introduction of the tumour necrosis factor gene into tumour infiltrating lymphocytes, which can then be return-ed to the patient, has been promoted as another approach for gene therapy in cancer. More recently, a proposal has been made to introduce what have been called *conditionally toxic genes* into cancer cells. An example is the thymidine kinase gene of the herpes simplex virus which allows the metabolism of the substance ganciclovir by cellular kinases into the triphosphate form which inhibits DNA polymerase resulting in the death of the cancer cells as well as surrounding cells by a 'bystander' effect.

Other modalities

These include the use of antisense oligonucleotides to block the gene products of oncogenes, as well as the introduction of genes into bone marrow cells to render them resistant to chemotherapeutic agents.

Coronary artery disease

It has been proposed that gene therapy could be used to introduce the LDL receptor into persons with a family history of early coronary artery disease even if they do not have familial hypercholesterolaemia.

Peripheral vascular disease

It has been suggested that in persons with peripheral vascular disease arterial vessel segments or vascular grafts could be resurfaced with endothelial or smooth muscle cells into which anticlotting agent genes have been introduced.

Rheumatoid arthritis

Interleukin-1 (IL-1) is an immune system signal which triggers inflammation. It has been proposed that gene therapy could be used to introduce genes for the IL-1 receptor antagonist protein into synovial cells in persons with rheumatoid arthritis, in which the inflammatory process is believed to play a key aetiological role.

Acquired immunodeficiency syndrome (AIDS)

It could be possible to render individuals resistant to infection with human immunodeficiency virus by using gene therapy to inhibit the release of viral progeny from infected cells in the disease process.

THE HUMAN GENOME PROJECT

The human genome project involves a major international collaborative effort to map and sequence the entire human genome. This is clearly a huge undertaking given that the haploid human genome contains between 50 000 and 100 000 genes and consists of approximately 3 000 000 000 base pairs.

Vast financial resources are being directed towards this enterprise. In the United States, the National Institutes of Health has a National Center for Human Genome Research (NCHGR). The budget for the NCHGR in 1994 will be in excess of US $100 000 000. This is only a small part of the planned expenditure which amounts to over $3 000 000 000 over a 15 year period!. Other nations including France, Japan and the United Kingdom are also investing large sums of public and charitable money in major gene mapping projects.

Understandably, opponents of the human genome project argue that expenditure of this magnitude could be better used in other medical and scientific research. Supporters of the project maintain that this research will be of major benefit by improving our understanding of disorders in which genetic factors are involved, thereby leading to the development of new strategies for their prevention and treatment.

At a practical level the project is overseen by the Human Genome Organisation (HUGO). Annual work-shops are held at which information is pooled and individual chromosome maps compiled. The results are published and are available to all interested parties.

GENE MAPPING STRATEGIES

The approach previously taken by participants at the Human Genome Mapping meetings (p. 62) involved mapping each individual chromosome. A major strategy being pursued by a number of centres participating in the human genome project, which can be viewed as a 'top end down' approach, involves the production of what are variously known as *index, framework,* or *skeleton* maps of the whole genome. This involves using highly polymorphic DNA markers such as di-, tri-, and tetranucleotide repeats (p. 55) situated less than 15 centiMorgans apart. These can be ordered either by linkage studies or by a combination of physical mapping techniques such as somatic cell hybridisation (p. 59), fluorescent in situ hybridisation (FISH) (p. 28) and the construction of overlapping YAC contigs (p. 61).

Once a gene associated with a disease is mapped to such an *index* or *framework map* of the human genome, it can then be isolated by conventional physical cloning methods. Alternatively there are now techniques such as exon trapping (p. 62) or identification of expressed sequences from cDNA libraries (p. 48) which will provide a source of what are known as *expressed sequence tags* (ESTs).

Sequencing of the human genome

Another approach to the human genome project is to sequence the whole of the human genome. This can be viewed as a 'small end up' strategy. Technically, this is difficult as the human genome contains large sections of repetitive DNA (p. 11) which are resistant to cloning and sequencing. In addition, a large amount of effort could be wasted as the regions likely to be of greatest importance, the expressed sequences or genes, only constitute a small fraction of the total genome (p. 11).

It is also important to consider the magnitude of this approach. Using conventional sequencing technology it is estimated that a single laboratory worker could sequence up to 2000 bp per day. This means that it would take 1.5×10^6 person days to sequence the whole of the human genome! Projects which involved sequencing in other organisms indicate just how much work is involved. For example, it took 35 laboratories in 17 countries to sequence the 315 000 bp of chromosome 3, one of the 16 chromosomes in yeast. The potential benefits of this approach can be demonstrated, however, by the fact that although 34 genes had previously been mapped to this yeast chromosome, sequence data revealed 182 sequences with open reading frames and appropriate regulatory elements, i.e. in excess of 140 new genes were identified by this means. Similar projects are being undertaken in other species, such as the round worm, *Caenorhabditis elegans,* which has 100×10^6 bp in its genome.

The human genome project is an ambitious undertaking which has generated heated discussion and debate. Given the rapid progress which is occurring in sequencing technology and data management, it is entirely plausible that the entire genome will have been mapped by the end of the millennium with enormous implications for the amelioration of human suffering.

ELEMENTS

1 Treatment of genetic disease by conventional means requires identification of the gene product and an understanding of the pathophysiology of the disease process. Therapeutic options can include dietary restriction or supplementation, drug therapy, replacement of an abnormal or deficient protein or enzyme and replacement or removal of an abnormal tissue.

2 Recombinant DNA technology has enabled human derived biosynthetic gene products such as human insulin and growth hormone to be produced for the treatment of human disease.

3 Before a trial of gene therapy is carried out in humans, the gene involved must be characterised, the particular cell type or tissue to be targeted must be identified, an efficient, reliable and safe vector system has to be developed which results in stable continued expression of the introduced gene, and the safety and effectiveness of the particular modality of gene therapy has to be demonstrated in an animal model.

4 Germ line gene therapy is universally viewed as ethically unacceptable, while somatic cell gene therapy is generally viewed as being acceptable, as this is seen as similar to existing treatments such as organ transplantation.

5 The human genome project is an international research effort, the purpose of which is to track down the genes responsible for inherited disease in humans and determine the sequence of the human genome. Although justification of the planned expenditure is controversial, this research is likely to pay dividends in our understanding of both genetic and non-genetic diseases.

FURTHER READING

Anderson W F 1992 Human gene therapy. Science 256: 808–813
A consideration of gene therapy by one of its main proponents.
Cappecchi M R 1994 Targeted gene replacement. Scientific American 270: 34–41
Review of the techniques to produce transgenic animal models for inherited diseases in humans.
Chumakov I, Rigault P, Guillou S et al 1992 Continuum of overlapping clones spanning the entire human chromosome 21q. Nature 39: 380–387
Overlapping clones of the entire long arm of chromosome 21!
Müller-Hill 1993 The shadow of genetic injustice. Nature 362: 491–492
A brief commentary urging caution against being caught up in the enthusiasm for the human genome project.
Mulligan R C 1993 The basic science of gene therapy. Science 260: 926–936

A considered review of the problems and approaches to gene therapy.
Cooperative Human Linkage Center: Murray J C, Buetow K H, Weber J L, Ludwigsen S, Scherpbier-Heddema T, Manion F, Quillen J, Sheffield V C, Sunden S, Duyk G M,; Genethon: Weissenbach J, Gyapay G, Dib C, Morrissette J, Lathrop G M, Vignal A; University of Utah: White R, Matsunami N, Gerken S, Melis R, Albertsen H, Plaetke R, Odelberg S,; Yale University; Ward D; Centre d'Etude du Polymorphisme Humain (CEPH); Dausset J, Cohen D, Cann H 1994 Comprehensive human linkage map with centimorgan density. Science 265: 2049–2054.
The human gene map based on highly polymorphic markers produced by collaboration between the Centre d'Etude de Polymorphisme Humain, the National Institutes of Health and Genethon.

Ethical considerations

INTRODUCTION

Ethical issues can be defined as those which involve moral questions and dilemmas. Traditionally they are approached by applying a set of moral principles, based usually on a synthesis of the philosophical and religious views of well-informed, respected, thinking members of society. In this way a code of practice evolves which is seen as reasonable and acceptable by a majority and which often forms the basis of professional guidelines or regulations.

Ethical issues arise in all branches of medicine but are particularly contentious in genetics because of the way this subject impinges not just on an individual but also on the extended family and on society in general. In the minds of the general public, clinical genetics and genetic counselling can be easily confused with *eugenics*, which can be defined as the science of 'improving' a species through breeding. It is important to emphasise that the modern specialty of clinical genetics has absolutely nothing in common with the totally unacceptable eugenic philosophies which were practised in Nazi Germany and, to a much lesser extent, in the United States between the two world wars. Genetic counselling is a **non-directive** and **non-judgmental** communication process whereby factual knowledge is imparted to facilitate informed personal choice.

Nevertheless clinical genetics is a subject which lends itself to ethical debate, not least because of the new opportunities provided by discoveries in molecular genetics. In this chapter some of the more controversial and difficult areas will be considered. It will soon become apparent that for many of these issues there is no right or wrong answer and individual views will vary widely. Sometimes in a clinical setting the best that can be hoped for is arrival at a mutually acceptable compromise with an explicit agreement that opposing views are respected and, personal conscience permitting, a patient's expressed wishes are carried out.

GENERAL PRINCIPLES

When undertaking any patient contact there are a number of important general principles to keep in mind.

INFORMED CONSENT

A patient is entitled to an honest and full explanation before any procedure or test is undertaken. Information should include details of the risks, limitations and implications of each procedure.

INFORMED CHOICE

A patient is entitled to full information about all options available including the option of not participating. Potential consequences should be discussed. No duress should be applied and the doctor or nurse should not have a vested interest in the patient pursuing any particular course of action.

AUTONOMY

The patient is in charge. At any stage he or she can decide to proceed no further.

CONFIDENTIALITY

A patient has a right to complete confidentiality which can only be breached under extreme circumstances, such as when it is deemed that a patient's behaviour could convey a high risk of harm to himself or to others.

Potential areas of conflict in clinical genetics include genetic testing in children (pp. 250, 289), the distinction between research and service, and the rights of the individual versus the rights of the extended family, the doctor and society. These points will be illustrated in the following situations.

PRENATAL DIAGNOSIS

Many methods are now widely available for diagnosing structural abnormalities and genetic disorders during the first and second trimesters (p. 261). The use of these techniques for monitoring pregnancies at risk generates little controversy. It is the ensuing possibility of termination of pregnancy on the grounds of fetal abnormality which causes unease and raises very sensitive issues surrounding the severity of abnormality which can be considered to justify termination as an option and the way in which society provides for children and adults with disability.

In the United Kingdom termination of pregnancy is permitted up to and beyond 24 weeks gestation if the fetus has a lethal condition such as anencephaly, or if there is a serious risk of major physical or mental handicap. Terms such as 'serious' are not defined in the relevant legislation.

Prenatal diagnosis and termination of pregnancy (p. 268), sometimes mistakenly called 'therapeutic' abortion, raise many difficult issues. The general principles of informed consent and informed choice are particularly pertinent. In the United Kingdom approximately 70% of all pregnancies are monitored for neural tube defects by measurement of alpha-fetoprotein in maternal serum at 16 weeks gestation (p. 269). It is unlikely that all of these women have a full understanding of all aspects of the test and resources are not always available to provide detailed counselling. Similarly, many women have a detailed ultrasound scan to assess fetal anatomy (pp. 262, 271) without realising that an abnormality could be detected which would lead to termination of pregnancy as an option. It is obvious that accurate and full information should be provided by unhurried staff who are well-informed, experienced and sympathetic.

The most difficult problems in prenatal diagnosis are those surrounding autonomy and individual rights. Parents have rights, doctors and nurses have rights, and the unborn fetus has rights but no means of expressing them. Medical staff have a legal right not to participate in termination of pregnancy on conscientious grounds but are expected to refer their patient to a colleague who has no such objections. At one end of the spectrum, there is widespread agreement that being of the 'wrong' sex is not an abnormality and does not provide grounds for termination of pregnancy.

Problems can arise when the fetus is found to have a relatively mild abnormality such as non-syndromal cleft lip and palate for which surgical correction usually achieves an excellent outcome. For some parents, particularly those who have themselves had an unhappy childhood because of being stigmatised for a similar problem, the prospect of having a similarly affected child can be unacceptable.

It is inevitable that a subject as emotive as termination of pregnancy will generate controversy. Proponents of choice argue that selective termination is the lesser of two evils when compared to a life time of pain and suffering. Usually prenatal diagnostic techniques provide reassurance and their availability allows many couples to embark upon a pregnancy from which they would otherwise have been deterred. When viewed in the context of abortion in general, termination on the grounds of fetal abnormality constitutes only a very small proportion of the total of well over 100 000 abortions carried out each year in the United Kingdom.

Those who hold opposing views argue on religious, moral or ethical grounds that selective termination is little less than legalised infanticide. There is also concern that prenatal diagnostic screening programmes will lead to a devaluing of handicapped individuals in society with a shift of resources away from their care to the funding of additional programmes aimed at 'preventing' their birth. The cost—benefit argument can be persuasive in cold financial terms but takes no account of the fundamental human and social issues which are involved.

POPULATION SCREENING

Population screening programmes offering carrier detection for common autosomal recessive disorders have been in operation for many years (p. 273). These have been well received for thalassaemia and Tay–Sachs disease, for which screening has been carefully planned with well-informed and highly motivated target populations. In contrast, efforts to introduce sickle-cell carrier detection in North America have generally been unsuccessful. Pilot studies assessing the responses to cystic fibrosis carrier screening in Caucasian populations have yielded conflicting results (p. 274).

The differing receptions to these various screening programmes illustrate the importance of informed consent and the difficulties of ensuring both autonomy and informed choice. For example, it has been suggested that screening for cystic fibrosis carrier status could be included in the neonatal screening programme or be introduced as an option for all school children at age 16 years. Clearly newborn infants cannot make an informed choice and it is doubtful whether all 16-year-olds are sufficiently mature to make a fully reasoned decision for themselves.

Consequently many pilot studies have focused on adults and their responses to the offer of carrier testing from either their general practitioner or in the antenatal clinic. This has raised the vexed question of whether an offer from a respected family doctor could be interpreted as a tacit recommendation to participate which cannot be easily refused. A personal 'opportunistic' invitation to participate from a general practitioner yields a much higher acceptance rate than a casual written invitation to attend for screening at a future date. This difference in rates of uptake could simply be a reflection of inertia but could also indicate that patients feel pressurised to agree to a test which they do not actually want.

It is therefore important that even the most well intended offer of carrier detection should be worded carefully so as to ensure that participation is entirely voluntary. Full counselling in the event of a positive result is also essential to minimise the risk of a feeling of stigmatisation or genetic inferiority.

In population screening confidentiality is also important. Many carriers will not wish their carrier status to be known amongst classmates or colleagues at work. The issue of confidentiality will become particularly difficult for individuals who are found to be genetically susceptible to a potential industrial hazard such as smoke or dust. There is concern that such individuals will be discriminated against by potential employers (p. 149) and doctors could find themselves in the invidious position of having to provide information which jeopardises their patient's employment prospects.

FAMILY SCREENING

It is widely agreed that the identification of a carrier of a condition which could have implications for other family members should lead to the offer of tests for the extended family. This applies particularly to carriers of balanced translocations and serious X-linked recessive disorders. In the case of translocations this is sometimes referred to as translocation 'chasing'. For an autosomal recessive disorder such as cystic fibrosis the term cascade screening is applied (p. 238).

The main ethical problem raised by family screening is that of confidentiality. A carrier of a translocation or serious X-linked recessive disorder is usually urged to alert close family relatives to the possibility that they could also be carriers and therefore be at risk of having affected children. Alternatively, permission can be sought for members of the genetics team to make these approaches. Occasionally a patient, for whatever reason, will refuse to allow this information to be disseminated.

Faced with this situation what should the clinical geneticist do? In practice most clinical geneticists would try to convince their patient of the importance of offering tests to relatives, possibly by providing an explanation of the consequences and ill-feeling which could result in the future if an affected baby were to be born in the family whose birth could have been predicted and perhaps avoided. Often skilled and sensitive counselling will lead to a satisfactory solution. Ultimately, however, most clinical geneticists would opt to respect their patient's confidentiality rather than break the trust which forms a cornerstone of the traditional doctor–patient relationship.

PREDICTIVE TESTING

The development of molecular techniques for diagnosing single gene disorders either by direct mutational analysis or indirectly using linkage (pp. 57, 247) has made it possible to offer predictive or presymptomatic testing for adult onset disorders such as familial adenomatous polyposis and Huntington's disease. This has raised several important ethical issues.

PREDICTIVE TESTING IN CHILDHOOD

Understandably, parents sometimes wish to know whether or not a child has inherited the gene for an adult onset autosomal dominant disorder which is in the family. It can be argued that this knowledge will help the parents guide their child towards the most appropriate educational and career opportunities and that to refuse their request is a denial of their rights as parents.

The problem with agreeing to this request is that it is a clear infringement of the child's own future autonomy. Increasingly, it is felt that testing should be delayed until the child reaches an age when he or she can make his or her own informed decision. There is also concern about the possible deleterious effects on a child of growing up with the certain knowledge of developing a serious adult onset hereditary disorder.

The situation is very different if predictive testing could be of direct medical benefit to the child. This applies to conditions such as familial hypercholesterolaemia (p. 134) for which early dietary management can be introduced and also to some of the familial cancer predisposing syndromes (p. 175) for which early screening is indicated.

PREDICTIVE TESTING WITH IMPLICATIONS FOR INTERMEDIATE FAMILY RELATIVES – 'DIAGNOSIS BY PROXY'

A positive test result in an individual can have major implications for close antecedent relatives who themselves do not wish to be informed of their disease status. Once again, consider Huntington's disease (HD) for which direct mutational analysis is now available. A young man aged 20 years requests predictive testing prior to starting his family. His fears are based on a confirmed diagnosis in his 65-year-old paternal grand-father. Predictive testing would be relatively straightforward were it not for the fact that his father, who is obviously at a prior risk of 1 in 2, specifically does not wish to know whether he will develop the disease.

Thus the young man has raised the difficult question of how to comply with his request without inadvertently carrying out a predictive test on his father. A negative result in the young man leaves scope for doubt so that in principle no harm would be done. A positive result in the son, however, would be difficult to conceal from an observant father who will be alert to his son's subsequent behaviour. Clearly a positive result in the son would indicate that the father must be heterozygous for the HD gene.

There is no easy solution to this particular problem. The son is entitled to have the test and the best compromise probably involves alerting both the son and his father to the sensitivities of their situation in the hope that they themselves can resolve it in a satisfactory manner.

PREDICTIVE TESTING AND THE INSURANCE INDUSTRY

The availability of predictive tests for adult onset disorders which convey a special health risk or the chance of a reduced life expectancy has opened up a public debate on the extent to which the results of these tests should be revealed to outside agencies such as life insurance companies. In countries with only limited public health care services, this will also be an issue for private health care insurance. Furthermore, if either life or health insurance are arranged by an employer, then there will also be implications for long-term career prospects.

The life insurance industry is competitive and profit driven. Understandably life insurers are concerned that individuals who receive a positive result from a predictive test will take out large policies without revealing their true risk status. This is referred to as 'adverse selection'. On the other hand there is a fear that those who test positive will find themselves victims of discrimination and that individuals with a family history of a late onset autosomal dominant disorder will be refused insurance unless they undergo predictive testing.

This is one of the most difficult ethical issues to emerge as a result of recent molecular discoveries and if anything the problems will be exacerbated as new tests are developed for susceptibility to common adult illnesses such as cancer and coronary artery disease (p. 181). The solution could lie in a voluntary agreement that those seeking life insurance up to an arbitrary limit should not have to undertake or reveal the results of predictive tests, but that such testing is acceptable for applications for cover for larger amounts.

GENE THERAPY

By far the most exciting potential benefit of recent progress in molecular biology is the prospect of gene

therapy (p. 278). It is understandable that both the general public and the health care professions should be concerned about the possible side-effects and abuse of gene therapy. To address these anxieties, advisory or regulatory committees have been established in several countries to assess the practical and ethical aspects of gene therapy research programmes.

Concern centres around two fundamental issues. The first relates to the practical aspects of ensuring informed consent on the part of patients who wish to participate in gene therapy research. Adult patients and parents of affected children could well be desperate to participate in gene therapy research given that their disease is otherwise incurable. Consequently they could be tempted to disregard the possible hazards of what is essentially a new and untried therapeutic approach.

In the United Kingdom, the Committee on the Ethics of Gene Therapy has recommended that until this is shown to be safe, all gene therapy programmes should be subjected to careful scrutiny by local hospital research ethical committees. In addition, they have recommended that a national supervisory body should be established to review all proposals to conduct gene therapy in humans. In this way it is anticipated that the rights of individual patients in terms of both consent and confidentiality will be safeguarded.

The second aspect of gene therapy which generates concern is the possibility that it could be used for eugenic purposes. On this point the British committee has recommended that genetic modification involving the germ-line (p. 279) should not be attempted. Therefore by limiting gene therapy to somatic cells it should not be possible for newly modified genes to be transmitted to future generations. This committee has also recommended that somatic cell gene therapy should only be used to try to treat serious diseases and not to alter human characteristics such as intelligence or athletic prowess.

The potential benefits of gene therapy are so great that it has been deemed reasonable that pilot studies be undertaken in small groups of patients with serious disorders such as cystic fibrosis. The degree of caution expressed by national committees considering the ethics of gene therapy illustrates the care which is being taken by medical and governing bodies to ensure that human gene manipulation will not be abused.

CONCLUSION

It is clear that ethical considerations are of major importance in clinical genetics. Each new discovery has potential for good or bad and raises new dilemmas for which there are often no easy answers. On a global scale the computerisation of medical records coupled with the widespread introduction of genetic screening make it essential that safeguards are introduced to ensure that future populations are not open to eugenic or dysgenic abuse. It is encouraging and important that these issues are the subject of continued open public debate and that society is alert to the dangers inherent in the misuse of the new genetic technology.

ELEMENTS

1 Ethical considerations impinge on almost every aspect of clinical genetics.

2 Subjects which can generate particularly difficult ethical problems include prenatal diagnosis, population and family screening, presymptomatic or predictive testing and the possible eugenic abuse of new developments such as gene therapy.

3 It is important that guidelines and regulations are established which recognise a patient's fundamental rights of informed consent, informed choice, autonomy and confidentiality.

FURTHER READING

Harper P S, 1993 Insurance and genetic testing. Lancet 341: 224–227
   A detailed review of the issues and potential problems raised by genetic testing in the context of life and health insurance.
Harper P S, Clarke A, 1990 Should we test children for 'adult' genetic diseases? Lancet 335: 1205–1206
   A thoughtful account of the rights and wrongs of predictive testing in children.
Report of the Committee on the Ethics of Gene Therapy. 1992 HMSO, London
   The recommendations of the committee chaired by Sir Cecil Clothier on the ethical aspects of somatic cell and germ-line gene therapy.

Glossary

A. Abbreviation for adenine.

Acetylation. The introduction of an acetyl group into a molecule; often used by the body to help eliminate substances by the liver.

Acrocentric. Term used to describe a chromosome where the centromere is near one end and the short arm usually consists of satellite material.

Adenine. A purine base in DNA and RNA.

Adenomatous polyposis coli (APC). See *Familial adenomatous polypsosis.*

AIDS. Acquired immunodeficiency syndrome.

Allele (= allelomorph). Alternative form of a gene found at the same locus on homologous chromosomes.

Allograft. A tissue graft between non-identical individuals.

Allotypes. Genetically determined variants.

Alternative pathway. One of the two pathways of the activation of complement which, in this instance, involves cell membranes of microorganisms.

Alu repeat. Short repeated DNA sequences which appear to have homology with transposable elements in other organisms.

Am. The group of genetic variants associated with the IgA heavy chain.

Amber. UAG, one of the three stop codons.

Amino acid. An organic compound containing both carboxyl (-COOH) and amino groups (-NH$_2$).

Amniocentesis. Procedure for obtaining amniotic fluid and cells for prenatal diagnosis.

Anaphase. The stage of cell division when the chromosomes leave the equatorial plate and migrate to opposite poles of the spindle.

Anaphase lag. Loss of a chromosome as it moves to the pole of the cell during anaphase which can lead to monosomy.

Aneuploid. A chromosome number which is not an exact multiple of the haploid number, i.e. $2N - 1$ or $2N + 1$ where N is the haploid number of chromosomes.

Anterior information. Information previously known which leads to the *prior probability.*

Antibody (= immunoglobulin). A serum protein which is formed in response to an antigenic stimulus and reacts specifically with that antigen.

Anticipation. The tendency for some autosomal dominant diseases to manifest at an earlier age and to increase in severity with each succeeding generation.

Anti-codon. The complementary triplet of the tRNA molecule which binds to it with a particular amino acid.

Antigen. A substance which elicits the synthesis of antibody with which it specifically reacts.

Antigen binding fragment (Fab). The fragment of the antibody molecule produced by papain digestion responsible for antigen binding.

Antiparallel. Opposite orientation of the two strands of a DNA duplex, one runs in the 3' to 5' direction, the other in the 5' to 3' direction.

Antisense oligonucleotide. A short oligonucleotide synthesised to bind to a particular RNA or DNA sequence to block its expression.

Apoptosis. Programmed involution or cell death of a developing tissue or organ of the body.

Arteriosclerosis. Hardening of the arterial medial wall.

Artificial insemination by donor (AID). Use of semen from a male donor as a reproductive option for couples at high risk of transmitting a genetic disorder.

Ascertainment. The finding and selection of families with a hereditary disorder.

Association. The occurrence of a particular allele in a group of patients more often than can be accounted for by chance.

Assortative mating (= non-random mating). The preferential selection of a spouse with a particular phenotype.

Atherosclerosis. The fatty degenerative plaque which accumulates in the intimal wall of blood vessels.

Autoradiography. Detection of radioactively labelled molecules on an X-ray film.

Autosomal inheritance. The pattern of inheritance shown by a disorder or trait determined by a gene on one of the non-sex chromosomes.

Autosome. Any of the 22 non-sex chromosomes.

Bacteriophage (= phage). A virus which infects bacteria.

Balanced polymorphism. Two different genetic variants which are stably present in a population, i.e. selective advantages and disadvantages cancel each other out.

Balanced translocation. See *Reciprocal translocation.*

Barr body. The condensation of the inactive X chromosome seen in the nucleus of certain types of cells from females. See *X-chromatin.*

Base. Short for the nitrogenous bases in nucleic acid molecules (A = adenine; T = thymine; U = uracil; C = cytosine, G = guanine).

Base pair (bp). A pair of complementary bases in DNA (A with T, G with C).

Bayes' theorem. Combining the prior and conditional probabilities of certain events or the results of specific tests to give a joint probability to derive the posterior or relative probability.

Bence-Jones protein. The antibody of a single species produced in large amounts by a person with multiple myeloma, a tumour of antibody-producing plasma cells.

Bias of ascertainment. An artefact, which must be taken into account in family studies when looking at segregation ratios, caused by families coming to attention because they have affected individual(s).

Biosynthesis. Use of recombinant DNA techniques to produce molecules of biological and medical importance in the laboratory.

Bivalent. A pair of synapsed homologous chromosomes.

Blastomere. A single cell of the early fertilised conceptus.

Blood chimaera. A mixture of cells of different genetic origin present in twins as result of an exchange of cells via the placenta between non-identical twins in utero.

Break point cluster (bcr). Region of chromosome 22 involved in the translocation seen in the majority of persons with chronic myeloid leukaemia.

C. Abbreviation for cytosine.

CA repeat. A short dinucleotide sequence present as tandem repeats at multiple sites in the human genome producing microsatellite polymorphisms.

Cancer family syndrome. A term used to describe the clustering in certain families of particular types of cancers, in which it has been proposed that the different types of malignancy could be due to a single dominant gene, specifically Lynch type II.

Cancer genetics. The study of the genetic causes of cancer.

Candidate gene. A gene whose function suggests that it is likely to be responsible for a genetic disease.

5' Cap. Modification of the nascent mRNA by the addition of a methylated guanine nucleotide to the 5' end of the molecule by an unusual 5' to 5' triphosphate linkage.

Cascade screening. Identification within a family of carriers for an autosomal recessive disorder or persons with an autosomal dominant gene following ascertainment of an index case.

CAT box. A conserved, non-coding, so-called 'promoter' sequence about 80 bp upstream from the start of transcription.

Cellular immunity. Immunity which involves the T lymphocytes, e.g. transplantation immunity and delayed hypersensitivity.

Cellular oncogene. See *Proto-oncogene.*

CentiMorgan (cM). Unit used to measure map distances, equivalent to a 1% chance of recombination (crossing-over).

Central dogma. The concept that genetic information is usually only transmitted from DNA to RNA to protein.

Centric fusion. The fusion of the centromeres of two acrocentric chromosomes to form a Robertsonian tranlocation.

Centriole. The cellular structure from which microtubules radiate in the mitotic spindle involved in the separation of chromsomes in mitosis.

Centromere (= kinetochore). The point at which the two chromatids of a chromosome are joined, and the region of the chromosome which becomes attached to the spindle during cell division.

Chemical cleavage mismatch. A DNA mutation detection system which involves the addition of the chemicals hydroxylamine and osmium tetroxide which react with free cytosine and thymine nucleotides respectively. By denaturing the double stranded DNA being screened and allowing it to hybridise with a single-stranded radiolabelled DNA probe, any mismatched cytosine or thymine nucleotides will be exposed and therefore be susceptible to reaction with the hydroxylamine and osmium tetroxide. The addition of piperidine results in cleavage of the DNA being screened at any such sites allowing identification of mutations.

Chiasmata. Cross-overs between chromosomes in meiosis.

Chimaera. An individual composed of two populations of cells with different genotypes.

Chorion. Layer of cells covering a fertilised ovum some of which, the chorion frondosum, will later form the placenta.

Chorionic villus sampling. Procedure using ultrasound guidance to obtain chorionic villi from the chorion frondosum for prenatal diagnosis.

Chromatid. During cell division each centromere divides longitudinally into two strands, or chromatids, which are held together by the centromere.

Chromatin. The tertiary coiling of the nucleosomes of the chromosomes with associated proteins.

Chromosomal analysis. The process of counting and analysing the banding pattern of the chromosomes of an individual.

Chromosomal fragments. Acentric chromosomes which can arise as a result of segregation of a paracentric inversion and which are usually incapable of replication.

Chromosome instability. The presence of breaks and gaps in the chromosomes from persons with a number of disorders associated with an increased risk of neoplasia.

Chromosome jumping or linking. A technique of chromosome mapping which involves circularisation of DNA fragments produced by restriction enzyme digestion in the presence of a plasmid sequence cut with the same restriction enzyme, followed by digestion with a second restriction enzyme, which does not cleave within the plasmid sequence, allowing deletion of the 'internal' DNA from these fragments. The plasmid sequence acts as an identifying 'tag' and allows cloning of the ends of the original DNA fragments which, with complementary libraries, can be used to map markers directionally which are hundreds of kilobases apart.

Chromosome mapping. Assigning a gene or DNA sequence to a specific chromosome or a particular region of a chromosome.

Chromosome-mediated gene-transfer. The technique of transferring chromosomes or parts of chromosomes to somatic cell hybrids to enable more detailed chromosome mapping.

Chromosome painting. The hybridisation in situ of fluorescent labelled probes to a chromosome preparation to allow identification of a particular chromosome(s).

Chromosomes. Thread-like, darkly-staining bodies within the nucleus, composed of DNA and chromatin which carry the genetic information.

Class switching. Term used for the normal change in antibody class from IgM to IgG in the immune response.

Classical pathway. One of the two ways of activation of complement, in this instance, involving antigen–antibody complexes.

Clone. A group of cells, all of which are derived from a single cell by repeated mitoses, all having the same genetic information.

cM. abbreviation for centiMorgan.

Codominance. When both alleles are expressed in the heterozygote.

Codon. A sequence of three adjacent nucleotides which codes for one amino acid or chain termination.

Common cancers. The cancers which occur commonly in humans, such as bowel and breast cancer.

Common diseases. The diseases which occur commonly in humans, e.g. cancer, coronary artery disease, diabetes, etc.

Community genetics. The branch of medical genetics concerned with screening and the prevention of genetic diseases on a population basis.

Complement. A series of at least ten serum proteins in humans (and other vertebrates) that can be activated by either the 'classical' or the 'alternative' pathways and which interact in sequence to bring about the destruction of cellular antigens.

Complementary DNA (cDNA). DNA synthesised from mRNA by the enzyme reverse transcriptase.

Complete ascertainment. A term used in segregation analysis for a type of study which identifies all affected individuals in a population.

Compound heterozygote. An individual who is affected with an autosomal recessive disorder having two different mutations in homologous alleles.

Concordance. When both members of a pair of twins exhibit the same trait they are said to be concordant. If only one twin has the trait they are said to be discordant.

Conditional probability. Observations or tests which can be used to modify prior probabilities using Bayesian calculation in risk estimations.

Conditionally toxic gene. Genes which are introduced in gene therapy which, under certain conditions or after the introduction of a certain substance, will kill the cell.

Confined placental mosaicism. The occurrence of a chromosomal abnormality in chorionic villus samples obtained for first trimester prenatal diagnosis in which the fetus has a normal chromosomal complement.

Congenital. Any abnormality, whether genetic or not, which is present at birth.

Congenital hypertrophy of the retinal pigment epithelium (CHRPE). Abnormal retinal pigmentation which, when present in persons at risk for familial adenomatous polyposis, is evidence of the heterozygous state.

Conjugation. A chemical process in which two molecules are joined, often used to describe the process by which certain drugs or chemicals can then be excreted by the body, e.g. acetylation of isoniazid by the liver.

Consanguineous marriage. A marriage between 'blood relatives', that is between persons who have one or more ancestors in common, most frequently between first cousins.

Consensus sequence. A GGGCGGG sequence promoter element to the 5' side of genes in eukaryotes involved in the control of gene expression.

Constant region. The portion of the light and heavy chains in which the amino acid sequence is relatively constant from molecule to molecule.

Constitutional. Present in the fertilised gamete.

Constitutional heterozygosity. The presence in an individual at the time of conception of obligate heterozygosity at a locus when the parents are homozygous at that locus for different alleles.

Consultand. The person presenting for genetic advice.

Contigs. Contiguous or overlapping DNA clones.

Continuous trait. A trait, such as height, for which there is a range of observations or findings, in contrast to traits which are all or none, cf. *discontinuous*, such as cleft lip and palate.

Control gene. A gene which can turn other genes on or off, i.e. regulate.

Cor pulmonale. Right-sided heart failure which can occur after serious lung disease, such as in persons with cystic fibrosis.

Cordocentesis. The procedure of obtaining fetal blood samples for prenatal diagnosis.

Corona radiata. Cellular layer surrounding the mature oocyte.

Correlation. Statistical measure of the degree of association or resemblance between two parameters.

Cosmid. A plasmid which has had the maximum DNA removed to allow the largest possible insert for cloning but still has the DNA sequences necessary for in vitro packaging into an infective phage particle.

Co-twins. Both members of a twin pair, whether dizygotic or monozygotic.

Counsellee. Person receiving genetic counselling.

Coupling. When a certain allele at a particular locus is on the same chromosome with a specific allele at a closely-linked locus.

Cross-over (= recombination). The exchange of genetic material between homologous chromosomes in meiosis.

Cross-reacting material (CRM). Immunologically detected protein or enzyme which is functionally inactive.

Cryptic splice site. A mutation in a gene leading to the creation of the sequence of a splice site which results in abnormal splicing of the mRNA.

Cystic fibrosis transmembrane conductance regulator (CFTR). The gene product of the cystic fibrosis gene responsible for chloride transport and mucin secretion.

Cytogenetics. A branch of genetics concerned principally with the study of chromosomes.

Cytoplasm. The ground substance of the cell in which are situated the nucleus, endoplasmic reticulum and mitochondria, etc.

Cytoplasmic inheritance. See *Mitochondrial inheritance.*

Cytosine. A pyrimidine base in DNA and RNA.

Cytotoxic lymphocytes (= killer). A group of T cells which specifically kill foreign or virus infected vertebrate cells.

Daltonism. A term given in the past to X-linked inheritance after John Dalton who noted this pattern of inheritance in colour blindness.

De novo. Literally 'from new', as opposed to inherited.

Deformation. A birth defect which results from an abnormal mechanical force which distorts an otherwise normal structure.

Deleted in colorectal carcinoma (DCC). A region on the long arm of chromosome 18 often found to be deleted in colorectal carcinomas.

Deletion. A type of chromosomal aberration or mutation at the DNA level in which there is loss of part of a chromosome or one or more nucleotides.

Delta-beta thalassaemia. A form of thalassaemia in which there is reduced production of both the delta and beta globin chains.

Denaturing gradient gel electrophoresis. A mutation detection system which involves mixing a radiolabelled single-stranded DNA probe with the double-stranded DNA being screened, which is heated to make it single stranded. This mixture is electrophoresed on a denaturing gradient gel. DNA which is identical with the sequence of the DNA probe will form a homoduplex, which under the denaturing conditions of the gel will remain hybridised. Any mismatches of the DNA being screened with the DNA probe will result in the formation of a heteroduplex which, as it is run down the denaturing gradient of the gel will become single stranded at a certain point resulting in a branched structure which has decreased mobility. This results in an altered position compared to the homoduplex which can be detected on an autoradiograph.

Deoxyribonucleic acid. See *DNA.*

Developmental field. A set of apparently unrelated embryonic primordia which react together to a single environmental or genetic insult to produce a particular pattern of birth defects.

Dictyotene. The stage in meiosis I in which primary oocytes are arrested in females until the time of ovulation.

Diploid. The condition in which the cell contains two sets of chromosomes. Normal state of somatic cells in humans where the diploid number (2*N*) is 46.

Discontinuous trait. A trait which is all or none, e.g. cleft lip and palate, in contrast to *continuous* traits such as height.

Discordant. Differing phenotypic features between individuals, classically used in twin pairs.

Disomy. The normal state of an individual having two homologous chromosomes.

Dispermic chimaera. Two separate sperm fertilise two separate ova and the resulting two zygotes fuse to form one embryo.

Dispermy. Fertilisation of an oocyte by two sperm.

Disruption. An abnormal structure of an organ or tissue as a result of external factors disturbing the normal developmental process.

Diversity region. DNA sequences coding for the segments of the hypervariable regions of antibodies.

Dizygotic (= fraternal). Type of twins produced by fertilisation of two ova by two sperm.

DNA (= deoxyribonucleic acid). The nucleic acid in chromosomes in which genetic information is coded.

DNA fingerprint. Pattern of hypervariable tandem DNA repeats of a core sequence which is unique to an individual.

DNA library. A collection of recombinant DNA molecules from a particular source, e.g. genomic or cDNA.

DNA ligase. An enzyme which catalyses the formation of a phosphodiester bond between a 3'-hydroxyl and a 5'-phosphate group in DNA thereby joining two DNA fragments.

DNA mapping. The physical relationships of flanking DNA sequence polymorphisms and the detailed structure of a gene.

DNA probes. A DNA sequence which is labelled, usually radioactively, which is used to identify a gene, e.g. a cDNA or genomic probe.

DNA sequence amplification. See *Polymerase chain reaction.*

Dominant. A trait which is expressed in individuals who are heterozygous for a particular allele.

Dosage compensation. The phenomenon in women who have two copies of genes on the X chromosome having the same level of the products of those genes as males who have a single X chromosome.

Dosimetry. The measurement of radiation exposure.

Double heterozygote. An individual who is heterozygous at two different loci.

Double-minute chromosomes. Amplified sequences of DNA in tumour cells which can occur as small extra chromosomes, as in neuroblastoma.

Drift (= random genetic drift). Fluctuations in gene frequencies which tend to occur in small isolated populations.

Duplication. A type of chromosomal aberration or mutation in DNA in which part of a chromosome or one or more nucleotides is duplicated.

Dysmorphology. The study of the definition, recognition and aetiology of multiple malformation syndromes.

Dysplasia. An abnormal organisation of cells into tissue.

Dystrophin. The product of the Duchenne muscular dystrophy gene.

Ecogenetics. The study of genetically determined differences in susceptibility to the action of physical, chemical and infectious agents in the environment.

Em. The group of genetic variants of the IgE heavy chain of immunoglobulins.

Empiric risks. Advice given in recurrence risk counselling for multifactorially determined disorders in which the inherited contribution is due to a number of genes, i.e. polygenic, based on observation and experience.

Endoplasmic reticulum. A system of minute tubules within the cell involved in the biosynthesis of macromolecules.

Endoreduplication. Duplication of a haploid sperm chromosome set.

Enhancer. DNA sequence which increases transcription of a related gene.

Enzyme. A protein which acts as a catalyst in biological systems.

Epidermal growth factor (EGF). A growth factor which stimulates a variety of cell types including epidermal cells.

Erythroblastosis fetalis. See *Haemolytic disease of the newborn.*

Euchromatin. Genetically active regions of the chromosomes.

Eugenics. The 'science' which promotes the improvement of the hereditary qualities of a race or a species.

Eukaryote. Higher organism with a well-defined nucleus.

Exon (= expressed sequence). Region of a gene which is not excised during transcription forming part of the mature mRNA and therefore specifying part of the primary structure of the gene product.

Exon trapping. A process by which a recombinant DNA vector which contains the DNA sequences of the splice site junctions is used to clone coding sequences or exons.

Expansion. Refers to the increase in the number of triplet repeat sequences in the various disorders due to dynamic or unstable mutations.

Expressed sequence tags (ESTs). PCR of mRNA to produce DNA sequences which can be used to map expressed sequences to the human genome.

Expressivity. Variation in the severity of the phenotypic features of a particular gene.

Extinguished. Loss of one allelic variant at a locus due to random genetic drift.

Extrinsic malformation. Term previously used for *Disruption.*

Fab. The two antigen binding fragments of an antibody molecule produced by digestion with the proteolytic enzyme papain.

False-negative. Affected cases missed by a diagnostic or screening test.

False-positive. Unaffected cases incorrectly diagnosed as affected by a screening or diagnostic test.

Familial adenomatous polyposis. A dominantly inherited cancer predisposing syndrome characterised by the presence of a large number of polyps of the large bowel with a high risk of developing malignant changes.

Familial cancer-predisposing syndrome. One of a number of syndromes in which persons are at risk of developing one or more types of cancer.

Favism. A haemolytic crisis due to G6PD deficiency occurring after eating fava beans.

Fc. The complement binding fragment of an antibody molecule produced by digestion with the proteolytic enzyme papain.

Fetoscopy. Procedure used to visualise the fetus and often to take skin and/or blood samples from the fetus for prenatal diagnosis.

Fetus. The name given to the unborn infant during the final stage of in utero development, usually from 12 weeks gestation to term.

Filial. Offspring.

First-degree relatives. Closest relatives, that is, parents, offspring, sibs, sharing on average 50% of their genes.

Fitness (= biological fitness). The number of offspring who reach reproductive age.

Five-prime (5') end. The end of a DNA or RNA strand with a free 5' phosphate group.

Fixed. The establishment of a single allelic variant at a locus due to random genetic drift.

Flanking DNA. Nucleotide sequence adjacent to the DNA sequence being considered.

Flow cytometry. See *Fluorescent activated cell sorting.*

Fluorescent activated cell sorting (FACS). A technique in which chromosomes are stained with a fluorescent dye which selectively binds to DNA, the differences in fluorescence of the various chromosomes allow them to be physically separated by a special laser.

Fluorescent in situ hybridisation (FISH). Use of single-stranded DNA sequence with a fluorescent label to hybridise with its complementary target sequence in the chromosomes allowing it to be visualised under ultraviolet light.

Founder effect. Certain genetic disorders can be relatively common in particular populations through all individuals being descended from a relatively small number of ancestors, one or a few of whom had a particular disorder.

Frameshift mutations. Mutations, such as insertions or deletions, which change the reading frame of the codon triplets.

Framework map. A set of markers distributed at defined approximately evenly spaced intervals along the chromosomes in the human genome.

Framework region. Parts of the variable regions of antibodies which are not hypervariable.

Fraternal twins. Non-identical twins.

Frequency. The number of times an event occurs in a period of time, e.g. 1000 cases per year.

Full ascertainment. See *Complete ascertainment.*

Fusion polypeptide. Genes which are physically near to each other and have DNA sequence homology can undergo a cross-over which leads to formation of a protein which has an amino acid sequence which is derived from both of the genes involved.

G. Abbreviation for the nucleotide guanine.

Gamete. A germ cell (sperm or ovum) containing a haploid (*N*) number of chromosomes.

Gastrulation. The formation of the bi- then tri-laminar disc of the inner cell mass which becomes the early embryo.

Gene. A part of the DNA molecule of a chromosome which directs the synthesis of a specific polypeptide chain.

Gene amplification. Process in tumour cells of the production of multiple copies of certain genes, the visible evidence of which are *homogeneously-staining regions* and *double-minute chromosomes.*

Gene flow. A term used to describe differences in allele frequencies between populations which reflect migration or contact between them.

Gene therapy. Treatment of inherited disease by addition, insertion or replacement of a normal gene or genes.

Genetic code. The triplets of DNA nucleotides which code for the various amino acids of proteins.

Genetic counselling. The process of providing information about a genetic disorder which includes information about the diagnosis, its cause, the risk of recurrence and options available for prevention.

Genetic dose. Term used in radiation dosimetry to describe the radiation exposure of a population.

Genetic heterogeneity. The phenomenon that a disorder can be caused by different allelic or non-allelic mutations.

Genetic isolates. Groups which are isolated for geographical, religious or ethnic reasons which often show differences in allele frequencies.

Genetic load. The total of all kinds of harmful alleles in a population.

Genetic register. A list of families and individuals who are either affected by or at risk of developing a serious hereditary disorder.

Genetic susceptibility. An inherited predisposition to a disease or disorder which is not due to a single gene cause and is usually the result of a complex interaction of the effects of multiple different genes, i.e. *polygenic inheritance.*

Genocopy. The same phenotype due to different genetic causes.

Genome. All the genes carried by a cell.

Genomic DNA. DNA sequences in the chromosomes.

Genomic imprinting. Differing expression of genetic material dependent on the sex of the transmitting parent.

Genotype. The genetic constitution of an individual.

Germ cells. The cells of the body which transmit genetic information to the next generation.

Germ-line gene therapy. The alteration or insertion of genetic material in the gametes.

Germ-line mosaicism. The presence in the germ-line or gonadal tissue of two populations of cells which differ genetically.

Germ-line mutation. A mutation in a gamete.

Gm. Genetic variants of the heavy chain of IgG immunoglobulins.

Goldberg–Hogness box. See *CAT box.*

Gonad dose. Term used in radiation dosimetry to describe the radiation exposure of an individual to a particular radiological investigation or exposure.

Gonadal mosaicism. See *Germ-line mosaicism.*

Gray (Gy). Equivalent to 100 rad.

Growth factor receptors. Receptors on the surfaces of cells for a growth factor.

Growth factors. A substance which must be present in culture medium to permit cell multiplication, or substances involved in promoting growth of certain cell types, tissues or parts of the body in development, e.g. fibroblast growth factor.

Guanine. A purine base in DNA and RNA.

Haemoglobinopathy. An inherited disorder of haemoglobin.

Haemolytic disease of the newborn. Anaemia due to antibody produced by a Rhesus-negative mother to the Rhesus-positive blood group of the fetus crossing the placenta and causing haemolysis. If this haemolytic process is severe, it can cause death of the fetus due to heart failure because of the anaemia or what is known as *Erythroblastosis fetalis.*

Haploid. The condition in which the cell contains one set of chromosomes, i.e. 23. This is the chromosome number in a normal gamete.

Haplotype. Conventionally used to refer to the particular alleles present at the four genes of the HLA complex on chromosome 6. The term is also used to describe DNA sequence variants on a particular chromosome adjacent to or closely flanking a locus of interest.

Hardy–Weinberg equilibrium. The maintenance of allele frequencies in a population with random mating and absence of selection.

Hardy–Weinberg formula. A simple binomial equation in population genetics which can be used to determine the frequency of the different genotypes from one of the phenotypes.

Hardy–Weinberg principle. The relative proportions of the different genotypes remain constant from one generation to the next.

Hb Barts. The tetramer of gamma globin chains found in the severe form of alpha thalassaemia, which causes hydrops fetalis.

Hb H. Tetramer of the beta globin chains found in the less severe form of alpha thalassaemia.

Helper lymphocytes. A subclass of T lymphocytes necessary for the production of antibodies by B lymphocytes.

Helper virus. A retroviral provirus engineered to remove all but the sequences necessary to produce copies of the viral RNA sequences along with the sequences necessary for packaging of the viral genomic RNA in retroviral mediated gene therapy.

Hemizygous. A term used when describing the genotype of a male with regard to an X-linked trait, since males have only one set of X-linked genes.

Hereditary non-polyposis colorectal cancer (HNPCC). A form of familial cancer in which persons are at risk of developing bowel cancer, not associated with a large number of polyps as in familial polyposis coli, in which the bowel cancer is usually proximal and right-sided.

Hereditary persistence of fetal Hb. Persistence of the production of fetal haemoglobin into childhood and adult life, one form of which can be due to a deletion.

Heritability. The proportion of the total variation of a character attributable to genetic as opposed to environmental factors.

Hermaphrodite. An individual with both male and female gonads often in association with ambiguous external genitalia.

Heterochromatin. Genetically inert or inactive regions of the chromosomes.

Heterogeneity. The phenomenon of there being more than a single cause for what appears to be a single entity. See *Genetic heterogeneity.*

Heteromorphism. An inherited structural polymorphism of a chromosome.

Heteropyknotic. Condensed darkly-staining chromosomal material, e.g. the inactivated X chromosome in females.

Heterozygote (= carrier). An individual who possesses two different alleles at one particular locus on a pair of homologous chromosomes.

Heterozygote advantage. An increase in biological fitness seen in unaffected heterozygotes compared to unaffected homozygotes, eg. sickle-cell trait and resistance to infection by the malarial parasite.

Heterozygous. The state of having different alleles at a locus on homologous chromosomes.

Histocompatibility. Antigenic similarity of donor and recipient in organ transplantation.

Histone. Type of protein rich in lysine and arginine found in association with DNA in chromosomes.

HIV. Human immunodeficiency virus.

HLA (human leucocyte antigen). Antigens present on the cell surfaces of various tissues, including leucocytes.

HLA complex. The genes on chromosome 6 responsible for determining the cell-surface antigens important in organ transplantation.

Hogness box (= TATA box). A conserved, non-coding, so-called 'promoter' sequence about 30 bp upstream from the start of transcription.

Holandric inheritance. The pattern of inheritance of genes on the Y chromosome: only males are affected and the trait is transmitted by affected males to their sons but to none of their daughters.

Homeobox. A stretch of approximately 180 base pairs found to be conserved in different homeotic genes.

Homeotic gene. Genes which are involved in controlling the development of a region or compartment of an organism producing proteins or factors which regulate gene expression by binding particular DNA sequences.

Homogeneously staining regions (HSR). Amplification of DNA sequences in tumour cells which can appear as extra or expanded areas of the chromosomes which stain evenly.

Homograft. Graft between individuals of the same species but with different genotypes.

Homologous chromosomes. Chromosomes which pair during meiosis and contain identical loci.

Homologous recombination. The process by which a DNA sequence can be replaced by one with a similar sequence to determine the effect of changes in DNA sequence in the process of site-directed mutagenesis.

Homozygote. An individual who possesses two identical alleles at one particular locus on a pair of homologous chromosomes.

HTF islands. Methylation-free clusters of CpG dinucleotides found near transcription initiation sites at the 5' end of many eukaryotic genes which can be detected by cutting with the restriction enzyme Hpa II producing tiny DNA fragments.

Human genome project. A major international collaborative effort to map and sequence the entire human genome.

Humoral immunity. Immunity which is due to circulating antibodies in the blood and other body fluids.

H–Y antigen. A histocompatibility antigen originally detected in the mouse and previously thought to be located on the Y chromosome, now thought to be coded for by a gene on chromosome 6 and controlled by a regulatory gene on the Y chromosome.

Hydatidiform mole. An abnormal conceptus which consists of abnormal tissues: a complete mole contains no fetus but can undergo malignant change and receives both sets of chromosomes from the father; a partial mole contains a chromosomally abnormal fetus with triploidy.

Hypervariable DNA length polymorphisms. A number of different types of variation in DNA sequence which are highly polymorphic, e.g. variable number tandem repeats, mini- and microsatellites.

Hypervariable region. A number of small regions present in the variable regions of the light and heavy chains of antibodies in which the majority of the variability in antibody sequence occurs.

Identical twins. See *Monozygotic.*

Idiogram. An idealised representation of an object, e.g. an idiogram of a karyotype.

Immunoglobulin. See *Antibody.*

Immunoglobulin allotypes. Genetically determined variants of the various antibody classes, e.g. the Gm system associated with the heavy chain of IgG.

Immunoglobulin superfamily. Eight multigene families involved in the immune response with structural and DNA sequence homology.

Immunoglobulins. An antibody.

Imprinting. The phenomenon of a gene or region of a chromosome showing different expression depending on the parent of origin.

Inborn error of metabolism. A genetically inherited metabolic defect which results in deficient production or synthesis of an abnormal enzyme.

Incest. Union between first-degree relatives.

Incidence. The rate at which new cases occur, e.g. 2 in 1000 births are affected by neural tube defects.

Incompatibility. A donor and host are incompatible if the latter rejects a graft from the former.

Incomplete ascertainment. A term used in segregation analysis to describe family studies in which complete ascertainment is not possible.

Index case. See *Proband.*

Index map. See *Framework map.*

Inducer. Small molecule which interacts with a regulator protein and triggers gene transcription.

Informative. Variation in a marker system in a family which enables a gene or inherited disease to be followed in that family.

Initiator. A gene which is part of a replicon which forms a product that interacts with the replicator to initiate DNA replication.

Insertion. Addition of chromosomal material or DNA sequence of one or more nucleotides within the genome.

Insertional mutagenesis. The introduction of mutations at specific sites to determine the effects of these changes.

In situ hybridisation. Hybridisation with a DNA probe carried out directly on a chromosome preparation or histological section.

Intermediate inheritance. See *Codominance.*

Interphase. The stage between two successive cell divisions during which DNA replication occurs.

Intersex. An individual with external genitalia not clearly male or female.

Intrinsic malformation. A malformation due to an inherent abnormality in development.

Intron (= intervening sequence). Region of DNA which generates that part of precursor RNA which is spliced out during transcription and does not form mature mRNA and therefore does not specify the primary structure of the gene product.

Inv. The group of genetic variants of the kappa light chains of immunoglobulins.

Inversion. A type of chromosomal aberration or mutation in which part of a chromosome or sequence of DNA is reversed in its order.

Inversion loop. The structure formed in meiosis I by a chromosome with either a para- or pericentric inversion.

In vitro. In the laboratory, literally 'in glass'.

In vivo. In the normal cell, literally 'in the living organism'.

Isochromosome. A type of chromosomal aberration in which one of the arms of a particular chromosome is duplicated because the centromere divides transversely and not longitudinally as normal during cell division. The two arms of an isochromosome are therefore of equal length and contain the same set of genes.

Isolate. A term used to describe a population or group of individuals who for religious, cultural or geographical reasons have remained separate from other groups of persons.

Isozymes. Enzymes which exist in multiple molecular forms which can be distinguished by biochemical methods.

Joining region. Short conserved sequence of nucleotides involved in somatic recombinational events in the production of antibody diversity.

Joint probability. The product of the prior and conditional probability for two events.

Karyotype. The number, size and shape of the chromosomes of an individual. Also used for the photomicrograph of an individual's chromosomes arranged in a standard manner.

Kb. Abbreviation for kilobase.

Killer lymphocytes. See *Cytotoxic lymphocytes.*

Kilobase. 1000 base pairs (bp).

Km. Genetic variants of the kappa light chain of immunoglobulins.

Law of addition. If two or more events are mutually exclusive then the probability that *either* one *or* the other will occur equals the *sum* of their individual probabilities.

Law of independent assortment. Members of different gene pairs segregate to offspring independently of one another.

Law of multiplication. If two or more events or outcomes are independent, then the probability that *both* the first *and* the second will occur equals the product of their individual probabilities.

Law of segregation. Each individual possesses two genes for a particular characteristic, only one of which can be transmitted at any one time.

Law of uniformity. When two homozygotes with different alleles are crossed, all the offspring in the F1 generation are identical and heterozygous, i.e. the characteristics do not blend and can reappear in later generations.

Lethal mutation. A mutation which leads to the premature death of an individual or organism.

Liability. A concept used in disorders which are multifactorially determined to take into account all possible causative factors.

Library. Set of cloned DNA fragments derived from a particular DNA source, e.g. a cDNA library from the transcript of particular tissue, or a genomic library.

Ligase. Enzyme used to join DNA molecules.

Ligation. Formation of phosphodiester bonds to link two nucleic acid molecules.

Linkage. Two loci situated close together on the same chromosome, the alleles at which are usually transmitted together in meiosis in gamete formation.

Linkage disequilibrium. The occurrence together of two or more alleles at closely linked loci more frequently than would be expected by chance.

Linking (jumping) library. A method of DNA cloning that directionally maps DNA sequences which can be hundreds of kilobases apart.

Liposomes. Artificially prepared cell-like structures in which one or more bimolecular layers of phospholipid enclose one or more aqueous compartments, which can include proteins.

Locus. The site of a gene on a chromosome.

Locus control region (LCR). A region near the beta-like globin genes involved in the timing and tissue specificity of their expression in development.

Locus heterogeneity. The phenomenon of a disorder being due to mutations in more than one gene or locus.

Lod score. A mathematical score of the relative likelihood of two loci being linked.

Long terminal repeat (LTR). One of two long sections of double-stranded DNA synthesised by reverse transcriptase from the RNA of a retrovirus involved in regulating viral expression.

Loss of constitutional heterozygosity (LOCH). Loss of an allele inherited from a parent frequently seen as evidence of a 'second hit' in tumorigenesis.

Lymphokines. A group of glycoproteins released from T lymphocytes after contact with an antigen which act upon other cells of the host immune system.

Lyonisation. The process of inactivation of one of the X chromosomes in females originally proposed by the geneticist Mary Lyon.

Major histocompatibility complex (MHC). A multigene locus which codes for the histocompatibility antigens involved in organ transplantation.

Malformation. A primary structural defect of an organ or part of an organ which results from an inherent abnormality in development.

Manifesting heterozygote or *carrier.* The phenomenon of a female carrier for an X-linked disorder having symptoms or signs of that disorder due to non-random X-inactivation, e.g. muscular weakness in a carrier for Duchenne muscular dystrophy.

Map unit. See *CentiMorgan.*

Marker. A loose term used for a blood group, biochemical or DNA polymorphism which, if shown to be linked to a disease locus of interest, can be used in presymptomatic diagnosis, determining carrier status and prenatal diagnosis.

Marker chromosome. A small extra structurally abnormal chromosome.

Maximum likelihood method. The calculation of the Lod score for various values of θ to determine the best estimate of the recombination fraction.

Meconium ileus. Blockage of the small bowel in the newborn period due to inspissated meconium, a presenting feature of cystic fibrosis.

Meiosis. The type of cell division which occurs in gamete formation with halving of the somatic number of chromosomes so that each gamete is haploid.

Mendelian inheritance. Inheritance which follows the laws of segregation and independent assortment as proposed by Mendel.

Messenger-RNA (mRNA). A single-stranded molecule complementary to one of the strands of double-stranded DNA which is synthesised during transcription and transmits the genetic information in the DNA to the ribosomes for protein synthesis.

Metacentric. Term used to describe chromosomes in which the centromere is central with both arms being of approximately equal length.

Metaphase. The stage of cell division when the chromosomes line up on the equatorial plate and the nuclear membrane disappears.

Metaphase spreads. The preparation of cells during the metaphase stage of mitosis in which they are condensed.

Methaemoglobin. A haemoglobin molecule in which the iron is oxidised.

Microdeletion. A small chromosomal deletion detectable by high resolution prometaphase chromosomal analysis.

Microsatellite. Polymorphic variation in DNA sequences due to a variable number of tandem repeats of the dinucleotide CA, or tri- or tetra-nucleotides.

Microtubules. Long cylindrical tubes composed of bundles of small filaments which are an important part of the cytoskeleton.

Minichromosomes. Artificially constructed chromosomes which contain centromeric and telomeric elements which allow replication of foreign DNA as a separate entity.

Minigene. A construct of a gene with the majority of the sequence removed which still remains functional, e.g. a dystrophin minigene.

Minisatellite. Polymorphic variation in DNA sequences due to a variable number of tandem repeats of a short DNA sequence.

Missense mutation. A point mutation which results in a change in an amino-acid-specifying codon.

Mitochondria. Minute structures situated within the cytoplasm which are concerned with cell respiration.

Mitochondrial DNA (mtDNA). Mitochondria possess their own genetic material which codes for enzymes involved in energy-yielding reactions, mutations in which are associated with certain diseases in humans.

Mitochondrial inheritance. Transmission of a mitochondrial trait exclusively through maternal relatives.

Mitosis. The type of cell division which occurs in replication of somatic cells.

Monosomy. Loss of one member of a homologous pair of chromosomes so that there is one less than the diploid number of chromosomes (2N–1).

Monozygotic (= identical). Type of twins derived from a single fertilised ovum.

Morphogen. A chemical or substance which determines a developmental process.

Morula. The 12 to 16 cell stage of the early embryo at 3 days post-conception.

Mosaic. An individual with two different cell lines derived from a single zygote.

Mucoviscidosis. An older term used for cystic fibrosis.

Multifactorial inheritance. Inheritance controlled by many genes with small additive effects (polygenic) plus the effects of the environment.

Multiple alleles. The existence of more than two alleles at a particular locus in a population.

Multipoint linkage analysis. Analysis of the segregation of alleles at a number of closely adjacent loci.

Mutant. A gene which has undergone a change or mutation.

Mutated in colorectal carcinoma (MCC). A gene involved in colorectal cancer as evidenced by loss of constitutional heterozygosity at 5q21.

Mutation. A change in genetic material, either of a single gene, or in the number or structure of the chromosomes. A mutation which occurs in the gametes is inherited, a mutation which occurs in the somatic cells (somatic mutation) is not inherited.

Mutation rate. The number of mutations at any one particular locus which occur per gamete per generation.

Myeloma. A tumour of the plasma or antibody-producing cells.

Neurofibromin. The protein of the gene for neurofibromatosis type 1.

Neutral gene. A gene which appears to have no obvious effect on the likelihood of an individual's ability to survive.

New mutation. The occurrence of a change in a gene arising as a new event.

Nick translation. In vitro method used to introduce radioactively labelled nucleotides into DNA.

Non-disjunction. The failure of two members of a homologous chromosome pair to separate during cell division so that both pass to the same daughter cell.

Non-identical twins. See *Dizygotic.*

Non-paternity. The biological father is not as stated.

Non-penetrance. The occurrence of an individual being heterozygous for an autosomal dominant gene but showing no signs of it.

Non-random mating. See *Assortative mating.*

Nonsense mutation. A mutation which results in one of the termination codons, which leads to premature termination of translation of a protein.

Northern blotting. Electrophoretic separation of messenger-RNA with subsequent transfer to a filter which can be localised with a radiolabelled probe.

Nucleolus. A structure within the nucleus concerned with protein synthesis.

Nucleosome. DNA-histone sub-unit of a chromosome.

Nucleotide. Nucleic acid is made up of many nucleotides, each of which consists of a nitrogenous base, a pentose sugar and a phosphate group.

Nucleus. A structure within the cell which contains the chromosomes and nucleolus.

Obligate carrier. An individual who, by pedigree analysis, must carry a particular gene, e.g. parents of a child with an autosomal recessive disorder.

Ochre codon. UAA, one of the three stop codons.

Oligonucleotide. A chain of, literally, a few nucleotides.

Oncogene. A gene affecting cell growth or development which can cause cancer.

Oncogenic. Literally, 'cancer causing'.

Operator gene. A gene which switches on adjacent structural gene(s).

Operon. A unit of gene action consisting of an operator gene and the closely linked structural gene(s) which it controls.

Ova. Mature haploid female gametes.

Oz. The group of genetic variants of the lambda light chain immunoglobulins.

Pachytene quadrivalent. The arrangement which the two pairs of chromosomes involved in a reciprocal translocation adopt in meiosis I when undergoing segregation.

Packaging cell line. A cell line which has been infected with a retrovirus in which the provirus is genetically engineered to lack the packaging sequence of the proviral DNA necessary to produce infectious viruses.

Packaging sequence. The DNA sequence of the proviral DNA of a retrovirus necessary for packaging of the retroviral RNA into an infectious virus.

Paint. Use of fluorescent labelled probes derived from a chromosome or region of a chromosome to hybridise with a chromosome in a metaphase spread.

Panmixis. See *Random mating.*

Paracentric inversion. A chromosomal inversion which does not include the centromere.

Parthenogenesis. The development of an organism from an unfertilised oocyte.

Partial sex-linkage. A term used to describe genes on the homologous or pseudoautosomal portion of the X and Y chromosomes.

Penetrance. The proportion of heterozygotes for a dominant gene who express a trait, even if mildly.

Peptide. An amino-acid chain, a portion of a protein.

Pericentric inversion. A chromosomal inversion which includes the centromere.

Phage. Abbreviation for *Bacteriophage.*

Pharmacogenetics. The study of genetically determined variation in drug metabolism.

Phase. Assignment of the chromosome on which a particular allele is in relation to alleles at other closely-linked marker loci.

Phenocopy. A condition which is due to environmental factors but resembles one which is genetic.

Phenol enhanced reassociation technique (pERT). Use of the chemical phenol to facilitate rehybridisation of slightly differing sources of double-stranded DNA to enable isolation of sequences which are absent from one of the two sources.

Phenotype. The appearance (physical, biochemical and physiological) of an individual which results from the interaction of the environment and the genotype.

Plasmid. Small, circular DNA duplex capable of autonomous replication within a bacterium.

Platelet derived growth factor (PDGF). A substance derived from platelets which stimulates growth of certain cell types.

Pleiotropy. The multiple effects of a gene.

Point mutation. A single base pair change.

Polar body. The daughter cell of gamete division in the female in meiosis I and II which does not go on to become a mature gamete.

Poly(A) tail. A sequence of 20 to 200 adenylic acid residues which is added to the 3'-end of most eukaryotic mRNAs increasing its stability by making it resistant to nuclease digestion.

Polygenic inheritance. A term used to describe the genetic contribution to the aetiology of disorders in which there are both environmental and genetic factors in causation.

Polymerase chain reaction (PCR). The repeated serial reaction involving the use of oligonucleotide primers and DNA polymerase which is used to amplify a particular DNA sequence of interest.

Polymorphic information content (PIC). The amount of variation at a particular site in the DNA.

Polymorphism. The occurrence in a population of two or more genetically determined forms in such frequencies that the rarest of them could not be maintained by mutation alone.

Polypeptide. An organic compound consisting of three or more amino acids.

Polyploid. Any multiple of the haploid number of chromosomes (e.g. 3N, 4N, etc.).

Polysome (= polyribosome). A group of ribosomes associated with the same molecule of messenger RNA.

Population genetics. The study of the distribution of alleles in populations.

Positional cloning. The localisation of a gene to a particular region of a chromosome which then leads to its isolation.

Posterior information. Information available for risk calculation from the results of tests or analysis of offspring in pedigrees.

Posterior probability. The joint probability for a particular event divided by the sum of all possible joint probabilities.

Post-translational modifications. Various modifications of protein which occur after their synthesis.

Predictive testing. Presymptomatic testing, often used in relation to testing of persons at risk for Huntington's disease.

Preimplantation diagnosis. The ability to detect the presence of an inherited disorder in an in vitro fertilised conceptus before reimplantation.

Prenatal diagnosis. The use of tests during a pregnancy to determine whether the unborn child is affected with a particular disorder.

Presymptomatic diagnosis. The use of tests to determine whether a person has inherited a gene for a disorder before he/she has any symptoms or signs.

Prevalence. At a point in time, the proportion of persons in a given population with a disorder or trait.

Prior probability. The initial probability of an event.

Probability. The proportion of times an outcome occurs in a large series of events.

Proband (= index case). An affected individual (irrespective of sex) through whom a family comes to the attention of an investigator. *Propositus* if male; *Proposita* if female.

Probe. A labelled, single-stranded DNA fragment which hybridises with, and thereby detects and locates, complementary sequences among DNA fragments on, for example, a nitrocellulose filter.

Processing. Alterations of mRNA which occur during transcription including splicing, capping and polyadenylation.

Prokaryotes. Lower organisms with no well-defined nucleus.

Promoter. Recognition sequence for the binding of RNA polymerase.

Promoter elements. DNA sequences which include the GGGCGGG *consensus sequence*, the AT-rich *TATA* or *Hogness box*, and the *CAT box* which are in a 100–300 base-pair region located 5' or upstream to the coding sequence of many structural genes in eukaryotic organisms which control individual gene expression.

Prometaphase. The stage of cell division when the nuclear membrane begins to disintegrate allowing the chromosomes to spread with each chromosome attached at its centromere to a microtubule of the mitotic spindle.

Pronuclei. The stage just after fertilisation of the oocyte with the nucleus of the oocyte and sperm present.

Prophase. The first visible stage of cell division when the chromosomes are contracted.

Proposita. A female individual as the presenting person in a family.

Propositus. A male individual as the presenting person in a family.

Protein. A complex organic compound composed of hundreds or thousands of amino acids.

Proto-oncogene. DNA genomic sequences with homology to viral oncogenes, which are involved in regulating cell turnover.

Pseudoautosomal. A term used to describe genes which behave like autosomal genes as a result of being located on the homologous portions of the X and Y chromosomes.

Pseudodominance. The apparent dominant transmission of a disorder when an individual homozygous for a recessive gene has children with an individual who is a carrier.

Pseudogene. DNA sequence homologous with a known gene but functionless.

Pseudohermaphrodite. An individual with ambiguous genitalia or external genitalia opposite to the chromosomal sex in which there is gonadal tissue of only one type.

Pseudohypertrophy. Literally, false enlargement. Seen in the calf muscles of boys with Duchenne muscular dystrophy.

Pseudomosaicism. False mosaicism seen occasionally as an artefact with cells in culture.

Pulsed field gel electrophoresis (PFGE). A technique of DNA analysis using electrophoretic methods to separate large DNA fragments, up to 2 million base pairs in size, produced by digesting DNA with restriction enzymes with relatively long DNA recognition sequences which, as a consequence, cut the DNA relatively infrequently.

Purine. A nitrogenous base with fused five- and six-member rings (adenine and guanine).

Pyrimidine. A nitrogenous base with a six-membered ring (cytosine, uracil, thymine).

Quantitative inheritance. See *Polygenic inheritance.*

Rad. A measure of the amount of any ionising radiation which is absorbed by the tissues. 1 rad is equivalent to 100 ergs of energy absorbed per gram of tissue.

Random genetic drift. The chance variation of allele frequencies from one generation to the next.

Random mating (= panmixis). Selection of a spouse regardless of the spouse's genotype.

Reading frame. The order of the triplets of nucleotides in the codons of a gene which are translated into the amino acids of the protein.

Recessive. A trait which is expressed in individuals who are homozygous for a particular allele but not in those who are heterozygous.

Reciprocal translocation. A structural rearrangement of the chromosomes in which material is exchanged between one homologue of each of two pairs of chromosomes. The rearrangement is balanced if there is no loss or gain of chromosome material.

Recombinant DNA. A union of two different DNA sequences from two different sources, e.g. a vector containing a 'foreign' DNA sequence.

Recombination. Cross-over between two linked loci.

Recombination fraction (θ). A measure of the distance separating two loci determined by the likelihood that a cross-over will occur between them.

Reductionist approach. The identification of families with a multifactorially determined disorder, such as schizophrenia, which show apparent single gene inheritance, used to carry out linkage studies leading to positional cloning of the gene(s) responsible.

Regulator gene. A regulator gene synthesises a repressor substance which inhibits the action of a particular operator gene.

Relative probability. See *Posterior probability.*

Relative risk. How frequently a disease occurs in an individual with a specific marker compared to those without the marker in the general population.

Rem. The dose of any radiation which has the same biological effect as one rad of X-rays.

Repetitive DNA. DNA sequences of variable length which are repeated up to 100 000 (middle repetitive) or over 100 000 (highly repetitive) copies per genome.

Replication. The process of copying the double-stranded DNA of the chromosomes.

Replication bubble. The structure formed by coalescence of two adjacent replication forks in copying the DNA molecule of a chromosome.

Replication fork. The structure formed at the site(s) of origin of replication of the double-stranded DNA molecule of chromosomes.

Replication units. Clusters of 20–80 sites of origin of DNA replication.

Replicons. A generic term for DNA vectors such as plasmids, phages and cosmids, which replicate in host bacterial cells.

Repressor. The product of the regulator gene of an operon which inhibits the operator gene.

Repulsion. When a certain allele at a locus is on the homologous chromosome for a specific allele at a closely linked locus.

Restriction endonucleases. Group of enzymes each of which cleaves double-stranded DNA at a specific nucleotide sequence and so produces fragments of DNA of different lengths.

Restriction fragment. DNA fragment produced by a restriction endonuclease.

Restriction fragment length polymorphism (RFLP). Polymorphism due to the presence or absence of a particular restriction site.

Restriction map. Linear arrangement of restriction enzyme sites.

Restriction site. Base sequence recognised by a restriction endonuclease.

Reticulocytes. Immature red blood cells which still contain messenger RNA.

Retrovirus. RNA virus which replicates via conversion into a DNA provirus.

Reverse genetics. The process of identifying a protein or enzyme through its gene using recombinant DNA techniques rather than the approach of identifying the gene through its gene product.

Reverse painting. Amplification using PCR of an unidentified portion of chromosomal material, such as a small duplication or marker chromosome, which is then used as a probe for hybridisation to a normal metaphase spread to identify its source of origin.

Reverse transcriptase. An enzyme which catalyses the synthesis of DNA from RNA.

Ribonucleic acid (RNA). See *RNA.*

Ribosomes. Minute spherical structures in the cytoplasm, rich in RNA; the location of protein synthesis.

Ring chromosome. An abnormal chromosome caused by a break in both arms of the chromosome, the ends of which unite leading to the formation of a ring.

RNA (= ribonucleic acid). The nucleic acid which is found mainly in the nucleolus and ribosomes. *Messenger-RNA* transfers genetic information from the nucleus to the ribosomes in the cytoplasm and also acts as a template for the synthesis of polypeptides. *Transfer-RNA* transfers activated amino acids from the cytoplasm to messenger-RNA.

Robertsonian translocation. A translocation between two acrocentric chromosomes with loss of satellite material from their short arms.

Satellite. A distal portion of the chromosome separated from the remainder of the chromosome by a narrowed segment or stalk.

Satellite DNA. A class of DNA sequences which separates out on density-gradient centrifugation as a shoulder or 'satellite' to the main peak of DNA and corresponds to 10–15% of the DNA of the human genome consisting of short tandemly repeated DNA sequences which code for ribosomal and transfer RNAs.

Screening. The identification of persons from a population with a particular disorder, or who could carry a gene for a particular disorder.

Secondary oocyte or spermatocyte. The intermediate stage of a female or male gamete in which the homologous duplicated chromosome pairs have separated.

Secretor gene. A gene in humans which results in the secretion of the ABO blood group antigens in saliva and other body fluids.

Secretor status. The presence or absence of excretion of the ABO blood groups antigens into various body fluids, e.g. saliva.

Segmental. Limited area of involvement, e.g. a somatic mutation limited to one area of embryonic development.

Segregation. The separation of alleles during meiosis so that each gamete contains only one member of each pair of alleles.

Segregation anlaysis. Study of the way in which a disorder is transmitted in families to establish the mode of inheritance.

Segregation ratio. The proportion of affected to unaffected individuals in family studies.

Selection. The forces which affect biological fitness and therefore the frequency of a particular condition within a given population.

Selfish DNA. DNA sequences which appear to have little function which, it has been proposed, preserve themselves as a result of selection within the genome.

Sensitivity. Refers to the proportion of cases which are detected. A measure of sensitivity can be made by determining the proportion of *false-negative* results, i.e. how many cases are missed.

Sequence. A stretch of DNA nucleotides. Also used in relation to birth defects or congenital abnormalities which occur as a consequence of a cascade of events initiated by a single primary factor, e.g. Potter's sequence which occurs as a consequence of renal agenesis.

Severe combined immunodeficiency. A genetically heterogeneous lethal form of inherited immunodeficiency with abnormal B and T cell function leading to increased susceptibility to both viral and bacterial infections.

Sex chromatin (= Barr body). A darkly-staining mass situated at the periphery of the nucleus during interphase which represents a single, inactive, condensed X chromosome. The number of sex chromatin masses is one less than the number of X chromosomes (e.g. none in normal males and in 45,X females, one in normal females and XXY males, etc.)

Sex chromosomes. The chromosomes responsible for sex determination (XX in women, XY in men).

Sex-determining region of the Y (SRY). The part of the Y chromosome which contains the testis-determining gene.

Sex influence. When a genetic trait is expressed more frequently in one sex than another. In the extreme when only one sex is affected this is called *sex limitation.*

Sex limitation. When a trait is only manifest in individuals of one sex.

Sex-linked inheritance. A disorder determined by a gene on one of the sex chromosomes.

Sex-linkage. The pattern of inheritance shown by genes carried on the sex chromosomes. Since there are very few Mendelising genes on the Y chromosome the term is often used synonymously for X-linkage.

Sex ratio. The number of male births divided by the number of female births.

Siamese twins. Conjoined identical twins.

Sib (= sibling). Brother or sister.

Sickle-cell crisis. An acute haemolytic episode in persons with sickle-cell disease associated with a sudden onset of chest, back, or limb pain, fever and dark urine due to the presence of free haemoglobin in the urine.

Sickle-cell disease. The homozygous state for haemoglobin S associated with anaemia and the risk of sickle-cell crises.

Sickle-cell trait. The heterozygous state for haemoglobin S which is not associated with any significant medical risks under ordinary conditions.

Sickling. The process of distortion of red blood cell morphology under low oxygenation conditions in persons with sickle-cell disease.

Sievert (Sv). Equivalent to 100 rem.

Signal transduction. A complex multi-step pathway from the cell membrane, through the cytoplasm to the nucleus with positive and negative feedback loops for accurate cell proliferation and differentiation.

Silencers. A negative *'enhancer'*, the normal action of which is to repress gene expression.

Silent mutation. A point mutation in a codon which, due to the degeneracy of the genetic code, still results in the same amino acid in the protein.

Single stranded conformational polymorphism (SSCP). A mutation detection system in which differences in the 3-dimensional structure of single stranded DNA result in differential gel electrophoresis mobility under special conditions.

Sister chromatid exchange. Exchange (crossing-over) of genetic material between two chromatids of any particular chromosome in mitosis.

Site directed mutagenesis. The ability to alter or modify DNA sequences or genes in a directed fashion by processes such as insertional mutagenesis or homologous recombination to determine the effect of these changes on their function.

Skeleton map. See *Framework map.*

Skewed X-inactivation. A non-random pattern of inactivation of one of the X chromosomes in a female which can arise through a variety of mechanisms, e.g. an X-autosome translocation.

Solenoid model. The complex model of the quaternary structure of chromosomes.

Somatic cell gene therapy. The alteration or replacement of a gene limited to the non-germ cells.

Somatic cell hybrid. A technique involving the fusion of cells from two different species which results in the loss of chromosomes from one of the cell types and which is used in assigning genes to particular chromosomes.

Somatic cells. The non-germ line cells of the body.

Somatic mutation. A mutation limited to the non-germ cells.

Southern blot. Technique for transferring DNA fragments from an agarose gel to a nitrocellulose filter on which they can be hybridised to a radiolabelled single-stranded complementary DNA sequence or probe.

Specificity. The extent to which a test detects only affected individuals. If unaffected persons are detected, these are referred to as *false-positives.*

Spermatid. Mature haploid male gamete.

Spindle. A structure responsible for the movement of the chromosomes during cell division.

Splicing. The removal of the introns and joining of exons in RNA during transcription with introns being spliced out and exons being spliced together.

Spontaneous mutation. A mutation which arises de novo.

Sporadic. When a disorder affects a single individual in a family.

SRY (sex-reversed Y). The sex-determining region of the Y chromosome which contains the testis-determining gene.

Stop codons. One of three codons (UAG, UAA and UGA) which cause termination of protein synthesis.

Submetacentric. Term used to describe chromosomes in which the centromere is slightly off-centre.

Suppressor lymphocytes. A subclass of T lymphocytes which regulates immune responses, particularly suppressing an immune response to 'self'.

Switching. Change in the type of beta- or alpha-like globin chains produced in embryonic and fetal development.

Synapsis. The pairing of homologous chromosomes during meiosis.

Synaptonemal complex. A complex protein structure which forms between two homologous chromosomes which pair during meiosis.

Syndrome. The complex of symptoms and signs which occur together in any particular disorder.

Syntenic genes. Two genes at different loci on the same chromosome.

T. Abbreviation for thymine.

T cell receptor. Antigenic receptor on the cell surface of T lymphocytes.

TATA (Hogness) box. See *Hogness box.*

Telomere. The distal portion of a chromosome arm.

Telophase. The stage of cell division when the chromosomes have completely separated into two groups and each group has become invested in a nuclear membrane.

Template strand. The strand of the DNA double helix which is transcribed into mRNA.

Teratogen. An agent which causes congenital abnormalities in the developing embryo or fetus.

Terminator. A sequence of nucleotides in DNA which codes for the termination of translation of messenger-RNA.

Tertiary trisomy. One of the abnormal outcomes of segregation of a balanced reciprocal translocation.

Tetraploidy. Twice the normal diploid number of chromosomes (4*N*).

Thalassaemia intermedia. A less severe form of beta thalassaemia which requires less frequent transfusions.

Thalassaemia major. An inherited disorder of human haemoglobin which is due to underproduction of one of the globin chains.

Thalassaemia minor. See *Thalassaemia trait.*

Thalassaemia trait. The heterozygous state for beta thalassaemia, associated with an asymptomatic mild microcytic, hypochromic anaemia.

Three-prime (3') end. The end of a DNA or RNA strand with a free 3' hydroxyl group.

Threshold. A concept used in disorders which exhibit multifactorial inheritance to explain a discontinuous phenotype in a process or trait which is continuous, e.g. cleft lip as a result of disturbances in the process of facial development.

Thymine. A pyrimidine base in DNA.

Tissue-typing. Cellular and serological testing to determine histocompatibility for organ transplantation.

Trait. Any detectable phenotypic property or character.

Transcription. The process whereby genetic information is transmitted from the DNA in the chromosomes to messenger RNA.

Transcription factors. Genes which include the *Hox, Pax,* and zinc finger containing genes which control RNA transcription by binding to specific DNA regulatory sequences forming complexes which initiate transcription by RNA polymerase.

Transduction. The transfer of DNA from a donor cell through a phage by recombination of the genetic material into a recipient cell or organism.

Transfection. The tranformation of bacterial cells by infection with phage to produce infectious phage particles. Also the introduction of foreign DNA into eukaryotic cells in culture.

Transformation. Genetic recombination in bacteria in which foreign DNA introduced into the bacterium is incorporated into the chromosome of the recipient bacteria. Also the change of a normal cell into a malignant cell, e.g. as results with infection of normal cells by oncogenic viruses.

Transgenic animal model. Use of techniques such as targeted gene replacement to introduce mutations into a particular gene in another animal species to study an inherited disorder in humans.

Transient polymorphism. Two different allelic variants present in a population whose relative frequencies are altering due to either selective advantage or disadvantage of one or the other.

Translation. The process whereby genetic information from messenger RNA is translated into protein.

Translocation. The transfer of genetic material from one chromosome to another chromosome. If there is an exchange of genetic material between two chromosomes then this is referred to as a *reciprocal translocation.* A translocation between two acrocentric chromosomes by fusion at the centromeres is referred to as a *Robertsonian translocation.*

Transposon. Mobile genetic element able to replicate and insert a copy of itself at a new location in the genome.

Triple test. The test which gives a risk for having a fetus with

Down's syndrome in mid-trimester as a function of age, serum alphafetoprotein, oestriol and human chorionic gonadotrophin levels.

Triplet. A series of three bases in the DNA or RNA molecule which codes for a specific amino acid.

Triplet amplification or *expansion.* Increase in the number of copies of triplet repeat sequences responsible for mutations in a number of single gene disorders.

Triploid. A cell with three times the haploid number of chromosomes, i.e. 3*N*.

Trisomy. The presence of a chromosome additional to the normal complement (i.e. 2*N* + 1) so that in each somatic nucleus one particular chromosome is represented three times rather than twice.

Trophoblast. The outer cell mass of the early embryo which gives rise to the placenta.

Truncate ascertainment. See *Incomplete ascertainment.*

Tumour suppressor gene. A term to describe genes which appear to prevent the development of certain types of tumour.

U. Abbreviation for uracil.

Ultrasound. Use of ultrasonic soundwaves to image objects at a distance, e.g. the developing fetus in utero.

Unbalanced translocation. A translocation in which there is an overall loss or gain of chromsomal material, e.g. partial monosomy of one of the portions involved and partial trisomy of the other portion involved.

Unifactorial (= Mendelising). Inheritance controlled by a single locus.

Uniparental disomy. When an individual inherits both chromosomes of a homologous pair from one parent.

Uniparental heterodisomy. Uniparental disomy due to inheritance of the two different homologues from one parent.

Uniparental isodisomy. Uniparental disomy due to inheritance of two copies of a single chromosome of a homologous pair from one parent.

Universal donor. A person of blood group O, Rhesus negative who can donate blood to any person irrespective of their blood group.

Universal recipient. A person of blood group AB, Rhesus positive who can receive blood from any donor irrespective of their blood group.

Uracil. A pyrimidine base in RNA.

Utrophin. A gene on chromosome 6 with homology to the dystrophin gene.

Variable expressivity. The variation in type of phenotypic features seen in persons with autosomal dominant disorders, e.g. variable number of cafe-au-lait spots or neurofibromata in neurofibromatosis type 1.

Variable region. The portion of the light and heavy chains of immunoglobulins which differs between molecules and which helps to determine antibody specificity.

Variants. Alleles which occur less frequently than in 1% of the population.

Vector. A plasmid, phage or cosmid into which foreign DNA can be inserted for cloning.

Virions. Infectious viral particles.

Virus. A protein-covered DNA or RNA containing organism which is only capable of replication within bacterial or eukaryotic cells.

X-chromatin. See *Barr body* or *Sex chromatin.*

X-inactivation. See *Lyonisation.*

X-inactivation centre. The part of the X chromosome responsible for the process of X-inactivation.

X-linkage. Genes carried on the X chromosome.

X-linked dominant lethals. Disorders which are seen only in females and not seen in males as they are thought to be incompatible with survival of the early embryo in hemizygous males, e.g. incontinentia pigmenti.

X-linked recessive. Genes which are carried by females and expressed in hemizygous males.

Xanthomata. Subcutaneous depositions of lipid, often around tendons; a physical sign associated with disordered lipid metabolism.

Yeast artificial chromosome (YAC). A plasmid-cloning vector which contains the DNA sequences for the centromere, telomere, and autonomous chromosome replication sites that enable cloning of large DNA fragments up to 2–3 million base pairs in length.

Y-linked inheritance. See *Holandric inheritance.*

Zinc finger. A finger-like projection formed by amino acids positioned between two separated cysteine residues which form a complex with a zinc ion, found in genes which have important developmental regulatory roles.

Zona pellucida. Cellular layer surrounding the mature unfertilised oocyte.

Zoo blot. A southern blot of DNA from a number of different species used to look for evidence of DNA sequences conserved during evolution.

Zygote. The fertilised ovum.

Index